ketoCONTINUUM

ketoCONTINUUM

Consistently Keto for Life

Annette Bosworth, M.D.

Dr. Boz®

MEDICAL DISCLAIMER

The information presented in this book is the result of years of practice experience. The information in this book is general in nature and not a substitute for an evaluation and advice by a competent medical specialist. The content provided is for educational purposes and does not take the place of the doctor-patient relationship. Every effort has been made to ensure that the content provided is accurate, helpful and understandable. However, this is not an exhaustive coverage of the subject. No liability is assumed. You are responsible for your own health.

The stories in this book are based on true stories. They were told in truth with the exception of their names and circumstances to protect their anonymity.

Dedication

This book is dedicated to my dad, Richard C. Bosworth
[March 21, 1943 - June 7, 2020]

Dad, thanks for teaching me leadership. You prayed for a boy and instead got a strong-willed girl. I needed no help learning how to push myself and work hard— a natural bulldozer. You taught me that leaders win when they "Pause and observe." Thank you for showing me when to hold back, and when to use my grit—that everything is teachable if you create the right attitude. Thank you for the memory of every hog-chore that kept me studying when I wanted to quit.

Your teachable moments forged courageous, faith-filled children. Your strength lives on in us.

Your kids,

Ann, Jess, & Peg

Praise for ketoCONTINUUM

Angela Earnheart: *Follower of Dr Boz who is now Dr Boz's Project Manager - aka "Angel from God"*

Great book! I wish I'd read this book before starting my keto journey. I've lost over 145 pounds following Dr. Boz and using a ketogenic diet. However, I had several stalls and multiple mistakes that wouldn't have happened if I'd had this book. Not only does Dr. Boz provide all the steps to achieve ketosis, she explains how to recover from plateauing in weight loss. I doubt that I could have ever achieved my goals without the knowledge contained in this book! It provides all of the Do's and Don'ts for a keto-genic lifestyle in a story format that keeps you enter-tained as you learn all things keto.

Patrick Vassar: *Age 63 Associate Industrial Engineer*

ketoCONTINUUM swept me into a story teaching about healing a man's broken brain and body. Dr Bosworth used David's story to teach about how keto chemistry healed him, but his story was as if I was reading about me. His story was hauntingly familiar-- I could not put it down. This amazingly detailed, yet very under-standable, science-based road map is exactly what I needed. It's like having a personal coach to guide me to my best health and well being, just like David. This step by step guide is a prize for those new to Keto and those with years of living it day to day.

John G. Johnson: *Age 51. Writer*

  I had the opportunity to pre-read ketoCONTINUUM. Think of it as the "sequel" to Dr. Boz's runaway bestseller, ANYWAY YOU CAN, which I also read and practiced what was taught within. Yes, I benefited—tremendously! As strange as this seems, there was a downside to my success—Questions. Yes. Questions arose that I wanted answers to. For example, 'where do I go from here after benefitting from the recommended steps in Anyway You Can?' and 'How do I go deeper to maintain what Dr. Boz skillfully argues is not a "diet", but a lifestyle, an attitude, a chemistry set coursing through one's veins'? Thankfully, ketoCONTINUUM answered those questions—and answers so much more. Dr. Boz's new book is the next step in one's "ketogenic-evolution." This book, without a doubt, will provoke the reader to change.

Lecersia Clark: *Age 57. Fortune 500 Aerospace Engineering Director (Retired)*

  I've started reading several keto books that I never finished, this one I read TO THE END. I even read the appendix TWICE. This book is for anyone who wants more energy and better health, regardless of whether or not weight loss is your goal! Dr. Boz's writing style will keep your attention while she shares her expertise from over 20 years of internal medicine as she applies it to one of her patients. She relates the adventures of David, who initially stumbles in his keto journey. You will cheer him on as he learns how to reject a typical, unhealthy American lifestyle and transforms into an energetic, confident, and happier man. Dr. Boz provides the science behind changing your body chemistry to remove fat, lower inflammation, increase energy, and improve your health. David's trials and successes keep you reading to find out how he does it. Above all, she convincingly showed me the tools I needed to improve my health. I hope someday I get to meet her and personally thank her for this gift of education.

ANONYMOUS YOUTUBE COMMENT:

Dr Boz, Thank you for for teaching this stuff. Briefly, I had a torn meniscus which was causing me a lot of pain and after trying to deal with it I finally went to see my orthopedic. First thing he said upon entering room was that I needed a knee replacement possibly both knee — to which I replied, "That is not happening." I went to my GP. He told me to start a keto lifestyle and told me to order your book, ANYWAY YOU CAN. He said to read that book before I began. Within 3 weeks the pain in my knee was gone and so was any arthritis. I began in Feb 2020 and am so grateful for the information you have taught me.

God invented man because he loves stories.

HASIDIC SAYING

Table Of Contents

PREFACE:

As a doctor the number one question I get from patients facing a scary choice in medicine, 'Doc, what would you do?' My first book, ANYWAY YOU CAN told the story of what happened when my 71-year-old mother, dying of cancer asked me that question. Her story of courage, faith, and tenacity sold nearly 100,000 copies and inspired many to improve their health through the lessons in that book.

ketoCONTINUUM arose from the protocol I use within my clinic to help patients stay consistently keto. I teach keto chemistry to achieve optimum health in my patients. My favorite way to teach is through story telling and keto support groups.

Storytelling matters. ANYWAY YOU CAN offered an excellent tool to introduce ketosis. Grandma Rose's intimate story filled the reader with compassion for her while they accidentally learned about ketones. ketoCONTINUUM takes the education to a higher level. Although the two stories are linked, ANYWAY YOU CAN is not a prerequisite for ketoCONTINUUM.

ketoCONTINUUM maps out the medical protocol for getting patients consistently keto. In an attempt to reach "students" through optimal forms of learning, ketoCONTINUUM is shared in paperback, eBook, and audiobook. Also, the condensed version of the information is taught in the online course, Consistently Keto through short videos and worksheets. The ketoCONTINUUM Workbook augments the content by facilitating the lessons. When a patient documents their progress, it helps them to take ownership of their keto-journey. Medical advisors appreciate the engaged, educated patient who presents with a workbook filled with helpful information. The more educated the patient, the stronger the medical team.

The publication of this book took longer than expected. 2020 swept pandemic and death through my community and my life. The setbacks seemed to multiply as the weeks turned into months. My motivation to persevere wavered. Through the grace of God and the applied neuroscience found in the pages of this book, my thoughts have been put into words.

If you are motivated to change your health, this book maps out the optimal plan for a life filled with energy, improved healing, and reversal of chronic inflammation. Use ketoCONTINUUM to improve the health of your community, one ketone at a time.

PART ONE

Chapter 1

DAVID

Friday afternoon. David's lazy eyes drifted towards the clock: 3:30 pm. How could the day drag like this? He considered leaving. Call it a week. Give up the fight for another week. The glamor of being boss for forty years, photographing Senators, presidents, priests, and thousands of families, had lost its luster. The grind wore the shine off that title.

David reigned as the best in the business, and had the Rolodex to prove it. You could document the influential people in the region just by looking through his pictures. From the famous to the ordinary, David knew their names, their titles, their relatives, social status, and their ex-wives. He knew every branch in their family tree and their history. Four decades had made him a bit of a legend.

Friday afternoon mass started in 30 minutes. He could use that excuse to escape - again. The last three masses — David fell asleep; but at least he got the chance to escape from the office. Away from the reality of his seventh decade of life. At the church pancake breakfast last week, Father had asked, "You okay, David?"

"Yep," David lied through the heaviness of his fatigue.

These days, David could fall asleep faster than his basset hound. In the minutes he played with these thoughts, his eyelids slouched half-open. He glanced at the stack of unfinished jobs needing attention. David hadn't touched them since Tuesday … of last week. He should have tackled the lurking problems hiding in that pile weeks ago. Maybe even longer. But David couldn't get his mind to focus. The sludge of pushing his thoughts to do the slow part of the job proved too heavy, not fun, daunting, burdensome, and most of all … boring. Aside from the creative part of his career, this process suffocated him.

"Buckle down," he scolded himself. "Just do it."

David muttered those internal words often; yet the unfinished work piled on. His business needed to push rewind. The focused, dynamic version of his mind had dissolved and his creativity slipped into history. Without a miracle, his photography doors would close.

Joy used to fill David's chest every time he ignored the world and peered through his lens. Until recently, the colors of life sprung alive inside the tunnel of a camera. Now, discouragement and gloom draped like a gray film over him. Shades of grim took hostage over every corner of his life.

Along with the muted color, his thoughts lost their way somewhere in his head. Was this what it felt like to be 61? Was it depression? Maybe the economy? Or was there something wrong inside him?

David sat there staring at his pile. Thoughts wandered to yesterday's photoshoot and embarrassment pushed away the memory of his mistake. "How could I have done that, " he growled to himself as the pit in his stomach jerked from the backside of his bellybutton. He'd called the Senator's wife Martha instead of Marcia. A mere slip of the tongue, except that Martha was the Senator's ex-wife's name. Ouch! He knew that. He pressed his hands to his cheeks, rubbing away the memory. The mistake betrayed his reputation. So out of character.

When David got nervous, he rambled. Nervous chatter would trot off his tongue like a prepubescent boy on his first date. But lately, he couldn't shut up. His mouth rattled out of control all the time as if possessing a mind of its own. Recently, a flash of anxiety wouldn't dissipate. Instead, it hijacked his thoughts and blocked all thinking. A whisper of fear galloped down his neural circuits and triggered his babbling talk-box. The world excused a prepubescent boy who talked out of control, but not David. The blessing of his acquired status mandated the control of his mind.

If you listened carefully, you could hear the rate of his speech slowdown as the thought formulated into words. Messages left one section of his brain and ran out of fuel before arriving at their destination. His ideas rambled at high speed, then faded before they fully formed. In the rare moments, when twitches of inspiration sprung into his head, they flickered away as fast as a hummingbird in June.

"Just be quiet. Shhh. Don't speak," David told himself.

The secret to a great picture: Shut up.

Listen.

Studying David's craft, you saw more than just a moment of a person's life. David possessed the gift of capturing thoughts onto a photograph. Thoughts his clients wanted the world to know, but couldn't articulate. In one perfectly, brilliantly timed click, the energy vibrating from the image spoke through the print. The key to the perfect photograph began with David's silence. His focused, calm demeanor relaxed the client. When he centered his mind, he led the way to a great photo with, "Tell me who you hope sees this photo."

Then silence. David's calm composure attracted the client's thoughts to arrive inside the emptiness. He allured them with the absence of sound. The art of that moment lived and breathed in the silence. He waited for their unspoken secrets to dance into the air. Click.

Most people broke the silence by 75 seconds. One man took six minutes— the best picture of David's career.

David's recent chatter left no empty space. Yesterday, his anxiety vibrated across the room destroying the picture. He swept away the calm when he uttered the one name that filled Mrs. Senator with dread, not peace. Without his 'silent skill,' his photos flopped—ordinary, plain pictures.

Where had the mature, masterful version of his mind gone? His brain acted fifteen. Undisciplined and unfocused. His greatness crumbled with the slightest distraction.

David added a fresh crunch of pretzel to the paste inside his mouth. He chewed mindlessly. Haunting tooth pain had recently nudged him to switch from candy to this healthy pretzel option.

Chewing. Thinking. Chewing. Regretting.

Afternoon mass had already started. Indecision won.

David considered his upcoming weekend. The thought of a couples-card night flexed the whisper of a smile. John and Darlene joined him and his wife, Kat, once a month. Saturday night mass kicked off their monthly ritual. The four adults met at the cathedral, enjoyed the service, and dined afterward. They capped the night around a dining room table with several pinochle games - men against the women. Seven years and they had not missed a month. Their friendship wove cards, mass, and good food into the decade's best memories. In January, playing cards until two in the morning granted the perfect excuse to sleep in on a cold South Dakota Sunday.

The anticipation of Saturday night cards pushed David to read that last email. One more email, then he'd call it a week. Unbeknownst to David, this last fateful email would forever change his life. "Dr. Boz," a local physician requested a professional image with her mother for a book she wrote — Dr. Boz's first book. And personal to her. David's reputation for knowing people's stories prompted Dr. Boz to send him the book's first three chapters.

David learned several things from skimming through these preview chapters: Dr. Boz's mother was dying from cancer and a weapon the doctor used to fight cancer was a ketone. A "ketone"? That word was foreign to David.

Dr. Boz and her mother scheduled a two-hour photoshoot. Conducting an obituary photo had proven unpredictable over the years. David knew his role. He needed to capture her sensitive memoir. Understanding his audience sorted his mediocre images from his masterpieces.

He looked through the chapters again in hopes of further understanding his audience. Cancer festered inside Grandma Rose for ten years. She was sick. Scanning the text, David stumbled upon this checklist at the end of Chapter 2:

"If you look down at your midsection and you can pinch fat, read this book."

David glanced down. Way more than a pinch swaddled his waist. More like a flat tire. He carried more than 170 pounds on his five-foot-three-inch frame.

"If your brain lacks focus, energy, and processing power, read this book."

David's recent hours of bouncing thoughts, swirling daydreams, and mental heaviness qualified him for the book. "Hook me up," he thought.

"If caffeine fuels your day, yet your brain slumps at 2 o'clock every afternoon, read this book."

David's energy came from candy or caffeine. These old friends had failed him for years, but what else was there?

"If you're over the hill and long to return your health to top performance, read this book."

Was this snake oil? It sounded too good to be true.

"If you'd like to cut down on the number of doctor visits, this book is for you."

David hadn't seen a physician in over a dozen years. Nothing hurt. Nothing bled. No broken parts.

The idea of a root canal sounded more attractive than someone mucking into his health. A decade ago, David's life insurance broker warned him about his high cholesterol. The broker still insured him - and he hadn't died yet!

Intrigued, David pushed print with the intent to read the rest of the chapters tomorrow. His exhausted body surrendered to the work-week. He closed the computer, grabbed the printed pages, and left.

Chapter 2

WHY SHOULD YOU CARE

David's health matched most Americans. For years his body hid the secret demon aging his cells. Those cells were aging faster than time. At first, he aged the usual way - one casual day at a time, without him noticing any change. Then that secret demon pushed fast forward on the aging timer. What's the demon? Hidden inflammation.

The same ten pounds had cycled on and off David's midsection over a dozen times. With under five and a half feet in height, those ten pounds shifted his suits from comfortably fitting to snug. He added weight, then went on a diet to lose it. In his younger years, a slight tweak of his habits removed most of his added pounds. Three or four times through this yo-yo dieting cycle left his body chemically different. His body kept track of the stress as his weight increased and decreased. The stress-induced chemistry shift pulled droplets of fluid into his cells. Each time the scale rose, millions of cells stretched with swelling. When he lost weight, some of that fluid wrung out, but not all the way. Deep within his cells, mistakes were happening. Some mistakes led to kinked DNA; others led to older looking cells. The rules had changed because of his stress. That change didn't come with a warning label, nor major symptoms. The altered chemistry allowed his health to drift further from ideal without telling him.

Each season of dieting ratcheted his cellular chemistry in the wrong direction. When he cut the calories way down in his attempt to shed the weight, his chemistry betrayed him. It locked his fat into place along with the extra fluid. Before age forty, David hauled fifty extra pounds on his 63-inch frame. His pudgy shape embarrassed him and sent a mismatched message. He led a successful company, had gained affection and respect within his community; but his rotundness spread the unspoken lies: lazy, selfish, secretive, fake, weak of mind, even weaker of spirit.

Years of trying to lose weight frustrated him.

He fought back with professional help. David's neighbor had slimmed down using a weight loss program. Inspired by the walking billboard for success, David entered the program with vigor and determination. He forked over the money and followed every rule. The expense helped him take the program seriously. Sure enough, he'd found his people: successful, busy, overweight men and women. Processed food wrapped in a plastic package became his idol. The program calculated his exact dose of calories. He picked up his weekly feedings and only ate those substances they called "food." Processed nonsense went down his gullet. Each week his scale dropped. So did everyone around him.

But hunger haunted him — always signaling his body for food. Buried within his DNA, his ancestors whispered, "Eat." Waves of this reptilian message washed over him, fighting against his primal signal to consume food. David used his faith to brace against the hidden force calling him to eat. Discipline held him from eating as his hunger spiked and then vanished. He prayed through the toughest parts. He pushed through pangs of hunger knowing life would restore if only he could lose the weight.

Each attempt to lose weight dialed down David's energy. With the subtraction of every pound, he felt weak and depressed. Clipping calories also turned down the thermostat on his cellular furnaces. Adjustments to managing his body with fewer resources happened with each plastic-wrapped packaged. Day after day, week after week, he set a deeper trap.

Wait a minute? Don't you have to cut calories to lose weight? Isn't that the rule?

Yes and no.

There are two ways to lose weight:

Cut DOWN your calories or

Shift UP your metabolism.

Two patients embark on losing weight.

Patient 1 eats fewer calories while ignoring the hormones of metabolism.

Patient 2 triggers her body-chemistry to surge her metabolism.

	Patient 1	Patient 2
Weight Loss Approach	Restrict Calories	Alter body chemistry
Metabolism	Slow	Fast
Energy	Decreases	Increases [Slowly at first, then spikes.]
Primary Fuel	Glucose	Ketone
Mitochondria	Conserves energy. Some "hibernate."	Burn ketones to deliver abundant energy.
Water retention	High - Water droplets inside and outside the cells.	Low
Brain	Slow. Increased risk of depression and other chronic illnesses.	Alert. Top concentration, mood, focus, & memory.
When you stop the diet	Easy to regain all the weight because insulin remains dysfunctional. Filling fat cells happens quickly.	Adding carbs increases swelling (water-weight.) Improved metabolism remains for weeks. Fat weight does not return quickly.

David knew little to nothing about his body's chemistry. Before meeting Dr Boz, he'd never heard the word ketosis. He believed weight loss happened if he ate fewer calories. His victory centered around the number on the scale. Restricted calories had worked before. He had lost weight. But low-calorie living sheathed David's body with stagnant droplets of fluid. Chronic swelling crippled his cells from fighting against invaders. His retained fluid blunted power to his muscles, aged his brain, and stiffened his heart. Inflammation creaked his joints and stole his creative mind. His deprived metabolism quickened his aging.

His cells had grown accustomed to the flames of his altered chemistry. Chronic inflammation invited the Grim Reaper to stay near. Without a restored chemistry set, David's destiny drifted toward a broken life. At 61, his cellular history slotted him for a slow death plagued with decades of lost vitality —a zombie of sorts, alive without life.

On Saturday afternoon, David read the pages sharing Grandma Rose's story. David didn't have cancer, but he related to her struggles of low energy and a wilted life. And it got better? How? Before joining his wife and friends for their Saturday night tradition, he tucked the pages into his bag. Three chapters from this inspiring story lassoed his desire for change. He sat through mass without hearing a word from outside his head. Internal dialog tuned out the universe as he daydreamed about his healthy, younger self.

As David slid into the booth at the diner, his inner Jerry Maguire blurted out, "I'm going to do what she did. I can't stop thinking about it. I want what she has. I want to do this. Will you do this with me?"

His wife and friends stared blankly, unaware of his recent mental tornado.

Reading a few pages of ANYWAY YOU CAN, David found hope in Grandma Rose's cancer story. Hacking her metabolism during a critical stage of life shared how ketones improved her health. Her health was way worse than David's and she resurrected it.

ANYWAY YOU CAN introduced the basic science lessons about ketogenic nutrition. David, along with thousands of other readers, found inspiration in Grandma Roses' triumph while learning about ketone chemistry.

ketoCONTINUUM builds upon those lessons on health, metabolism, and longevity. Learn why ketones carve back vitality by supercharging your mitochondria. ketoCONTINUUM teaches you how to grab hold of the rules needed to reset your body chemistry and add more than just days to your life. You will learn the roadmap to the fountain of youth. Together we will coax your mitochondria out of their dormant, sleepy phase, and reverse time.

Read what happens when David's broken 61-year-old body uses ketones to shoo away the dingy shadows of fatigue, depression, diabetes, and obesity. David uses the ketoCONTINUUM to recharge his life and take back his health.

You can do this too. Learn how to stay consistently keto. Track your progress using the accompanying workbook.

Like Grandma Rose, David will inspire you to step into the best chapter of your health - one ketone at a time.

Chapter 3

WRITE DOWN YOUR WHY

On Sunday, David awoke determined to renew his health. His slumber from last night's card game vaporized as he re-read the first few chapters about Grandma Rose. He mentally drafted his action plan for a new beginning.

Rejuvenation. Energy. Happiness. David wanted THAT.

Motivation for Improved Health

What motivates you to improve your health? This is not a rhetorical or flippant question. A casual answer to this question guarantees failure.

Grandma Rose wanted to live to see her grand-children thrive. Her motivation to change did not come from her hatred of cancer. She drew power from her love of family.

My catalyst to pump ketones through my blood bloomed from Grandma Rose. My mother needed a partner to help endure the changes associated with ketogenic living. During the most difficult stage in her life, I walked with her. Changed with her. This choice stirred my deepest motivation. When temptations and frustrations arose, I thought of Grandma Rose. My struggle paled in comparison to her sacrifices. My per-sistence and success all but guaranteed hers.

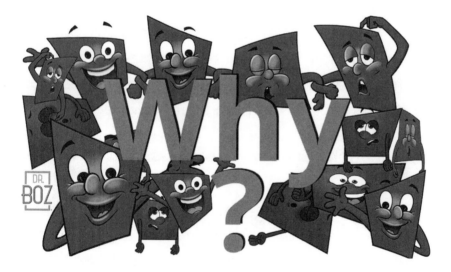

Improved health begins with finding your WHY. Why do you want better health?

Changing your health does not just happen by accident. All the money in the world won't buy you a healthier life. With or without insurance, you can choose to have rotten health. I have seen first hand that when insurance steps in as the broker for your health, everyone loses —the insurance company, the patient, and the doctor. Tides turn only when the patient shows genuine interest in their improved health. Change begins when the motivation to improve your life stirs within YOU, the patient.

Simon Sinek motivates leaders across the globe to find their WHY. He says, "People don't buy what you do; They buy **why** you do it." *"Why"* you do something is a lot more important than *what* you do, or even how you do it. Your WHY can carry you through adversities. Finding your WHY connects with your truest love. As cliche as this sounds, do it. Find the authentic source of your motivation using the exercises in the workbook.

You are looking for your passion. You'll know you're close to the truth when the verbs in you're journaling come alive. If your reason for going keto is to get rid of diabetes or high blood pressure, try again. Keep journaling your thoughts until words similar to these emerge:

"I long for the day when I sit up in the morning without pain. I dream of walking down the street with my husband to join our friends. My loss of energy, motivation, and joy have crippled my desire. I do keto to restore the living back into my life."

David's WHY

In 1972, David wanted a job. With the courage of a 15-year-old boy, he walked into Harold's Photography and asked to shadow the owner. The name on the sign told you who was the boss. Harold ran everything from cameras, to the cash register, to the broomstick. His peppered hair and beady eyes advertised his wisdom and maturity. David's jolly youth lowered the median age at the office by nearly three decades. His chaotic energy and unfocused enthusiasm met with Harold's pensive force of calm. Like a whirlwind meeting a cold front, these opposites clashed.

David saw Harold as someone who'd figured it out. Wise. Calm. Successful. Smart. Harold's large physical size and confidence attracted people. The old and young wanted to be around him. Harold made a living from that attraction.

David's unfiltered impulsivity walked into Harold's creative universe that Thursday afternoon in 1972. He watched the mastermind perform, and something switched alive inside. The most casual observer could not miss Harold's passion for the perfect picture. He connected effortlessly, smoothly, and intimately. His magnetic charisma melted the distance between him and his clients. Each photo shoot was a puzzle to solve and Harold had mastered the puzzles.

Despite the lack of skills in David and their contrasting characteristics, Harold offered him the studio's summer job. At $1 an hour, his first paycheck cashed out at $20. David siphoned his energy into useful places like sweeping, organizing, and setting up photoshoots. These odd jobs kept David close enough to the action to observe and learn. High School resumed that Fall. David continued working for Harold most days after school throughout his junior and senior years.

Harold taught, "Find out what makes them tick? What gets them talking? Help them share their stories. Listen. Don't speak. That's where the magic happens."

The lens captured perfect moments if they felt a real connection. Each photoshoot became a treasure hunt to find and unlock their story. People wanted to tell their secrets. They hid their secrets in casual conversations about their life. "Get them to tell their story, and the pictures communicate their secrets without words."

David learned the game. He liked the puzzles and the art of finding their connection. He connected. Not just with the photographed clients, but to Harold. Every time he walked into the studio and watched the master at work, David felt excitement. He had found his calling.

The next eight years David followed that calling and learned as much about human psychology as he did about the art of capturing their images. In 1980, at the young age of 23, David acquired Harold's business. Many successes showered David as he clicked his shutter and solved human puzzles. His creative mind threaded his social skills into the profitable tapestry of photography. Harold had seared the critical lessons into David's mind before the age of 25. David locked that thinking pattern into his memory, and a cash cow paid out for almost three decades.

But not recently. He no longer felt the thrill. Even when the secrets landed in his lap, he ignored them. Photography had morphed into a "job" that paid some bills.

David's business success depended on his brain, specifically the creative side. When his brain worked, he succeeded. David struggled with a secret. His brain had slowed down. Wilted. His business followed. He struggled with his performance during the shoots.

David's mental flexibility faded along with his connection to people. The outside world might not have noticed; but David did. His mistakes were the proof. With each flaw, his confidence wavered, and business died a little.

Photography businesses failed when they either couldn't adapt, or refused to, or were too slow to blend with modern times. Physically printed photos transitioned into digital ones. David's creative mind kept his company nimble which helped him to survive the industry changes. Recently, each mistake clouded his mind with insecure thoughts, gloom, fears, and flashbacks dating back to 1972. Symptoms of depression moved in. David needed to fix his sluggish brain or get out of the business.

I asked, "David, why do you want to do keto?"

He answered with a lie. He didn't mean to, but he lied. "My good friend John needs to lose weight. So do I. If I do it, he will do it too," he pledged.

That will not work.

David certainly wanted to help John. The Grim Reaper loomed around his friend, weighing 170 pounds over ideal body weight. If John failed to shed pounds, his weakened heart would not lift the burden.

John had suffered at least two heart attacks. A third one wouldn't fair well.

David told the truth when he pledged his commitment to his friend. The lie snuck in when he thought that was his highest motivation. John was not David's real motivation.

The thought of his company imploding paralyzed David. These thoughts caused a visceral pain to rise from his loins to his gut. He could not let his business fail; it succeeded when his brain succeeded. David wanted what Grandma Rose had: A vibrant mind!

David's WHY was his sincere desire to save his business. This desire woke him in the middle of the night and drove him into action.

Find your WHY.

Don't stop until you find the VERBS. Passion has action. A strong WHY sparks action.

Now, use the workbook to help find your WHY. Answer the questions leading to your WHY.

Chapter 4

FORM YOUR TRIBE

T hat night, David had shared carbs and cards with his oldest and most trusted friends. This meal marked a critical step towards David's success: Form Your Tribe.

David didn't know what I knew about his health. But he knew he needed to lose weight. He knew something had sucked away his vibrance.

Their evening dining ended with a mound of gooey chocolate topped with vanilla ice cream. Four spoons divided the sugar and pleasure. With a heaping scoop of courage, David channeled his inner Jerry Maguire and said, "I've had enough. I have to change. This 71-year-old lady ate fat and lost weight. I'm gonna do what she did. Do it with me?" The absurdity of eating fat to lose weight clashed in their minds as laughter erupted from his circle of trust.

Grandma Rose had lost weight, fought cancer, and restored her energy without a program or pills. Her struggle inspired him to take control of his health, mind, and weight. His circle of friends at the table needed the same improvements.

With a mouth full of dessert, John comically added, "This has lots of fat. I will do *this* diet with you, David!"

No one comprehended. David's mind swirled, wondering how to communicate what he wanted them to know. Thoughts of his revived health flickered in his mental whirlwind. The gap between what he said and what he meant spread too far. They were right. He sounded ridiculous. "Lose weight by eating fat?" Panic crept into the moment as he wondered how to get his friends to think like him.

He grabbed the printed pages of the book and began reading aloud. The words left David's mouth with the pressure of desperation. By the end of his first breath, the laughter had stopped. Not because they believed the words he read. It was the way he said it. His tone begged them to listen. The spoons returned to their plate of origin, leaving most of the chocolate delight uneaten.

"No!" David proclaimed. "Let's do this TOGETHER!" Captured by the desperate cry of their friend, they acquiesced. Little did David know that he had just created his support group. His accountability partners. His tribe. This critical step would lift him through the first several weeks of his ketogenic journey. David's desire to improve his health pulled his friends into the vortex for change. Their sincere interest in changing their health trailed David's by a mile. Their commitment would waiver over the next few months, while David's would grow stronger.

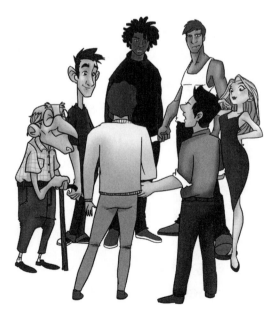

Have you ever created a support group?

Most people haven't. Starting a group sounds daunting and bizarre. When I mention support groups, most conjure trope images of a room with folding chairs as folks pledge to curb their addiction. That isn't the wrong image, but it is one of many options that work. Support groups start with the connection of wanting the same thing.

David's support group all wanted the same thing: To help David. That was their beginning. Sure, they could all stand to improve their health; but that wasn't why they started. David started the journey because he wanted better health. The other three started because they wanted to help David. Good enough.

When transitioning from one behavior to another, lean on a tribe. Even if the tribe doesn't appear to be supportive, it provides the platform to learn. Don't do it alone. Strength in numbers isn't a metaphor. As you pull away from one set of rules and start a new list, struggles will sabotage progress. Support fuels perseverance. Your tribe provides a place to hash out what you're going through. Helping one another sounds like a kumbaya moment from a childhood summer camp. This campy cliche works in times of crisis. Social connections keep you accountable and inspire you to continue despite setbacks. Quitting is easy when no one else knows you even started. Together wins.

If this is the third time you're starting the keto-genic diet, I will warn you now: the reason you're fail-ing is your WHY and your TRIBE.

I deliver expert advice on how to improve chron-ic health issues. Thousands of patient interactions taught me how to succeed at the long-game. Support groups are part of the long-game plan. They matter. They might seem to do little at first; yet, such groups are critical once you graduate from Beginner's Me-tabolism.

Obstacles complicate everyone's journey. If you wait for the troubles to arise before creating your sup-port group, you will fall short. You need support in place when the struggle happens. Creating a group while juggling the vulnerable phase of the transition plots the course to failure. Building a tribe sounds stressful and weird, but your tribe outlines the founda-tion for success - even when your tribe looks as messy as David's. The others who join you on this journey re-inforce your commitment when you need it the most. Sharing your struggle lightens the burden. Falling off the wagon, constipation, diarrhea, carb-cravings, de-pression, or a weight-loss plateau feels lonely without support. In a huff, people give up. With eyes shadowed and head down, they lurk through the next days hop-ing no one challenges them about the fleeting change in eating habits. There's no substitute for a support group. Emotions run high when changing the way you eat. These relationships forge you through the struggle.

I personally host a support group in my community. It's free to attend and takes place once a week. This support group remains one of my weekly highlights. People participate at different stages of their keto journey. Some people come for one season, others show up every week. Some join the group during a tough phase and then break away once they feel supported. Later, they come back offering support to a newcomer. Some branch to lead their own support groups. Part of the motivation to write this book came from the drive to create hundreds (dare I dream of thousands) of support groups.

The Opposite of Addiction is Not Sobriety: It's COMMUNITY

Like most, David ate to feel better. A valley in his life got him down, and food filled that emptiness. Eating had become his routine to self-soothing. In addition to his tribe of four, David attended our weekly support group. This helped him see options he never considered. David saw people use a different approach. New options filtered into his awareness after he heard others share their mistakes. The more genuine their testimony, the better that example came to mind during his own struggle. Their wins and losses created a Rolodex of options unknown to him - until now. David learned from the shared life. His stages of change followed some members and offered an example to newer ones.

Joy energized the room when someone broke through their struggle. Tiny successes like, "I said no to the potatoes at the office potluck last week" drew honest praise from the group. David used those observations to frame his expectations. The whole room related to how tempted he could feel. When people tried and failed, everyone learned. The value of the group resided in their sharing.

Pleasure washed over David's body when he ate. The comfort found in food traced back to his most primitive emotions. David had become addicted to the rise in his blood sugar at a young age. He used carb-filled food to feel pleasure. As with any addiction, David's satisfaction from food had weakened over the years. Like tobacco, cocaine, or pornography, the attrition of pleasure happened the longer and more often he used food to comfort himself.

Conquering an addiction begins with substituting an alternative for your favorite vice. Tobacco smokers chew nicotine gum. Alcoholics drink soda instead of strong liquor. The urgent desire for their vice gets filled with the substitution. Forging a new pattern may take years, but it begins with that replacement. The changed behavior sticks if the pleasure from the substitution exceeds the old option.

Support groups substitute relationships as their new source of pleasure. These groups switch out old addicted-habits for people-habits. The community of support provides a thread of connection at first. But these threads become life-ropes over time. Relationships fill that vacuum left behind from food-pleasure.

When trying to reverse a bad habit, no matter the vice, relapse happens on some level to every single person. This is because the wires inside their brain have practiced this habit many times. When I notice a patient stop connecting at group, it's a warning that their substitution—the people-habits— are wilting. The old wires in their brain are longing for the addicted habit to comfort and soothe. It's also just as dangerous when someone follows the "perfect" set of rules without exception. The overreach for perfection often accompanies self-shaming or scolding when a rule gets broken. One slip of their newly formed, rigorous regulations, and they fail. They give up entirely as they chastise themselves.

Their brains recorded this authoritative behavior from a ghost in their past. With little conscious prompting, they repeat the behavior they saw and modeled. Addiction floods back into their life as guilt deflates their drive. They feel so defeated, they don't want to try again. Support groups offer a chance to learn a different approach.

Mirror neurons get credit for learning this new behavior. These special nerves thread deep within the brains of all primates. Connection toward long term change starts within the signal of mirror neurons nestled in the grey matter. These particular nerves grant advanced learning to humans and monkeys. Through these neurons, we learn behavior by watching. We mirror behavior using mirror neurons. This is why support groups work— they activate mirror neurons.

When teaching skills from one generation to the next, a parent teaches behavior by performing the skill in front of their offspring. The simple act of witnessing behavior lays the foundation for that skill to be used later.

For example, the children of professional dancers grew up watching their parents dance. Hours spent watching Mom and Dad glide across the dance floor wired the brains of their offspring. Fifth-grade gym classes offered an early opportunity for the children to dance. They performed remarkably well. Why? Were they genetically enhanced dancers? No. They outperformed their peers in beginner's dance-class because of mirror neurons. Even though their bodies had rarely danced, their brains readily used the memories captured by mirror neurons. Subsequently, other fifth-graders ignited their mirror neurons as they watched their classmates dance. To a small degree, everyone watching the behavior improved their ability to dance thanks to mirror neurons' presence. Watching initiated mirror learning.

A support group utilizes this mirror-neuron learning strategy when attendees share examples of their behavior. Sharing stories allow onlookers to learn by watching how others deal with challenging situations. The example provides missing education via stimulation to their mirror neurons.

Brains suffering from addiction resist change. The drive to stay the same dictates their lives. They rely on substances or behaviors to escape undesirable thoughts or feelings. These choices delivered positive results early in their learning and, initially, served them well. Black and white rules provided important boundaries in their developing brains. Addiction wired their circuits when a rigid checklists offered no alternatives. These nerve pathways begin to soften when they watch examples of options they'd never seen before. In the critical choice-moment, they never considered some possibilities because they've never seen them.

When mirror neurons witness a new behavior, addiction weakens.

Watching others adapt to the next best idea offers freedom when life goes wrong. Choosing alternate coping skills during times of stress awakens a new arena. Each new idea triggered a mirror neuron to escape the otherwise trapped situation.

Shared struggles offer new learning through mirror neurons. Unlike reading a list of coping skills in a book, human brains learn better through watching someone else. Witnessing a group member admit their mistake and try again helps everyone in the group. It dramatically helps those with few examples of that behavior from their past. Demonstrating behaviors filled with grace and forgiveness profoundly impact success for brains that have never witnessed those gifts.

Do not underestimate the value of a support group. At first glance, support groups offer seemingly trivial examples. People delay starting a group for several reasons. For example: They lack strong committed leaders, The group has no directing, causing members to revert to old unhealthy patterns, Or the group lacks a ketone expert. Do not get distracted by forming the perfect group, at the ideal time, in the most luxurious setting. You need willing members to share their stories of success and failure. The learning unfolds by way of sharing. This is the secret. Sharing also strengthens mirror-neurons. Stories of falling off-track, getting stuck in a pattern, or tripping over old traditions teaches others. This simple, minor act gets overlooked and under-appreciated.

5 Steps to Form Your Group

David invited the people he connected to emotionally. This was his circle of trust. His tribe started with his wife and best `friends. These close relationships supported him for the first few weeks. Everyone in his tribe started out with a strong desire to use keto-chemistry. Each person lost weight. However, their commitment rose and fell based on other stressors. When life overflowed, only David's WHY persevered. He joined our local support group in search of additional support, attending most weeks. He even invited his tribe to come along.

1. Post signup at work, worship, or social media

Write down these words: "I am starting a keto support group to improve my health. Please join me every Tuesday at 5:30 PM to 6:30 PM in the conference room."

Focus first on attracting people, not the location. The people in your support group do not need to be your besties. Much like David, it's tempting to coerce your loved ones into this new way of health. Offer them an invite and then stop. Let them choose the next step. Changing others' behaviors fails more than it succeeds. Only two options have withstood the test of time to influence people you love to change behavior:

1) Keep working on yourself.

2) Stay connected to them.

Efforts of coercion, bribery, guilt, or down-right threatening folks will fail. Save your energy and the relationships—focus on improving you. The healthier you get, the more attracted they will be toward a new way of life.

A group from Michigan formed a tribe using a conference room at work. A woman in her 60s sought relief from chronic joint and back pain. She advertised at her place of work. Surprisingly, her boss joined and provided the space for the weekly meeting. Not long after, everyone in the group lost weight. Others shaved away several prescription medications. The boss saw layers of benefits to those who stayed the course. To strengthen the group's attraction, he rewarded any employee who attended the support group for 12 weeks. Better health spread throughout the company as the tribe grew. Attraction won.

Ketones & Faith

Ketones and faith make great partners. Fasting and enlightenment are not new words to religious leaders. Ketones calm the mind offering a higher level of meditation. Post a signup in your place of worship. You may attract others to join your K`eto support-group and enhance their prayerfulness. Call it theology for your mitochondria.

Eyeball to Eyeball

Online groups share continuous communication, but they do not replace your in-person meetings. Keep your connections face to face. If a pandemic sweeps the globe, meet outside to lower the chances of infection.

Mirror neurons work best when you physically meet—your brain changes with human interaction. I offer virtual attendance to my meetings after someone has attended at least one in-person meeting. Their commitment improves after they've attended one meeting. Mirror neurons happen because of the relationship. Without the relationship, the awakening of newly learned behavior fades.

2. Weekly meetings

Give yourself and your teammates the dependability of a weekly meeting. If they fall off the wagon for three weeks in a row, they know the time and place where the meeting happens. Meeting routinely creates a culture of accountability and consistency. Together you can reach your goals. The acronym T.E.A.M. means **T**ogether **E**ach **A**chieves **M**ore. Find encouragement and stability in your weekly gatherings. The stories of success and struggles will hold the group together. The psychology of change in any behavior begins with relating to others. Honor the moments of struggle and triumph with equal value. Long term change is difficult. In a few months, when commitment waivers, you will be thankful for your support group.

3. No food at keto group

The skill you hope to forge at a keto-group revolves around your relationship with food. Similarly, Alcoholics Anonymous centers on the relationship with alcohol. Much like no alcohol is allowed at an AA meeting, no food is permitted at the keto group.

4. Top tips for a successful meeting

Start each meeting on time. Even if no one arrives, honor yourself with timely starts and stops. Use the science of mirror neurons by politely asking newcomers to watch. Their questions can quickly take over a meeting. Prevent that by announcing this rule. Veterans check-in first. Offer them the center stage to share the best part of their past week and one recent struggle. Discussions can slide off-topic, yet still prove relevant. Struggles with food frequently arise from stressors in life. Allow the topic to drift towards those stressors. Bring the conversations back on topic if the focus drifts too far.

5. Revisit your WHY

A few gatherings quickly demonstrate how easy it is to forget your motivation. Leaders feel stressed and lose focus on why they started. Remind one another it is not about having all the answers - but rather having support. Fill meetings with words of forgiveness when you screw it up. Show one another how to start over, and keep trying.

My First Keto Group

Grandma Rose blossomed from the support I gave her. At the start of her story, her life expectancy spanned six months. Forming our tiny tribe of 2 soon grew to 3. Then 4. At first, we changed behavior, and we were all in. Despite the gravity of her situation, we fell off the wagon after 8 weeks. Yes, we did.

We harnessed the intense drive to change our behavior at the dreadful thought of a looming funeral. The imagery of her in a coffin heightened our focus. Thoughts of her cancer cells growing pushed off poor choices for a total of 8 weeks. I've seen this mistake over and over with the management of chronic problems. We made the same mistake. The urgency faded after we met one of our goals. Her 6-week cancer report came back with a WIN … and we celebrated. Then, we mentally started to relax.

Our resolve faded. My support group got us back on track to help Grandma Rose. When we fell off the wagon, we shared our failure. That disappointment connected us. Sharing our stress decreased the burden for both of us. We acknowledged our choices. We forgave one another — mostly ourselves— and we tried again. This was critical.

Patients often reach out to me for their family members saying, "I want you to help my loved one because they have cancer." My response, "Start your tribe. Begin hosting a meeting once a week. Invite your family."

When I deliver that message in person, I often get a look of shock. "You want me to do that?"

Yes! Your loved one receives something much more powerful from you than they will get from me - LOVE. Love them with the courage to start a support group. Even if they never come, make a commitment to do this for 3 months. You will not regret it. At the end of that time, ask someone else to lead the group for a season.

Be Humble at Times of Failure

When failure happens, announce you're trying again. Humility and vulnerability attract the right kind of people. Mess ups in life happen to all of us. Sharing those authentic moments where you try again inspires any decent human being. They will help you. They will want you to succeed. Somewhere your success at trying still means they succeeded too.

It's easy to trick yourself into thinking you can do it on your own. In the beginning, you probably can. I have walked hundreds of patients through changes in their behavior—the only ones with stable, persistent change connected to others throughout their evolution. Don't be afraid. Be brave.

Go to the workbook. Follow these steps to forming your tribe. Do not skip this. Don't make it complicated, but don't continue until you've done these steps within the workbook. The creation of a support group cannot be emphasized enough. You will need a cup of courage, but the rewards will overflow.

The power hides in "together."

Chapter 5

THROW AWAY THE PINE NEEDLES

What you consume dictates your body's chemistry and energy. A campfire provides an excellent analogy for how different foods result in different energy types fueling our body. Imagine starting a campfire. The fire could be made from logs, small sticks, or kindling such as pine needles or dried leaves. Your choice of fuel for the fire results in different types of campfires.

Food fuels our body much like the logs, sticks, and pine needles fuel a campfire. Our foods have a combination of carbohydrates, proteins, or fats. That's it. Period. These three nutrients categorize the fuels used by our body. We only have three options that combine in various ways within our food.

Notice what you had for your first meal today. That meal broke your overnight fast—hence the name 'break fast' or breakfast. Sort your first meal's items into these three nutrient categories:

Carbohydrates

Proteins

Fats

For example, if you had two eggs and buttered toast for breakfast, you would have satisfied all three nutrient categories:

Eggs = Protein and Fat;

Butter = Fat;

Toast = Carbohydrates.

On the other hand, if you had a bowl of oatmeal with milk, it was mostly carbohydrates with a little protein and fat.

Your daily energy depends on two things:

1) What type of fuel went into your body?
2) What chemistry was happening inside your body before you added that fuel?

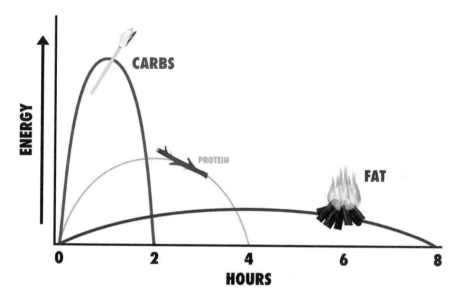

PRIMARY FUEL COMPARISON

CARBS:
Used first before fat
Spikes quickly
Lasts up to 2 hours

PROTEIN:
Broken into amino acids
Accounts for minimal energy
Lasts up to 4 hours

FAT:
Energy starts out slowly
Lasts the longest
Most sustainable form

Fuel Fast & Short - CARBS

After you raked a season's worth of pine needles together and piled them into a fire pit, you barely needed to add a flame to watch the mound ignite. The dead pine needles and leaves curled from the nearby heat and burst into flames. Some flew into the air because the process was so rapid. And then it's over. The fuel was gone.

That's how carbohydrates (carbs) fuel our body. Carbs break down into three types of sugars inside our body: glucose, fructose, and galactose. They spike with ease as their energy intensely burns. Hot and short. That's a sugar rush. What does this feel like? This sounds like a silly question, right?

Yes, it may seem silly until you spend time in a clinic with patients unaware of their high sugar levels. These patients can drink or eat a tremendous amount of sugar without experiencing any rush. Chronically elevated blood sugars leave folks unaware of this burst of added sugar. The sugar rush should be easy for you to feel.

Are you one of these patients? David was.

To better understand a sugar rush, imagine gulping down one cup of orange juice first thing in the morning. This sends blood sugars soaring. When your blood sugar peaks, you should feel a surge of energy. You should feel the pine needles burning. David lived unaware of his increased blood sugars, and didn't notice much when he drank a cup of orange juice. The juice added only a tiny fraction of fuel to his total blood glucose.

The downside of this quick carb-fuel hit David when the energy ran out. Carbs produced hot, fast energy. Much like the fire from dried pine needles, this sugar-energy spiked and then crashed within a short timeframe. That blazing hot flame rushed through his system. Then his campfire fizzled out, leaving him in the dark. Chilly. And tired. This recurring, fast-burning source of energy repeated the cycle of hot, then cold — never delivering stable energy. Flashes of flames from oscillating blood sugar did more damage than good as they peaked and fell over and over.

Fuel Slow & Long - FAT

The second type of fuel is fat.

Fat fuels your body the same way a brick or a solid, dense log feeds a fire. If you've tried to start a campfire with a thick tree trunk, you probably spent the night staring at a dark fire pit in the cold. Before the log would burn, it needed the right environment in the fire pit.

The hardest part about burning a log was getting it started. Once it finally ignited, a steady source of heat, light, and energy bathed over you for the rest of the night. The pine needles always burned long before the log burned. If handfuls of pine needles were thrown on the fire over and over, it was fun to watch, but often the log never caught fire. That's how fat works inside your body — and inside David's.

Fat, like the log, can be a tricky bugger to get started. But once your body starts burning fat for fuel, steady, sustainable, and long-lasting energy flows throughout the body. The heat from one burning log can spread to the next, releasing even more fuel.

How does fat energy feel?

Our campfire comparison fits here too. Many people struggle to ignite their first flame fueled by ketones, the body's molecule of fuel made from fat. The chemical environment needed for that first ketone-flame happens in the near-absence of pine needles. Once the carb-fuel has dwindled, our body recruits ketones into the campfire. The first keto-log may then ignite the next keto-log. Mitochondria are the human campfires found inside our cells. Only when several mitochondria burn ketones, will someone feel the benefit of fat-energy. As more cells move away from the flash flames of carbs in trade for ketones, their energy grows more abundant and reliable. When fat energy percolates through the body, a solid foundation of warmth and energy is felt.

Fuel Medium & Moderate - PROTEIN

Protein-energy acts like a campfire built from twigs or sticks. Sometimes sticks ember up in smoke without kindling. If you time the added sticks just right, there's enough heat to spread throughout the campfire. The sticks burn longer than the pine needles but not as well as the logs. Maintaining a campfire on sticks alone demands resupplying fuel over and over at the right time. Before too long, the flame-tender grows exhausted, and the fire dwindles out without the log's presence.

Similarly, when protein powers the body in the absence of fat, our energy runs low. Compared to pine needles [carbs] and the twigs [protein], logs [fat] win the blue ribbon for the most sustainable energy. Fat lasts the longest, delivers the highest amount of energy, and requires the least maintenance to sustain.

When our body fuels itself from fat, our mitochondria manufacture long-lasting, abundant energy with minimal refueling.

Why doesn't everyone burn ketones in their mitochondria?

ANSWER: It's hard to get that fat-fire started.

Ketones burn after the carbs incinerate. Just like pine needles flash through the fire before the logs will start, the carbs rush through the mitochondria before the ketones.

When you eat carbohydrates, sugar molecules appear in your blood. Sugars flow through your bloodstream into your cellular campfires and combust into hot, fast, pine-needle energy. Sugars deliver that quick power and then a crash. Those flames provide the highest heat, followed by plummeting energy as fuel (glucose) runs out. Ideally, your campfires would spark up the logs and burn ketones right away, but that's not how it works. Those ketones, like the logs, required a proper chemistry, or environment, to ignite. That environment takes time to create. ketoCONTINUUM teaches you how to create and maintain that chemistry.

Throw Away The Pine Needles:

Don't begin your ketogenic journey with a shopping spree for food. Instead, start with a garbage can. Remove sweet, carb-filled temptations and clean out your cupboards. Throw away your pine needles. Don't stop until your pantry shelves shine with emptiness. Your fridge should sparkle with blank spaces.

When patients join my local support group, I "encourage" them to complete this task within two days. They can pick:

1) Send me a picture of your cupboards and fridge.

Or

2) I will visit your home to see your pantry by the end of the week.

That's what accountability looks like. You live in a world filled with tempting carbs. They are everywhere. Give yourself a safe zone for your brain to retreat. Removing temptations from your home creates a sanctuary. Sharing your clean cupboard forces you to take action. This cleansing breaks the first bond of food addiction. Remove temptations.

Most people are addicted to carbs. When you eat carbs, your brain releases a 'feel-good' chemical called dopamine. The more sugar you eat, the more you feel good. This becomes a trap. Remember gulping down that orange juice? That joy during your sugar-rush came from rising dopamine.

Like with any addiction, when you abuse that joy, your brain and body adapt. It changes you. Eat too many carbs for too long — then suddenly take them away. OUCH! Your brain craves for the fix. That's withdrawal.

The first days of ketogenic eating feels like withdrawal. Do not underestimate the power of craving something within your reach. Hence, the importance of cleaning out your cupboards while you still feel "normal," before withdrawal sets in. It may take several days before your body ignites the first fat-burning logs inside your campfire. This will be the start to feeling better, but it takes time.

Show your support group the photographs of the pantry before and after your purge. Make light of this situation and describe the pantry items as your "drug of choice." The term "drug of choice" rings true for people fueled by pine needles for years. Like many addiction patients, this process is often described as throwing away "good old friends." Unfortunately, these friends harmed you. They burned hot, wicked flames inside your cells and torched your mitochondria.

You may be reluctant to clean out the cupboards—fear of your family's reaction when they discover the missing items. Be brave. Boldly have an upfront conversation about removing your addiction from the tempting zone, your home. Remove them from YOUR ENTIRE HOME.

My advice for patients struggling with addiction to heroin begins with removing access to their dealers. Alcoholics must remove all the booze from their homes. Carb-lovers, I implore you to throw away the carbs in your home before you start. Your family has plenty of places to find carbs. Clean out your home.

This step will make or break your next three weeks. Address this before you begin eating a ketogenic menu. You won't feel well during the next few days. Prepare your environment. That wonderful feeling folks brag about on a ketogenic diet will come, but not in these first few days.

Grandma Rose's Apocalyptic Pantry

I recall emptying Grandma Rose's apocalyptic pantry. Her health was in crisis and we needed the perfect ketogenic-chemistry. We had tears over how much food we threw away. TEARS OVER GARBAGE FOOD. It seemed sacrilegious to throw away jars of homemade comfort we had made together. But we did it.

We filled trash bags with cans of corn, peas, green beans, black beans, and lots of canned fruit. We tossed Bisquick, crackers, cornmeal, oatmeal, and rice. Out went wheat flour, white flour, rice flour, brown sugar, powdered sugar, white sugar, and farm-grown honey. We purged her fridge of carbohydrates hiding in ketchup, mayo, BBQ sauce, peanut butter, and low-fat milk. All the low-fat stuff like salad dressings, coffee creamers, and low-fat cheese got chucked as well. Next, we removed all baking goods like chocolate chips, evaporated milk, sweetened condensed milk, and cornstarch. Gone. All of it.

When we were done, we had three boxes of canned goods for the local charity and four trash bags full of food that no human should eat. The pantry and storage shelves in the basement went from overflowing to barren. What was left? Beef bouillon. Pecans. Macadamia nuts. Pickles made the cut. So did green olives in oil.

How do you know which food to throw away?

Lose anything with high sugar content - Look at the label. Any item with high carbs or sugars needs to go. Period.

A rule of thumb when it comes to highly processed foods? Trash them. My family removed everything made with flour, rice, corn, or sugar. Also, get rid of foods with more than eight ingredients. The closer to whole food, the better off you are.

Throwing away food can be very stressful. Do this with a friend, and make sure you don't quit until it's done.

Wipe out the dust mites and crumbs from those shelves. Wash out the cupboards when done.

The next day when you open those cupboards looking for your friends, a therapeutic moment happens. Those fickle friends are gone.

Don't turn this page until you have a picture on your phone to celebrate your success. [See workbook for where to post the picture.]

Chapter 6

INSULIN IS KING

When David looked into the mirror and imagined the slimmer version of himself, he mentally erased all of his extra fat. He imagined the flabby parts gone. Not smaller muscles or lighter bones, but less fat. He wanted his fat removed — all of it.

David's fat cells labored under the commanding leadership of the all mighty ruler — INSULIN. Heaps of energy squished inside this blubbery substance called — fat. Pound for pound, nothing held more stored-fuel than fat. Removing David's fat meant repurposing that energy swaddling his body.

To liberate this fuel, David needed permission from the king: Insulin. Why? Because none of David's fat cells could relinquish their storehouse without approval from King-Insulin. David's insulin had grown to the level of an abusive dictatorship that dominated his chemistry. This narcissistic, overpowering ruler needed to be addressed before David could successfully lose fat.

INSULIN IS KING

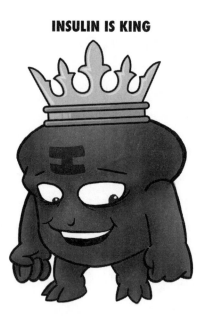

When David felt tired and desperately needed an energy boost, King Insulin refused to open the gold-mine of power locked within his fat. Insulin's commanding voice could not be overruled.

In fairness, David created this energy problem. For nearly half of a century, glucose was his primary fuel.

Years of a steadily eating carbs had boosted his insulin from regular functioning insulin to its current abusive dictatorship. David's insulin had grown to dominate his bloodstream.

Insulin shooed glucose from the bloodstream while locking away other combustible fuel from the burning campfires. Sweeping excess glucose out of his circulation saved David's life. Insulin kept track of the circulating glucose in his bloodstream. If Insulin failed, death occurred. Insulin knew when David's glucose was too high and kept ahead of the carbs that David ingested. Insulin knew the price of excess glucose would kill him. Insulin instructed glucose to disappear from the bloodstream by burning it or storing it.

GLUCOSE AS FUEL: Insulin could siphon the glucose from the bloodstream and shovel it into the human campfires inside his cells. This fueled David for a flash flame of energy.

GLUCOSE AS STORAGE: Insulin also stuffed glucose into storage as glycogen or fat. David's extra glucose could also quickly be strung into his liver and muscle cells. Strings with hundreds of glucose molecules wound together and spun into glycogen. Glycogen rapidly wound up hundreds of glucose molecules to be used later. During moments of plummeting glucose, glycogen will be the first storage to offer its strings of resources.

When every campfire burned glucose at full capacity, and all the storage spaces in the liver and muscle cells bulged with glycogen, Insulin spun the rest into fat. Thousands of glucose molecules found their home tucked into strands of fat. Most of David's excess glucose converted to newly made fat. Making fat took longer than assembling the glycogen. And once the body converted the extra glucose into fat, the only way out of the body would be through a ketone.

In addition to shooing glucose into the flames of mitochondria, stringing it into glycogen, or converting it to strands of fat, Insulin instructed all nearby fat cells to lock their exits. Insulin barked, *"Vacuum the sugars from the bloodstream!"* and, *"Fat Cells, lock your exits!"* until the glucose returned to normal. The origin of David's glucose mattered not. His fat cells followed the commands from the mighty dictator whenever it was present. When David drank healthy apple juice or ate an apple, Insulin sent the same message: "Store whatever can't be burnt."

Years of high insulin sung an evil song as it lingered around David's body. It increased his risk for diabetes, cancer, memory problems, mood problems, failing immune systems, and pain. David had all of these problems to some degree. Without reducing in his insulin, poor health paved the path to his coffin.

Insulin is not *all* evil. It plays a fundamental role in healthy, non-overweight bodies. Cells need insulin to trade, store, and exchange energy. If you don't produce it, you must inject it, or die an untimely death.

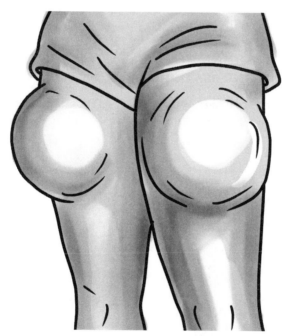

This artist drew inspiration from an old medical textbook. The picture showed a man whose body didn't produce insulin. Thankfully, he lived during a time when insulin-on-demand, via injection, existed. This patient has two large mounds of fatty tissue on each thigh, where he regularly injected insulin throughout the years. Shot, after shot, after shot, that hormone spoke to the cells of his body as it went into the muscle. Those shots saved his life since his pancreas failed to produce insulin.

The drawings above (and on the following page) demonstrate what happened in those areas near the injection sites. Fat grew! And grew and grew and grew. Insulin commanded that growth. The thigh muscles were not designed to store fat. But under the constant control of insulin, the tissue adapted. The cells followed insulin's orders as they mercilessly sucked, pulled, and trapped extra glucose and lipids into storage. These fat cells grew hundreds of times more massive than usual. Those rounded mounds are over-stuffed, over-grown fat cells.

The people in the pictures never went more than 24 hours without giving an insulin shot. The stored fat in those cells remained for decades due to the con-

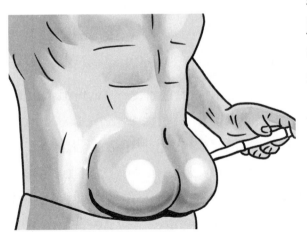

stant supply of injected insulin. This next picture tells a similar story.

This patient injected insulin into the same two spots in his abdomen. Insulin commanded those cells to store fat. Years of insulin injections chemically instructed those cells to overgrow and fill with adipose.

David's chronically elevated insulin instructed his storage cells to use a one-way door: Energy entered and never left. Unless David ran out of insulin for several days, he could not use the stored power in his fat cells. Those exit doors only opened if insulin returned to normal.

Before the invention of insulin injections, persons classified as Type 1 Diabetics, had to adhere to a strict low-carbohydrate menu.

Here's an example of their recommended daily nutrient breakdown from 1915:

>   10 grams of carbs, 40 calories
>
>   75 grams of protein, 300 calories
>
>   150 grams fat, 1350 calories.
>
>   15 grams of distilled alcohol

Almost all the calories came from fat. Fat swallowed in the absence of carbohydrates needed very little insulin.

Fifteen grams of alcohol might leave you scratching your head as to why the doctor recommended that. THE ANSWER: Distilled alcohol contains no carbohydrates. Also, an excessive buildup of ketones, called ketoacidosis, is dangerous and can happen in people that don't make insulin. Distilled alcohol halts the liver's production of ketones. Both alcohol and ketones can enter cells without the help of insulin. Glucose, on the other hand, requires insulin's assistance to enter most cells. If glucose can't get inside the liver's cells, those cells slowly ramp up their ketone factories. Within days, the cells are a maximum capacity making gobs and gobs of ketones. That's how ketoacidosis happens. Two molecules pump the brakes for manufacturing ketones: glucose and alcohol. Once inside the liver cells, glucose and alcohol stop liver cells from making ketones. Without insulin to carry the glucose inside those cells, these 1915 diabetics had no means to stop ketone production, except by drinking alcohol in carefully prescribed amounts.

The pancreas secretes insulin every time your gut comes into contact with carbohydrates. For example, milk contains a sugar called lactose — a carbohydrate, that when consumed, instructs the pancreas to secrete insulin. Insulin then permeates the body, and commands the cells to burn glucose, or store it.

David wanted empty fat cells. But in order to do that he had to turn off the vacuum that pulled energy (fat) into them. The on/off switch to that vacuum listened to insulin. How do you stop producing so much insulin? Eat fat, not carbs.

David loved carbohydrates. David's body burned almost 100% glucose as his fuel. He added pine-needles every couple of hours to power his body. His sluggish brain, wilting creativity, and distracted mind worsened due to inefficient brain-fuel. Throwing fistfuls of pine needles into his human campfires led to years of inflammation inside his noggin. This crippled his astrocytes and aged his mitochondria. The reversal required an alternate fuel. To shift his chemistry and repair his brain, he learned these rules about ketone chemistry.

Rule #1: Ketosis Can't Begin if Excess Blood Sugar is Present

David's biochemistry required him to deal with his abundant glucose first. His body could not burn fat when excess sugars lingered around his campfires.

David's insulin quickly ordered those units of sugar-energy to be burnt or rapidly stored. He scooped piles of glucose into his campfires and spun strings of glycogen. His pine needles burnt hot and fast; frying his mitochondria from the inside out with the constant presence of excess glucose.

If he stopped burning glucose, his blood-glucose levels would rise further. This would damage his body too. King Insulin protected him from toxic blood-sugar levels. At all costs, David's biochemistry saved him from death by sugar toxicity.

How could sugar be toxic?

Each sugar molecule attracted dozens of water molecules to stay circulating in his system. In many ways, abundant sugar acted like tiny sponges trapping water inside David's blood. Glucose absorbed toxic amounts of fluid and kept it from leaving his circulation. This excess fluid, called *inflammation*, injured the tissues as the fluid stretched each cell to its limits. Failure to reduce David's sugar not only expanded the volume of liquid pumping through his veins, it inflamed *every cell* that used sugar.

Elevated blood sugars populated David's brain the same way they swamped his blood. His increased blood sugar correlated with increasing glucose within his brain. David's mind became toxic from that increased amount of sugar sponged with water. Plumped up thinking cells were bogged down with too much glucose and the accompanying fluid. Swollen brain cells clouded David's thinking, much like a concussion. He couldn't focus as the electrical messages short-circuited in this swamp of sugar-water. His thoughts drifted away, and sometimes his speech slurred. If David recruited most of his brain cells into this toxicity, he would have slipped into a coma and died. It's true!

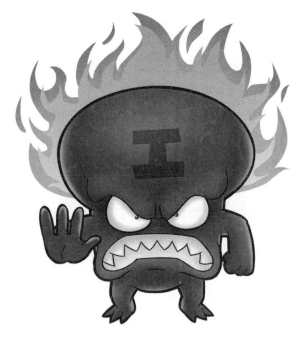

Burning glucose lowered the toxicity and protected him. However, fueling with only glucose increased his risk of toxic inflammation. Surges of glucose offered spikes of energy that plummeted as quickly as they rose. The rise and fall plunged inflammation in and out of his tissues. The inward wave stretched cells to their tearing point. The outward wave never completely removed the grimy residue of inflammation.

Rule #2: Ketosis Can't Begin with High Insulin

David's blood sugar naturally spiked after he drank orange juice. This automatically rang the alarm of insulin throughout his body. Rapidly rising glucose could shift his chemistry to that deadly level mentioned earlier. The counter-acting chemical to prevent that death was Insulin.

Insulin protected David. Nothing spoke louder, ruled over more parts of his body, or dominated all other messages. When insulin circulated in the blood, sugars disappeared. Insulin signaled the alarm until the levels returned to 'normal.'

Before ketone's power could rescue David, his sugars AND his insulin had to fall. How long did it take before David's campfires switched from using mostly carbs to burning fat for energy? The answer depended upon his insulin. It could take several days. Yes!

"Doc, this sounds like a starvation nightmare! I have to go days without eating before my body will switch to ketones?"

Hang on . . . Keep reading.

Rule #3: Eat Fat to Burn Fat

David's glucose levels and insulin production lowered a few days after eliminating carbs. First, his existing glucose in circulation burned away. Remaining stored glucose, those strings of glycogen in his liver and muscle cells, sat waiting for the opportunity to be freed. As soon as his blood glucose dropped, those supplies happily unwound their strings of storage. A steady stream of pine-needles flooded from these storage sites back into his circulation. In fact, David had so much stored glycogen, he could have fasted for a month and not emptied them all. Only after reducing his stored sugar could his campfires grow adapted to burning logs. There was no chance David would stop eating long enough to burn through all of his pine-needle-storage. There was so much. Years of storage. Instead, he could unlock his fat cells by - eating fat.

Look carefully at the graph charting insulin blood-levels after eating fat, protein, or carbs. This research did not study obese patients, like David; instead it focused on healthy, lean people. Insulin barely rose after consuming fat relative to the massive spike after eating carbs. David's most abundant supply of ketones hid inside his locked fat cells. But he couldn't get access until his insulin lowered. Eating fat instead of carbs reduced his insulin production dramatically, which, in turn, unlocked a few fat cells.

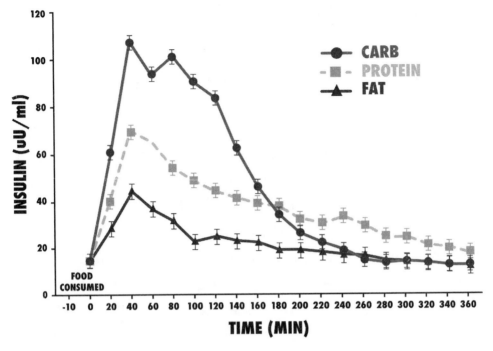

The Journal of Clinical Endocrinology & Metabolism | Volume 93, Issue 5, 1 May 2008, Pages 1971–1979
https://doi.org/10.1210/jc.2007-2289

In other words - ingesting fat cracked the code to less insulin. To lose his fat, David ate fat.

Rule #4: Measure Ketones

How would David know when his campfires switched fuels? Easy. He measured it.

This time David would measure his weight loss success with more precision than a bathroom scale. He would measure his keto-chemistry by detecting his ketones in his urine or blood.

Listed below are certain common foods and their impact on ketosis. If you want less fat insulating your body, stop making so much insulin. Less insulin means weight loss—specifically fat loss. The following fattening foods lock down your fat cells from releasing any of your stored fat.

FATTENING FOOD: Eat these to add fat to your body

Bread: Anything made from wheat flour, white flour, pumpernickel flour, rye flour, tortillas, waffles, rolls, pasta, raisin bread. Use finely ground almonds (almond flour) or coconuts (coconut flour) as a substitution. Be careful with these substitution flours. They stimulate insulin more than you'd think.

Cereals and Grains: bran cereals, cooked cereals, stuffing, unsweetened cereals, cornmeal, couscous, granola, grape-nuts, grits, pasta, quinoa, rice, brown rice, shredded wheat, sugar cereals.

Fruit Juices: All juices associated with fruit, except lemon or lime juice in small quantities.

Fruit: apple, applesauce, dried apples, apricots, bananas, cantaloupe, cherries, grapefruit, grapes, kiwi, honeydew, mangoes, mandarin oranges, nectarines, oranges, papaya, peaches, pears, pineapples, raisins, tangerines, dried fruit.

<u>Beans, Peas, and Nuts</u>: baked beans, black beans, peas, garbanzo beans, pinto beans, kidney beans, white beans, split beans, black-eyed beans, lima beans, cashew nuts, chestnuts, tofu, soybeans.

<u>Milk</u>: nonfat milk, chocolate milk, evaporated milk, skim milk, whole milk, soy milk, nonfat yogurt.

<u>High Carb-Vegetables</u>: corn, peas, potatoes, squash, yams, sweet potatoes.

<u>Snacks</u>: animal crackers, goldfish crackers, graham crackers, oyster crackers, popped popcorn, pretzels, sandwich crackers, chips, tortilla chips, potato chips, french fries.

<u>Sweets</u>: Anything with sugar, honey, or other sweeteners. Cake, biscuits, brownies, candy, chocolate, cookies, sauces, donuts, ice cream, jams, jellies, ketchup, pie, frosting.

WEIGHT LOSS FOOD: Eat these for fat loss

<u>Fat</u>: Ironically enough, to lose flab, you need to eat fat. Why? There are no carbs found in fat. The lowest amount of insulin is produced when you consume fat. Make sure not to add sugar (or other carbohydrates) to your fat.

<u>Meat</u>: beef, pork, ham, lamb, veal, bacon, pork belly, canned sardines in oil, or any game meat (rabbit, moose, elk, venison.)

WARNING: Excess protein can trigger insulin production. This is not a high protein diet. This is a high FAT menu. Once your mitochondria practice using ketones for several weeks, we can relax this rule a bit. At the onset, eat high-fat meats. Add some extra fat. The chemistry-shift within your body will transform you from the inside out.

<u>Processed Meat</u>: salami, pepperoni, sausage, Spam, liverwurst, bologna, hot dogs, bacon, ham. Make sure these are loaded with fat and not 'light' or 'lean' versions.

NOTE: Processed meat is not as inflammatory as carbs. Use pepperoni, hotdogs, or Spam. All of these are better than carbs. The salt in these foods helps too.

<u>Poultry</u>: chicken, turkey, duck, pheasant, or any game birds.

NOTE: Eat the skin - that's where the fat is. Looking for breading without carbs? Use pork rinds.

Seafood: As a "flat-lander" far away from the ocean, I encourage the locals to eat canned fish in oil, such as mackerel, sardines, or tuna. If you can find canned fish in fish oil, that is best. Fish packed in olive oil comes in a close second. Dried fish works too, as does smoked fish. Eat the skin. That's where the fat is. Your options grow significantly when near the coasts: salmon, halibut, cod, crab, prawns, clams, oysters, mussels, squid, octopus, smoked fish, dried fish.

Eggs: Whole eggs. When in doubt, add more yolks. That's where the fat is.

Allergic to eggs? (See the section at the end of this chapter.)

Salad/Leaves: (range from 0.5–5 carbs per 1 cup) leafy greens, dandelion, beet greens, collards, mustard greens, turnip, arugula, chicory, endive, escarole, fennel, radicchio, romaine lettuce, sorrel, spinach, kale, chard, parsley, lettuce, onion tops, leeks, broccoli sprouts, microgreens, alfalfa sprouts, seaweed. (Yuck!)

Cruciferous vegetables: (3–6 grams of carbs per 1 cup) brussels sprouts, broccoli, cabbage, cauliflower, turnips, watercress. Coat these vegetables with lard or bacon grease. Add salt and broil them. Yum! Think of these foods as carriers for delivering fat to your gut.

Uncooked vegetables that grow above ground: (2–4 grams of carbs per 1 cup) celery, cucumber, zucchini, chives, leeks, asparagus, eggplant.

Uncooked vegetables higher in carbs- only in moderation: (3–7 grams of carbs per 1 cup) mushrooms, bamboo shoots, bean sprouts, bell pepper, sugar snap peas, water chestnuts, radishes, jicama, green beans, wax beans, tomatoes.

Cooked Vegetables: (15–25 grams of carbs per 1 cup) sweet peas, artichokes, okra, carrots, beets, and parsnips.

WARNING: These vegetables throw most people out of ketosis. Eat once every 6 weeks. Don't go overboard with vegetables. They contain carbohydrates. Instead, think of them as nutritional 'vehicles' that carry fat to your gut. Add olive oil, sour cream, butter, or other fats to your vegetables. Don't overcook them.

Cheese: Choose full-fat cheeses, not low-fat. The high-fat, hard cheeses have the least amount of carbs.

Full-fat cheeses: (0.5–1.5 grams carbs per one ounce or about 1/4 cup) Gouda, Brie, Edam, Cheddar, Colby, Goat cheese, Swiss.

<u>Aged cheeses</u>: Cheddar, Gruyere, Manchego, Gouda, Parmesan (Parmigiano-Reggiano / Grana Padano.)

<u>Soft Cheeses</u>: Camembert, Brie, Blue, Feta, Swiss, Goat cheese, Monterey Jack, Mozzarella.

<u>Dairy</u>: heavy whipping cream, sour cream, cream cheese.

If you want to empty your fat cells, change your body's chemistry. Unlock the exit doors of your fat cells by decreasing insulin by eating fat

ALLERGIC TO EGGS

If you're allergic to eggs, consider eating only YOLKS. Egg-allergies come from a protein found in the white part of the egg. Remove the whites and eat only the yolks if you're allergic to eggs.

A number my patients with life-long egg allergies have calmed their reaction after eating ketogenic nutrition.

How is that possible? Allergies don't just go away?

No they don't *just* go away. But they fade when immune systems heal. A healthy, resilient immune system defends against foreign invaders.

Viruses, bacteria, and fungus offer easy examples to imagine an invasion causing a cold or a toilet full of dysentery. Food is also an invader. It enters through the gut lining and invades the body. Immune systems protect you. As a rule, your immune system should not attack itself. It should only attack invaders from the outside.

Allergies to food particles represent your immune system's overreaction. The intrusion of that food triggered cytokines to signal an alarm. In a way, it freaked out. Instead of seeing the nutrients in the food, your immune system went wild spewing off chemical warnings, "The sky is falling! The sky is falling! Everybody run for your lives." In *ANYWAY YOU CAN*, you read about the reversal of my mother's cancer invading her white blood cells. That rescue unfolded because of the chemistry linked to ketogenic nutrition.

Keto-chemistry repaired and strengthened her white blood cells that didn't have cancer. Keto-chemistry also restored the white blood cells of many allergy patients. As their white blood cells healed, their cells properly attacked invaders and stopped over reacting to normal food proteins. Their allergies faded. Many ketogenic patients struck out their allergies, one after another.

.

Chapter 7

SHOW ME YOUR MITOCHONDRIA

Your mitochondria's health predicts the quality of your life. Mitochondria are the furnaces or campfires inside cells. Sadly, they don't get enough spotlight. Mitochondria produce the cell's energy to perform their function. Simply put, they deliver life. Healthy mitochondria equals a healthy person. Every degenerative disease that wears down the human body links back to poorly functioning mitochondria. Every stinkin' one.

The day David snapped the photos of Grandma Rose, he knew nothing of his rusty and broken mitochondria. His campfires burned 100% pine needles. No logs. The medical clues that exposed his weakened mitochondria included:

- limited attention span,
- swelling around the sock line just above his ankles,
- and a depressed, monotone voice.

David's mitochondria shuffled straight glucose through his energy factories. Shoveling pine needles into his mitochondria every two to three hours for several decades had fried a few parts. Flames flashed through his mitochondria, trying to deliver enough fuel to keep him going. Volatile spikes of heat, followed by chilly valleys left grimy soot inside his cellular furnaces. This grungy film dusted the insides of his mitochondria with inflammation. They grew crippled from the drastic swings in energy flowing through the walls of his mitochondria. The end result was a crop of unhealthy campfires.

David's swollen ankles warned of his weakened state. The ring around his socks advertised years of mismatched supply and demand for energy. Healthy mitochondria flushed away unwanted fluid swamping between cells. Repeated surges of glucose sucked inflammation into that environment. His body would rid that excess fluid in no time if he healed his mitochondria.

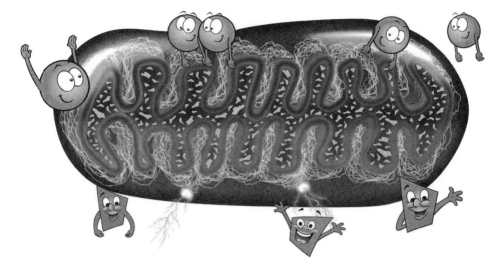

Healthy Mitochondria Use FLEX Fuel

Much like a hybrid car uses electrical fuel and then gas, healthy mitochondria easily go back and forth between glucose and ketones for fuel. Years of solo sugar-fuel left David's mitochondria deprived of flexibility.

Patients with healthy mitochondria radiate health - inside and out. On a microscopic level, their cells function efficiently without wasting energy or resources. Hardy mitochondria prevent rogue electrons from escaping as flying free-radicals. Instead, they produce ample power for the cell without wasting energy. An environment devoid of free-radicals ensures the cell will clone an exact, perfect, flawless copy. Healthy mitochondria populate the cells of lean, energetic people. They demonstrate proof of their superiority by the way a healthy person performs. Focused brains, glowing skin, and radiant energy occur when mitochondria stay soot-free. Those patients don't suffer from swollen joints or sluggish thinking — this sounds like a dream, right? These people did not magically possess healthy mitochondria. Their campfires burned logs —ketones— to gain the advantage from this stable, reliable fuel. Their mitochondria used ketones as the primary fuel, with a sprinkle of glucose.

Let's take a closer look at the health of David's cells. Specifically, imagine being inside of one of his muscle cells. First, take notice of the nucleus. The nucleus acts as the cell's central processing unit, and is responsible for the cell's optimal performance. As we swing past his nucleus, threads of protein lace the length of his muscle cells. These strings contract and expand, causing the muscle to squeeze and stretch. Macrophages act as dump trucks and scuttle about vacuuming trash from his cell. David's muscle cells have lots of trash cluttering inside his cells. Storage bins filled with fuel populate his cell. Some bins store glucose while others store fat.

While standing inside his muscle cell observing all of this, your attention would be drawn to several matching structures with electrical sparks coming from them. Energy flows out of these sparkling powerhouses with electric blue light. These magical sources producing light are David's mitochondria. That light is

David's life. Literally. Without energy leaving his power stations, he would die. Healthy muscle cells generate lots of electrical power. We could measure David's health by the amount of energy generated in his mitochondria. The energy flowing from of his mitochondria predicted his body's ability to defend against infection, repair from injury, and power the cells throughout the day. Was he feeling lazy or sluggish? He should ask his mitochondria to generate more heat.

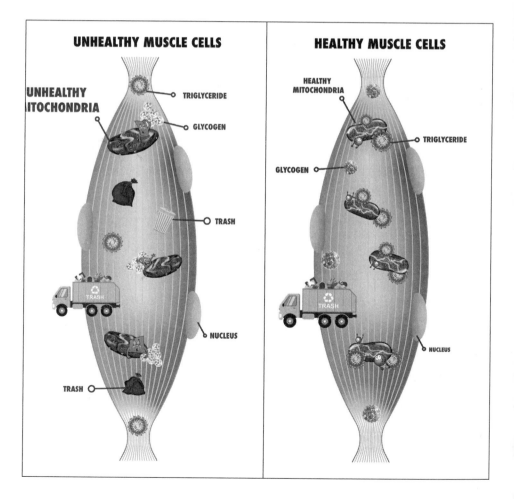

Can he do that?

Yes. As we zoom in for a closer look, David's mitochondria glitter from inside his cells. The sparkle comes from his delicate, valuable mitochondrial inner membrane. This meandering ribbon folds back and forth inside his mitochondrion. Magic happens in the space between the outside wall of his mitochondria and the inner membrane. David's mitochondria trades carbon, hydrogen, and oxygen for energy to produce the spark of life. The quantity of his energy depends upon which fuel donates the carbon and hydrogen. For fast, hot power, carbs bolt between those membranes. This works fine in a pinch, but repeated use destroyed his delicate inner ribbon.

As a young man, David seemed to have and maintain "normal" energy levels. He swallowed a few dozen carbs, and his mitochondria pulled glucose into that electrical bliss. A puff of energy smoked out as those carbs transformed. This worked well because he never ran out of carbs, and his mitochondria hadn't suffered any damage. They were young and perfect. A steady stream of pine needles [glucose] puffed repeated flames through his campfires [mitochondria.]

UNHEALTHY MITOCHONDRIA
Fueled by mostly glucose
Leaks energy
Less internal folds
Reduced volume

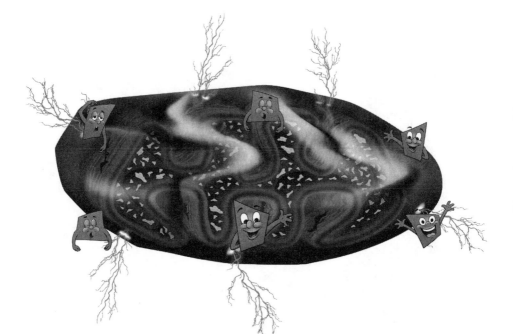

If David wanted steady energy from carbs only, he must maintain a low constant flame. In campfire terms, continuously dropping one pine needle at a time into the fire pit maintained a measured flow of warmth from kindling. Steadily, each needle burned from one end to the other. When one needle had sizzled most of the way, he added another to catch the flame at the end of the previous one. He could sustain his energy with mandatory attention toward dripping fuel into his pristine, youthful mitochondria. A slow constant drip caused little damage. A few bites of carbs every couple of hours did the trick.

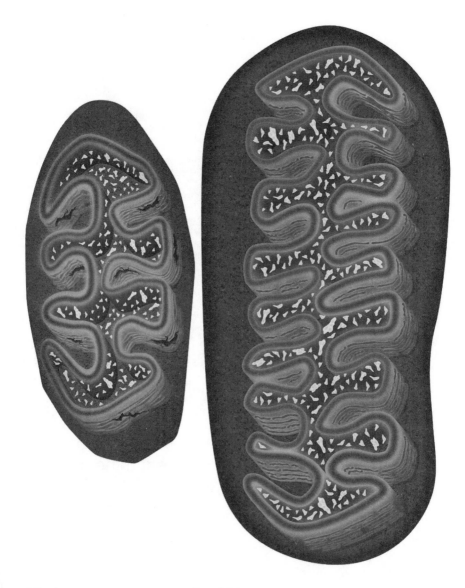

Over the years, David made the common mistake of adding more to each bite. Looking for increased energy, he ate a little more and a little more — until eventually he dumped buckets of pine needles into the hopper. Wheelbarrows full of carbs rushed lightning through his cells. Instead of a delicate little flame, repeated volts of energy cracked apart his perfect mitochondria. Blasts of heat seared his inner membrane and it no longer oscillate back and forth with a flowing twinkle. In fact, it crinkled. The outer shell declined too as the walls stiffened and splintered. His plump, youthful mitochondria were now crumpled and deflated. Fewer folds within his internal ribbon left him with an inefficient furnace. Flexibility traded out for stiff, brittle, weakened membranes. In some places you could see a hole through the wall. Wasted energy in the form of free-radicals seeped through those cracks. This wasteful process left David with a predictable afternoon slump in his energy. David's defective mitochondria coughed out soot-filled electrons, sending free-radicals to further destroy his cells. The more damaged his mitochondria, the older his cells looked — and the older he looked. Some furnaces imploded altogether. POOF. Gone.

David's mitochondria were rusty, swollen, old, and broken. That's cellular inflammation.

Liver Mitochondria

Specialized mitochondria inside liver cells made most of David's ketones. His ketones were MADE by mitochondria inside liver cells and BURNED by mitochondria throughout the body. The health of David's liver determined how quickly he made ketones in the absence of carbs. Healthy liver cells quickly produced ketones. Those cells stuffed with sugar and inflammation couldn't flip that switch on as fast or as powerfully. Over-stretched or fatty livers struggle when transitioning from sugar-fuel to fat-fuel. David's liver was 50% bigger than it should have been. Why? It's not from years of drinking alcohol. It's from years of consuming just too many carbs.

It's incorrect to believe that patients with the largest livers are alcoholics. The biggest livers belong to patients addicted to carbs. If they aren't yet diabetics, they soon will be. They abused their livers with years, possible decades, of ingesting constant carbs. Like David, folks with livers crammed with sugars don't allow enough time to eliminate their existing stored sugars before eating more.

Long before the label of diabetes, liver cells stretched to the max, storing the extra strings of carbs. Once those cells overflowed, the body made more liver cells. That's right.   Insulin grew liver cells. Insulin triggered the growth of more liver cells to divide and replicate in hopes to meet the storage demands. Rarely could the liver clone new cells as fast as the wheelbarrows of carbs arrived. Sugar remained in the bloodstream longer, waiting for storage space. Insulin worked overtime, whipping glucose out of the blood and into the cells. Some burned through the mito-chondria for a flash of energy, but much of his excess glucose bundled into glycogen-storage for later use. The screaming alarm of insulin became a constant noise. Eventually, the body grew deaf to the warning of insulin, and blood sugars rose. That's diabetes.

From Failure to Keto-Adapted

David's jolly tummy, ring around his ankles, and rising blood sugars all confirmed his unhealthy desti-nation. Excess insulin burned scars into his mitochon-dria. These microscopic burns were the root to David's lost creativity, low energy, and failing immune system. At the microscopic level, years of flames damaged his mitochondria. The flames erased some inner mem-brane folds, shrunk the overall size of his mitochondria by 25%, and deleted nearly a third of them altogether. His remaining stiff mitochondria cracked with the slightest strain and wasted his dwindling energy. His future guaranteed fatigue, accompanied by declining memory and mood. He was doomed.

HEALTHY MITOCHONDRIA

Ability to flex between fuels. Switching from glucose to ketones.

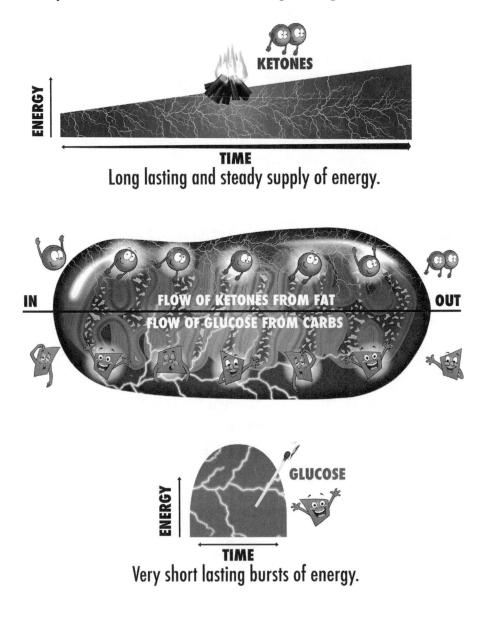

Long lasting and steady supply of energy.

Very short lasting bursts of energy.

If he left behind his life of extra carbs smothered with insulin, he could expect changes. Sure, weight loss would happen. But if he reversed the inflammation by way of keto-chemistry, he could repair his cells from the inside out.

Restoring his mitochondrial function would reduce his chances of Alzheimer's, depression, Parkinson's, multiple sclerosis, and Lou Gehrig's disease — just to name a few.

David's Mitochondria Flexed

David swallowed fat in the absence of carbs. As his glucose fuel burned away, his crusty mitochondria quivered in search of the next morsel of energy. David felt hungry and shaky as the cells craved for glucose. Glucose smoked through his dysfunctional mitochondria draining his abundance. As his sugar supplies dwindled, ketone fuel arrived onto the scene.

At first, his overall energy was rotten. His fat cells had rusted the doors shut after being locked for so long. Eating fatty foods withOUT carbs turned down his insulin spigot. Lower insulin allowed the fat he ate to churn through those specialized mitochondria in his liver. In went the fat, and out dripped ketones. Drip by drip, his crusty cells nursed ketones into energy.

Keto-chemistry greased his rusty old cells and plastered some of those breaks in the mitochondrial membranes. Soon David's mitochondria no longer sparked off wasted zaps from rogue electrons. Fewer free-radicals bouncing around resulted in less damage to his cells and his DNA. Ketones transformed the soot-covered dents, wrinkles, and cracks into glistening machines again. The magic of fat shined up his cellular junkyard.

Gently and slowly, David's cells transitioned. Instead of craving glucose, some cells now depended upon ketones. His real badge of health arrived weeks later when his cells preferred to burn ketones instead of glucose. These cells were now *keto-adapted.* They had adapted to using ketones as fuel.

Keto-adapted cells look different under the microscope. David's keto-adapted cells had swept away piles of trash and replaced the worn-out proteins around the cell. His wilted mitochondria had returned to their full, plump state, flaunting ample folds in the inner membrane, again. Keto-adapted cells also stored energy differently than the insulin-soaked ones. His unhealthy cells had piled a bunch of glucose just outside the mitochondria for quick shoveling. But months of burning ketones traded out sugar-storage for fat-storage. His healthy, fat-burning cells now organized the stored fat right next to the campfires.

Within 48 hours of eliminating carbs from his diet, David produced his first ketone. The following days enhanced the depth of his sleep and he stopped quivering from the withdrawal of carbs.

Weeks later, keto-adaption had stitched his cells back together and convinced David that this high-fat diet had sprinkled magic back into his life. This magical weapon was a ketone. Its most significant power took place between the folds inside his mitochondria.

Let's repair your mitochondria.

Chapter 8

BEFORE YOU START

Even though daydreams of better health swirled through David's mind like a reckless tornado, he had no thoughts about preparation. He had no worries. Oblivious to any downsides, he held nothing back and followed the steps Grandma Rose took to enter ketosis. If a 70-year-old lady filled with cancer could do it, he could too. How hard could it be?

But over the next few weeks, David stumbled — unaware of his high insulin, overstuffed liver cells, or crusty mitochondria. His lack of awareness offered the advantage of his untethered charge ahead. Blinded to his chronic inflammation, he fought quixotic windmills called low blood pressure, diarrhea, low magnesium, and depressed hormones.

Don't do what David did. Before you start, <u>read this chapter.</u>

Do not start with grocery shopping. Rushing towards the grocery store puts your focus in the wrong direction. Instead, read through this list of supplies. Buy the MUST-HAVES, Consider buying the SHOULD-HAVES, and read the few warnings. If David had approached keto this way, he'd have suffered far less.

MUST HAVES

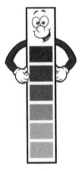

- PeeTone strips.

- Cronometer Application

- Food guide

- A dozen eggs

PeeTone Strips

PeeTone strips, also called urine ketone strips, reveal the hidden chemistry in your urine. These dandy tools test for the presence of ketones in the urine. When urine ketones soak into the sponge, the grey color turns maroon. Find these strips at your local pharmacy. No prescription needed. Grab the bottle with several dozen strips for $15. This will get you through the beginner's learning curve.

Ketosis is not a diet. It is a state of chemistry in your blood; it's measurable. This state of chemistry is measurable — I can't say this enough. Don't guess about your chemistry, measure it. Keto-chemistry starts with ketones flowing out your liver into your blood. Strings of fat unzip into ketones. These molecules bounce around your blood, looking for a cell hungry for keto-fuel.

Strangely, the first waves of ketones catch cells off guard, going mostly unused. These ketones get expelled by the kidney and flushed down the toilet. But eventually the cells adapt.

The secret is to measure the presence of ketones by peeing on PeeTone strips. Cheap and portable, these strips reliably sort those who made ketones versus those who didn't.

Pink or NOT Pink.

• Pink = producing ketones.

• NOT Pink = not producing ketones.

Cronometer Application

Have you ever counted the number of carbohydrates you eat? When I prescribe insulin injections for patients, they need to possess this skill. Mismatched insulin dosages relative to the number of carbs can be lethal. To help them through the intimidating part of this education, I assign a diabetic educator to teach carb-counting. Patients struggle at first to sort food and drinks containing carbs. The teacher and the patient work together to identify foods, estimate the number of carbs, and practice carb-counting with different types of foods and various serving sizes. Within a couple of weeks, the patient can look at a meal and estimate the total carbohydrates within 5 grams.

Starting the ketogenic diet means you need to count carbs. To succeed, you must invest time to gain knowledge about the foods you eat.

After sampling dozens of tools, I recommend CRONOMETER. Here is why:

1)The data behind the tool matters. Cronometer reigns supreme as the most accurate databank for food-nutrients. Many apps gift their application with a free version of their tool. Open access is traded for the expectation that you will enter nutritional data missing from their list.

The mammoth task of entering all foods into the databank gets shared with everyone that uses it. This strategy is not only brilliant, but cost-effective, too.

Cronometer crowdsources this task just like the others. Cronometer stands alone as the only application that verifies all incoming data. Their team fills the gaps of missing nutrients and confirms the correct information — before accepting it into their databank. This accuracy has literally meant the difference between life or death for some patients.

2) Cronometer tracks more nutrients than any other database. Micronutrients, like zinc, copper, or magnesium, will not matter to you unless you have a deficiency in your diet. Cronometer's accuracy delivers the best nutritional tracker. Period.

3) Cronometer starts with a free version. In the first weeks of a keto-menu, every beginner learns about their new food. Don't waste this education on a sloppy, misinformed tool. Cronometer accurately educates newbies and avoids the pitfalls from other databanks. This free application launches proficiency in carb-counting and nutrient awareness.

[See the workbook for screenshots to the recommended Cronometer settings. The screenshots will save you hours of frustration. Take a look and keep calm.]

Keto Food Guide

The rules of ketogenic nutrition are simple, but odd when compared to the standard American eating habits. You don't need a book as thick as this one to learn the rules. Bullet points will do. The Dr. Boz Keto Food Guide lists foods commonly eaten to achieve ketosis. Within two short weeks, you will look at a menu and know the dos and don'ts. When starting out, keep it simple (K.I.S.) The food guide sorts foods into good, better, and best choices. It outlines which foods fit into these categories. At first, reach for 'good' choices. Months from now, you will graduate to better decisions. Ultimately, I encourage choosing the 'best' options as outlined in the guide. [See workbook]

BEST choices are not for beginners. Don't start there. Instead, find the foods you like to eat. Circle them as you scan the list. Consistently eat these foods. I supply patients with a version that magnetizes to their fridge and a pocket-sized booklet. The most teachable moments happen when hunger strikes. No time for long paragraphs of wordy advice. This quick reference becomes a bible with reliable, timely information. When grocery shopping, ordering from a menu, or scrounging the fridge, this guide fits into those critical moments.

Within weeks of eating this way, your pallet will crave keto-friendly foods. Partnered with urine Pee-

Tone strips, these tools pave the path towards success. Once you master the information on the guide, share it. Hang the fridge guide at work, school, or church. Pass the pocket guide onto another newbie—the act of sharing benefits the giver and the receiver. You'll be reminded of the rules when you show someone how the guide works. You may even find a few choices you skipped over. With a season of keto behind you, helping someone else strengthens your resolve and adds accountability.

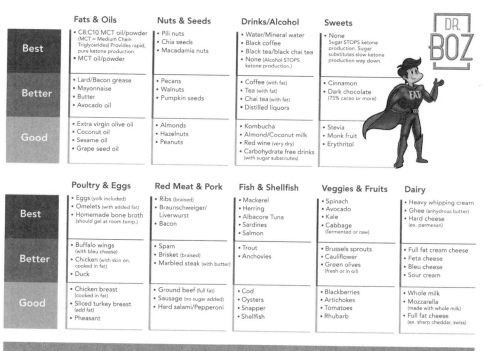

	Fats & Oils	Nuts & Seeds	Drinks/Alcohol	Sweets
Best	• C8:C10 MCT oil/powder (MCT = Medium Chain Triglycerides) Provides rapid, pure ketone production. • MCT oil/powder	• Pili nuts • Chia seeds • Macadamia nuts	• Water/Mineral water • Black coffee • Black tea/black chai tea • None (Alcohol STOPS ketone production.)	• None Sugar STOPS ketone production. Sugar substitutes slow ketone production way down.
Better	• Lard/Bacon grease • Mayonnaise • Butter • Avocado oil	• Pecans • Walnuts • Pumpkin seeds	• Coffee (with fat) • Tea (with fat) • Chai tea (with fat) • Distilled liquors	• Cinnamon • Dark chocolate (75% cacao or more)
Good	• Extra virgin olive oil • Coconut oil • Sesame oil • Grape seed oil	• Almonds • Hazelnuts • Peanuts	• Kombucha • Almond/Coconut milk • Red wine (very dry) • Carbohydrate free drinks (with sugar substitutes)	• Stevia • Monk fruit • Erythritol

	Poultry & Eggs	Red Meat & Pork	Fish & Shellfish	Veggies & Fruits	Dairy
Best	• Eggs (yolk included) • Omelets (with added fat) • Homemade bone broth (should gel at room temp.)	• Ribs (braised) • Braunschweiger/ Liverwurst • Bacon	• Mackerel • Herring • Albacore Tuna • Sardines • Salmon	• Spinach • Avocado • Kale • Cabbage (fermented or raw)	• Heavy whipping cream • Ghee (anhydrous butter) • Hard cheese (ex. parmesan)
Better	• Buffalo wings (with bleu cheese) • Chicken (with skin on, cooked in fat) • Duck	• Spam • Brisket (braised) • Marbled steak (with butter)	• Trout • Anchovies	• Brussels sprouts • Cauliflower • Green olives (fresh or in oil)	• Full fat cream cheese • Feta cheese • Bleu cheese • Sour cream
Good	• Chicken breast (cooked in fat) • Sliced turkey breast (add fat) • Pheasant	• Ground beef (full fat) • Sausage (no sugar added) • Hard salami/Pepperoni	• Cod • Oysters • Snapper • Shellfish	• Blackberries • Artichokes • Tomatoes • Rhubarb	• Whole milk • Mozzarella (made with whole milk) • Full fat cheese (ex. sharp cheddar, swiss)

optimal ketosis nutritional guide   BozMD.com

A Dozen Eggs

Eggs provide the perfect introduction to keto. Eggs taste great, are easy to cook, and are found everywhere. Avoid going inside your grocery store to buy them. Instead, pick up a dozen at a local gas station or convenient store. Grab some meat sticks, pepperoni slices, canned meat (like Spam), or hotdogs while you're there. These add variety to your eggs. Make sure to select the high-fat meat sticks. That's all I'd allow into your home right now.

Lima Bean Story

"Doc, I am a picky eater."

"I don't eat eggs?"

"I DON'T LIKE IT."

The restoration of your body begins with nutrient-dense foods. The egg of a chicken wins awards for its dense nourishment.

In my second year of practicing medicine, I had a case about a man's broken palate. Yes, his palate. Not the kind of pallet found in a storage shed, or the tool used to mix clay. I mean that word describing the kinds of foods he liked. His wife was my patient, first. After multiple visits, she was delighted with her care and announced that she was going to bring her husband to the next visit. Several months later, she arrived at the visit accompanied by her husband. I remind myself of her situation as I enter the room scrolling through the chart. She introduced her husband and shocked both of us when she said, "I've brought him for you to help fix him."

Sensing the tension in the room, she quickly explained that her husband had a terrible problem. Every time she added vegetables to his food, he gagged. She confessed that she'd been sneaking vegetables into his food through pancake batter, soups, smoothies, and even brownies. Each time, he gagged as soon as he tasted the first bite.

An awkward silence filled the room as several witty responses crossed my mind. After a long pause, her husband, feeling the embarrassment, tried to come to her rescue. "I've never liked vegetables. I know they're good for me but as soon as I taste them, my body rejects them. I gag and start to retch. Sometimes I do throw up."

I took a deep breath as I considered my options. Then I asked him, "If I stranded you on a desert island in the middle of nowhere for a year and the only food growing on that island was lima beans, what do you think would happen?"

The couple looked at each other, then back at me. You could almost sense the wave of nausea flickering across his face as he thought about lima beans.

I let the silence linger. He swallowed, afraid to answer. After the proper length of silence, I answered my own question. "You would learn to like lima beans. In fact, after months of eating lima beans, your palate would detect lima beans harvested on the 14th day versus those from the 18th day of harvest. You would be a world expert in lima beans."

The first part of improving and expanding one's palate is personal desire. Desire wouldn't show up on that desert island on the first day. However, hunger would eventually motivate the stranded person. The desire for food wires deeply into our psychology to survive. Hunger would motivate him to eat lima beans. Survival-thinking would win over his taste preferences. Before long, he would crave them. Yes! Really!

Attraction to a type of food is learned. Your family and your culture taught you what foods to like. People in China don't accidentally like rice more than people in America. They eat an abundance of rice from a young age. Their brains practice liking it. As adults, they like it and feed it to their children.

The finicky husband trapped on a deserted island would learn to like lima beans . . . when he starts to eat them. The first step happens inside his mind, not his tongue. He first must entertain the option of eating it. As long as his mind locked his identity as someone who never ate vegetables, there was nothing I could do. His mindset would always win. I asked him to imagine that extreme, isolated, starved setting — and then consider eating his forbidden food. He struggled to even consider the thought. Without his mindset shifting, there is no beginning.

When switching from a standard American diet to a keto diet, allow your palate to taste foods that you have sworn off. Open the idea of eating foods you've rarely tasted. Your palate is teachable. It will adapt once exposed. The only way to teach your palate to like foods is to eat them repeatedly.

Our first-world-problems deny us the pain of our primal survival instinct called hunger. Sugary, processed foods, with abundant carbohydrates have hypnotized our taste buds. Eating every 2-3 hours for a quick dose of pleasure repeatedly wired a bad habit. Swallow "healthy" orange juice and the blood sugars rise like a rocket, only to crash 2 hours later. This decline in sugar sparked a craving. Feed the craving and you feed the addiction.

Liver and canned sardines lose to fruit juices or processed carbs. The ketogenic menu introduces foods that have disappeared from most meals. If you don't like a food, I can't make you want it. You hold the power of choice. If you have never tasted some of these foods, allow yourself the chance.

One bite. That's where it starts. Next, set your expectations appropriately. You will not find your tongue dripping to try new high-fat low-carb foods. Unlike eating processed carbs, you must train your brain to want some of these foods. Teaching an addict to find a different outlet for their pain, involves acquiring a new skill. They will not reflexively strum a guitar as they process through a craving. They learn how to do that through practicing. You must practice with new flavors.

SHOULD HAVES

- Beta-Hydroxybutyrate Powder (Exogenous Ketones)

- Medium Chain Triglycerides C8:C10 Oil

BHB [Beta HydroxyButyrate]

BHB is commonly called exogenous ketones, but I prefer the term, *"Ketones-In-A-Can."* With luck on your side, you may find this powdered drink-mix at your local specialty vitamin store. I rarely see it sold in grocery stores. Type Dr Boz BHB into your internet browser. Push order. They should arrive about the time you really need them.

MCT C8:C10

This is a keto nutritional supplement that is vital in the first 1-2 months of keto living. I prefer the supplement in the soft gels allowing a slow titration of the dose and the portability of the product. One container of soft gels should last you through the tough season. The healthier you get, the less you will need MCT C8:C10 and BHB.

I will explain these more in a later section. Beginners, don't skip this list.

200 Club

The 200 Club is for those who eat more than 200 carbohydrates per day. Don't confuse this club with folks weighing more than 200 pounds.

In the perfect world, David would have counted carbs for three days before starting keto. Had he done this, he would have undoubtedly joined most Americans as part of the 200 Club.

Before keto, David began each morning with orange juice. Between meals, he munched on several handfuls of pretzels or hard candy for an energy boost. Bam! Those habits, alone, put him over the edge; he didn't even need to include his meals.

Sorting out the 200 Club has everything to do with chronic inflammation. Years of extra carbs pushed David's pancreas to squeeze out enough insulin to keep his blood sugar under 110 mg/dL. Excess insulin formed a thick rind of inflammation throughout his body. Counting carbs before starting would have warned David of the hidden danger ahead. Unaware and inspired, David followed Grandma Rose's lead. His grit carried him through an impending struggle that lasted two weeks. Most people would have given up.

Avoid the roadblock. Use Cronometer to count carbs for 3 days before you start.

Did you consume more than 200 carbs per day? If so, pause! This transition will trip your system without warning. This disaster is preventable. Before you cut carbs, count them. No matter your age or your size, this single metric sorts those who struggle the most.

Doctor Club

For 15 years, David avoided doctors. The absence of a check-up left him clueless to his rising blood pressure and elevated blood sugars. He chalked up his fatigue and foggy brain to "getting old."

Use this list of six warnings to avoid the troubles David encountered:

#1 If you take blood pressure medications, see your doctor before starting keto.

This is not a trick question. You got those prescriptions from your doctor. If you take blood pressure meds and want to get off them, this lifestyle will amaze your doctor. However, the transition can be dangerous. Prepare yourself. When I prescribe medication for high blood pressure, I instruct patients to check their pressures at home.

David infrequently checked his blood pressure. Recently, his numbers ranged on the high side at 130-140/ 75-90. He could have benefitted from a blood pressure medication. Instead, David transitioned into the keto diet and reversed one factor causing his elevated blood pressure: He lowered his blood sugar by eliminating carbs. Yes. Lowering blood sugar reduces the pressure inside the arteries. He was not diabetic — or so he thought.

As glucose molecules floated merrily down his bloodstream, they attracted nearby water molecules. With fewer glucose molecules came fewer water molecules. In the first week of removing carbs from his diet, David's excess water left his body. This meant less blood volume. Not because he lost red blood cells, but because he lost some of the blood's fluid. Less volume pushing on the walls of his arteries meant lower pressure within them.

Low carbs → Low sugar → Low water circulation → Low blood pressure

David didn't think his blood pressure warranted concern, nor did he think he was diabetic. If we pulled back the veil hiding David's reality, we'd see that he ate over 300 carbs per day, he had high blood pressure, and, for all practical purposes, was diabetic. Standard medical treatment would have added at least one medicine for his blood pressure and another one for high blood sugars.

Honestly, in this setting, it was a blessing that he didn't go to the doctor. The doctor would have told him to avoid eggs, bacon, and the hearty dose of salted butter. David did all those 'wrong' things during his transition to keto-chemistry.

Read more about what I teach my patients in Chapter 12: High Blood Pressure Medication.

#2 If you have less than 25% of your kidney function, see your doctor before starting the keto diet.

If 3/4ths of your kidney function is gone due to years of high blood sugars, high blood pressure, or other kidney-crushing problems, be sure your doctor knows you are doing this. Sadly, many could have prevented their kidneys' death had they used ketogenic nutrition sooner.

To find out if your kidneys are in danger, look at recent lab reports from your doctor. Find the section that says 'creatinine clearance'. Not just the word creatinine. Look for the words Creatinine Clearance. This refers to the percentage of waste cleared by the kidneys. An ideal score is 100%. You want 100% of the trash in your blood removed by your kidneys. Some of my healthy young patients clean their blood so well, their calculations compute to over 100%. A Creatinine Clearance of 25%, means 75% of the waste still circulates in the blood. A calculation of 110% means they cleared out more waste than expected. Patients with chronic problems like high blood pressure, diabetes, and other chronic inflammation sacrifice kidney cells leading to a reduced creatinine clearance. Thankfully, it takes years to go from a healthy 70-80% to under 50%. Keto-chemistry can repair early problems within the kidneys. At the very least, circulating ketones will slow the decline of kidneys. If your calculation is around 25%, you must closely align with your physician as you begin ketogenic nutrition.

#3 If you take Coumadin, see your doctor before starting a keto diet.

Not much explanation needed. The other name for this medication is warfarin. See your doctor if you are starting the Keto diet while taking Coumadin. Your blood levels will need to be checked more frequently while you transition.

#4 If you take a diuretic prescription— commonly known as a pee pill, see your doctor before starting the keto diet.

Diuretics, or pee pills, make you pee. They pull water out of your system. The first week of the ketogenic diet also makes you pee. You flush out extra fluid as you transition from pine-needles to logs. Adding keto-chemistry to the pill is double trouble. If you take a medication that makes you pee, your doctor will likely want you to decrease the dose or stop it altogether for the transition.

#5 If you inject insulin on a daily basis, see your doctor before starting the keto menu.

I can boldly state that keto chemistry will improve many of your health problems. You need this more than any other, but don't do this alone. Talk to your doctor. Low blood sugars kill quickly. High blood sugars kill slowly. With fewer carbs, you need less insulin. Reduce insulin proportional to your carbs. If you give too much insulin in the setting of too few carbs, it could suppress your glucose to dangerous levels. Do not do this alone.

#6 If you drink alcohol daily, beware.

Limit your alcohol for the first 6 weeks of a ketogenic menu. I recommend a complete halt. If no alcohol for six weeks seems over the top, I caution you to start the keto diet. Alcohol stops mitochondria from burning ketones as fuel. In other words, ketones will burn when available, unless alcohol is present. You will gain the most significant improvements in metabolism if no alcohol enters your keto-chemistry equation.

The struggle to surrender alcohol mirrors those who struggle with eating too many carbs. Patients dependent upon alcohol often have high carb intake too. I don't recommend tackling both carbs and alcohol at the same time. Start with booze. Once you can go two-weeks without a drink, then focus on carbs.

If you matched any of the 6, STOP.

If you matched any of those six categories, you are in the Doctor Club. You need closer observation than just reading a book. Take this book to your doctor. Fill out as much of the workbook as possible. Upon arrival, share the documents in the workbook with your doctor.

Also, I recommend folks in the Doctor Club drink BHB for the next 10-14 days. Sip on the supplement while you fill out sections inside the workbook. Sip on it as you cut back on your carbs.

Your body will find the transition more manageable if you "drip in" some ketones for several weeks. This golden tip has helped many of my fragile patients smoothly adapt to keto chemistry. They desperately needed ketosis. A transition like David's blocked their prior attempts. Titrating in ketones-in-a-can safely bridged them across the transition.

If you're in the 200 Club, SLOW DOWN.

If you eat more than 200 carbs per day, you do not need to see a physician before you start, but you need to take some precautions. Slow down.

Use the two-week countdown covered thoroughly in Chapter 12.

Just like the Doctor Club, I recommend drinking BHB for the next two weeks. Sipping on that supplement makes transitioning from pine needles to logs much easier.

MEASUREMENTS THAT MATTER:

Take a few measurements before tomorrow. Write them down inside your workbook with the date.

Carbs Consumed in 24 Hours

Add them up. Please do not skip this. It is profoundly important in predicting how well your transition will go. Make Cronometer your best helper for 3 days before starting.

Weight & Height

Hop on the scale. Even if you are not doing this for weight loss, measure your weight. It's fascinating to see how much weight slips out over the first two weeks. Patients using keto to help with their cancer or metabolic issues often worry about unwanted weight loss. Rest assured, most weight lost over the first 14 days comes from inflammation. This is not the weight you want on your body. Keeping track helps the medical team.

Add your height to the measurements in your Cronometer app and jot down your BMI. [See workbook.] Body Mass Index is calculated from your height and weight. Among the many metrics, BMI continues to be an excellent indicator of metabolic health. BMI predicts insulin resistance better than most blood tests, metabolic calculators, or stress tests. The few exceptions where BMI failed to predict insulin resistance happened when the number sunk under 18.

Waistline

Measure your waistline. Don't complicate this with questions, "Where on my waist should I measure?" It's not that complicated. You don't have to measure like a professional tailor. The pants you have on right now encircle your waist. Put the measuring tape or string over that waistband. Ladies wearing a dress - use the waistline around the top of your underpants or hosiery.

Neck Circumference

Measure the distance in inches around your neck. Your neck circumference predicts several health markers. Keto-chemistry will improve these. Seventeen inches is the magical cutoff. A neck size greater than 17 inches adds risk to your health. Document in the chart-workbook where you start.

Shin-Thumb Print

Finally, check to see if you have swelling over your shinbone. In doctor-speak, we call this peripheral edema. In the real world, it's better known as 'ring around the socks.' The shin-thumbprint measures how much inflammation you store in your lower legs. I do this on every physical exam in my clinic. This teaches me as much about their health as the blood pressure. I instruct medical students to do this as one of the best parameters for measuring chronic diseases.

"How inflamed is the patient?"

"Check the shinbone."

The area over your shinbone does not have any fat cells between the skin and bone. Healthy people with no inflammation have skin and connective tissues without extra fluid over the shin. Moisture should not swamp between the cells in the body. There should never be space between the cells. If fluid is squeezing into that hidden area, you have problems. Your body uses the potential space between cells as a ditch to pool extra fluid. Gravity pulls it to the lower leg, and we can squish it out of the way with a Shin-thumbprint. In fairness, it is a better storage location for extra fluid than in your lungs. Or your brain. I think of this fluid between cells as lighter fluid for inflamma-tion—that flame sweeps through the body traveling in this hidden space. See if you have lighter fluid waiting to ignite between your cells.

Here is how it is done. Start by looking at the thumbnail on your thumb. You should see a slightly pink color as you look through your thumbnail. Next, press your thumb firmly in to the paper on this page. Watch the tip of your thumb turn from pink to white as you apply pressure. Be sure you are looking at the very tip. The pink turns to white because the pressure stopped the blood from entering those tiny blood vessels in your thumbnail. Lift your thumb and it will turn pink again. If nail polish covers your nail, you can focus on the flesh on either side of the nail. Repeat that a couple of times to be sure you understand how much pressure you need to turn the tip of your thumb white. It's okay if you press too hard for this exercise. Pushing too little will not correctly measure your inflammation. The pressure you used to turn your thumb white is the same pressure needed for the Shin-Thumbprint test.

Now place your thumb onto your shin bone about 3-5 inches above your ankle. Be sure you are directly over the bone. Press firmly enough to blanch your thumbnail. Hold this pressure for thirty seconds. If it hurts too much when you first push onto the shin, slow down. Start with a little pressure, and gradually increase the amount you press. Don't start the 30-second clock until the tip of your thumbnail is white.

Hold for 30 seconds.

Then lift away. Is there an impression left in your shin from your thumb? If not ... do a little dance. Your inflammation hovers around ZERO. That's normal to have no hidden moisture in the ditches between cells. If there's a slight indentation, you have mild inflammation. If you buried your thumb up to the first knuckle, you have ditches full of lighter fluid. In**FLAME**d tissue.

Take a picture. You'll want to compare this to your results in 3 weeks.

The tissue between your skin and your shinbone is not fat. It is the connective tissue that should not have extra fluid soaking around. The pressure from your thumb pushed the water out of that area. You can not push fat around like that. Fatty tissue leaves no dimple — only extra water does. Ketogenic chemistry reverses inflammation and "wrings out" much of the unwanted fluid in the body. This concept is difficult for patients to grasp until I show them their Shin-Thumbprint. If you left a divot in your shin from this test, you will benefit significantly from ketones in circulation.

Chapter 9

DAVID'S DAY 1

Monday morning, David arrived at his office determined to write a brand new chapter. Sunday's whirlwind purging cupboards, primed his mind for success. He and his wife had emptied out their pantry and found bare shelves on Monday morning. The emptiness threw him out of his habit of cereal with orange juice before leaving the house.

Gone. Bare cupboards.

High fat. No carbs.

How hard can this be?

David added heavy cream to his coffee, hopped into his car, and drove to work. On his way, he drove through McDonald's, "Three eggs with three sausage patties. No bread. Just the eggs and sausage," he ordered.

David parked his car, and heartily ate breakfast. Now filled with a belly full of fat, he dashed across the street and into the drug store to buy PeeTone strips.

David and his wife worked together. He knew she'd arrive 90 minutes after him. The office atmosphere had different food-rules than his house. Removing the landmines of temptations hiding at the studio topped off his to-do list. He wanted them gone, just like his home. With a little luck, he could have the place carb-free by the time Kat got there.

"I've got this," he coaxed himself.

David's mind replayed the scene from last Friday as his eyes locked onto the pretzels claiming his desk. The pretzels held the familiarity of a good friend—a dangerous one. For years his friendship with food bridged him through the loneliest chapters. "Garbage! Don't allow one into your mouth," he muttered. The memory of comfort would win if he took one bite.

Armed with a large black garbage bag, he dumped the glass dish holding the salty snacks. Somehow the bowl was guilty too. Out went the candy he had for "the customers." Keeping people energized for a photoshoot meant dosing them with sugar at every turn. Truthfully, most of those treats ended up in his mouth. Beyond the pretzel bowl, the office concealed dozens of sweets. Like a war zone, a craving could randomly explode at any moment. The pretzels were tossed without remorse. The old bag of hard candy on the top shelf had aged beyond appealing. "Dump it."

Suckers with the string handle held fond memories, and had made it into a few of his favorite photos. Many adolescent moods had settled down, thanks to those. "It's a trap. Throw them away!" Sugar melted fears; quieted anxiety. "Dump them." Tootsie rolls. "Gone as well."

David rounded the corner to the office pantry with shelves of fast foods, just in case. "Just in case of what?" he thought. Ramen noodles for lunch. Cans of soup. Tossed.

His eyes locked onto a travel camera-bag housing the gear that he always took to photoshoots outside the office. It was his bag, no one else's. But secretly lining his "good bag," hiding along the side of the inside pocket... were his favorite treats. David's mouth watered as he remembered the last time he savored his favorite chocolate bar containing chunky bits of toffee.

The smooth chocolate on his tongue. The crunch of the toffee. The seal of the sugar as it glued his teeth together after a few bites. This was David's stash. Chocolate, like a temptress, called his hand towards the bag. He thought, "One last bite. I don't want them to go to waste. This is the end. Eat them. Be done. Forever."

"Let me help you," said a soft voice coming from behind David. This soothing voice yanked him out of his chocolate fantasy and back to reality. It was his wife. The voice of a savior.

"Hey, er, awm... You're early! Ah, help with what?" David said, while still getting his mind re-oriented to the here and now.

"Think I don't know about your secret stash." She said with a wry smile.

They both laughed. Her being there, at his side made David's temptation vanish. With someone watching, the right answer easily slid into place. He emptied the bag in front of her. She helped to empty the other hiding spots.

She approved the cleansed cupboards. The success of a clean work environment occurred at the dumpster. David and Kat simultaneously tossed their bags. That's a win. David breathed a sigh of relief, knowing that all of his temptations were out of the way. He could now take on the day.

Hunger chimed from the pit of his stomach a few hours later. Usually, he snacked on a few bits of "just in case" two hours after his cereal, and then again a few hours later. But today cheese and pepperoni were his snacks. Anytime the slightest hint of hunger quivered through him, he had a few more bites of these high-fat foods. He washed it down with his creamed coffee. A trip to the bathroom mid-afternoon offered his first chance to check urine ketones.

BAM! The sponge on the tip of the strip showed the slightest hint of pink. Positive. WOW! That was easy. He couldn't stop smiling. He was there.

In a flash, his afternoon photoshoot with Dr. Boz and Grandma Rose arrived. Excitedly he awaited their arrival. Grandma Rose was the focus of the chapters Dr. Boz had shared. Her words painted a grim picture: An elderly woman fighting cancer for over a decade. He imagined a frail, lady suffering from the deadly issues lurking inside her body.

David had photographed many folks preparing for their obituaries. A professional photo during times of illness could be tricky. An obituary photo often added closure. Even though the email never mentioned it, David knew the scene well. Years in the business taught him what the obit-requests looked like.

Midwesterners of Norwegian descent inherited the cultural etiquette too lovely to talk about the need for an obit-pic.

It is always assumed, never spoken.

David played the scene in his mind as he waited. The elder usually arrived dressed in their Sunday best with an heirloom of jewelry fastened in plain view, and escorted by the next generation. David found the photoshoots intimate. He often assessed his own mortality as he studied the pictures afterward. He was ready.

David looked up as two sisters walked into the studio. "Hi. May I help you?"

The two women removed their coats as they approached. "Hi, David. I'm Dr. Bosworth. This is Grandma Rose."

David arrested all movement. His attempt to speak came out in a stutter instead. He processed what he saw and sorted away from the idea these were sisters. Mother and daughter? He expected a crippled, debilitated, and wilted 73-year old woman. Instead walked in a thin, vibrant, energized lady who looked way, way younger than her age. Her skin glowed; her smile radiated energy into the whole room. She looked incredible.

After what felt like minutes, David finally delivered the proper welcoming words. "Come on in. Wow! It's so nice to meet you."

David compared the woman talking to him to the one he'd read about in those chapters, and the photo of Grandma Rose from 18 months ago. That picture matched all the words of illness, cancerous disease, and impending death. The photo looked normal for a 71-year-old woman with ten years of cancer. For all the wrong reasons, her image was South-Dakota-normal. She carried the 50 pudgy pounds expected in every Grandma. Her eyes shared her fatigue and fragility. Deeply creased wrinkles diving outward from her eyes advertised her age. Blood vessels roped under thin skin in the photo. The wilted look in her eyes was merely standard. You would call it normal too unless you met her today.

Grandma Rose glided into the office with the magic of Mary Poppins. As if a vacuum had sucked away 50 pounds of fat swaddling her cheeks, arms, and neck, she looked decades younger than the woman in the photo. Her flow of energy made the lights brighter, and the mood lighter. Happiness signaled David's eardrums as her strong voice said, "It's nice to meet you, David."

How could this person come from the words he'd read in those chapters? David chased away his pre-conceived image of Grandma Rose dancing around in his head. His thoughts swirled, dragging a million questions along:

How is this possible?

What did you eat today?

How long did it take to get the energy?

What happened to the cancer?

Are your cupboards still empty?

How did you reverse your age?

Can I do this?

She answered between snaps of the camera, "Steak, bacon, hamburgers - extra cheese and gua-camole, no bun. Burrito bowls without the rice or beans, extra sour cream."

David's questions ping-ponged back and forth, filling the photoshoot with genuine attraction and cu-riosity. Grandma Rose hypnotized and infused David with the hope that he, too, could restore his health the way she had. Meeting her motivated him. To see her with his own eyes cut through his haze of wishing.

David was in. He wanted what she had, "Send me a bottle of whatever she drank."

Before we left, I invited David to attend the local keto support group, "Just come. You'll learn so much. Just come."

David looked at his wife as the door closed, "Well, that certainly was not an obit-pic."

"Right!" Kat replied, "She isn't headed for a coffin anytime soon. What a remarkable story."

The invitation to the keto group saturated David's mind as he left the office that evening. He and Kat drove to the diner nearby. Images of Grandma Rose dazzled their thoughts as husband and wife ate as many Buffalo Wings as possible.

Supper passed in near silence while the wings disappeared.

Step 1: No sugar. No starch. High fat.

The best summary of this way of eating is "no sugar, no starch, high fat." Say those words out loud. Again. *"No sugar. No starch. High fat."*

Start your day with eggs & bacon. If you scramble the eggs, add FULL-fat cheese, not low-fat. Substitute a bowl of ground hamburger soaked in butter if you don't want bacon. Eat until you are full.

Do not skip breakfast. Most keto-beginners have no desire for breakfast on day one. For now, force yourself to eat breakfast. This won't be a permanent rule. But eating food filled with fat and flavor prepares the mind and body for success. This first week matters the most for eating a high-fat, low-carb breakfast.

You're about to burst into the big evil world of temptations. DO NOT walk out the door hungry. Fill your belly with fatty foods without sugar or starch— *just fat.*

In just a few days, David threw his brain into a fit of disruption as he transitioned fuels from 100% glucose to fat. Like most Americans, David had plenty of stored fat, but he couldn't access that until his insulin lowered. The way to do this is: No sugar. No starch. *High fat.*

Step 2: Twenty. 20.

Twenty is the magic number. The only number to focus on is 20. The only thing I want you to count is carbs. Not calories. Not grams of fiber, or fat, or protein. Not pounds or inches. Only carbs. Start your path to ketosis with no more than 20 grams of carbs per day.

Use the <u>Cronometer app.</u> Once you've set up the app, it will guide you by suggesting foods that fall within your settings. This works far better than a planned pre-packaged menu.

The Standard American Diet (SAD) loads plates with 60% carbs. SAD packs more than 200 grams of sugar-based fuel into your body. Every single cell burns glucose when you eat this way. From your brain to your skin, your system uses sugar for energy. Pine needles smoke through mitochondria at every turn.

As you exchange logs for pine needles, a mismatch in energy occurs. The glucose falls faster than the ketones can be used. This energy gap produces a mighty crabby mood. Beware. Hang in there.

If your BMI (body mass index) slides over 25.0, your endocrine system overshoots insulin. Your pancreas dispatches insulin to address excess carbs. Insulin locks fat inside that layer of pudginess. Stored fat remains locked until insulin sinks. Continuously elevated insulin sparks your cravings to eat carbs. You live in a constant cycle where insulin chases carbs.

Break that cycle. Cut your carbs. When you reduce your carb count to less than 20, your body shifts hormones with insulin leading the way.

Do not get distracted by dietary fiber, net carbs, counting sugars, or adding up calories.

Just remember the number 20 and count only total carbs!

Step 3: Pee on a PeeTone stick

Transitioning people's behavior starts with clear instructions and something measurable.

Clear Measurable Instruction: Limit your carb intake to 20. Pee on Peetone sticks to detect the presence of ketones.

Step 4: Grocery Shop

WARNING: Use brain chemistry to help you when entering the grocery store. How? Feel FULL....Very FULL. Satiated with FAT!

David and his wife left the diner with bellies stuffed full of BONE-IN hot wings before grocery shopping. Those little chicken wings had so much going for them. They contain a minimal amount of chicken meat surrounded by skin and fat. They took time to eat, and the spices prompted them to dip every bite into the fat-filled dressings of ranch or blue cheese.

They waddled into the grocery store with a hint of nausea from stuffing their guts.

Nausea communicated the fact that they were chemically satiated. That's the best way to go food shopping on the first days of keto.

The Paradox of Choice

Abundant choices derail newly formed habits. So take advantage of another behavioral hack. Our brains like routines with limited options. We act predictably inside our routines. During the first few weeks, limit your food choices by sticking to foods on this shopping list (below). These foods will pave a path toward success.

Extra food options act as a flickering neon sign, "TEMPTATION!" Temptations lead to failure. This is especially true during the early stages. Think of the first two-weeks as refining your behavior. Reset the food rules. Keep food choices straightforward.

Grocery List

RESTOCK your egg supply. Buy 5 dozen.

Bacon or Sausage Patties

Heavy Whipping Cream (HWC)

Pink Salt Crystals

Epsom Salt

Full-fat Hamburger

Butter

Pepperoni Slices

Meat Sticks

Sardines In Olive or Fish Oil (Just Do It)

Mayonnaise LOW CARB

Mustard

Olive Salad In A Jar (Muffuletta)

Onion

Pork Rinds

Fatty Cheese .. wrapped in wax.

Feta Cheese

Walnuts, Macadamia Nuts, or Pine Nuts

Bag of Chia Seeds.

WHILE AT the grocery store - check blood pressure.

Other General Rules to Follow

No Sweet Drinks

Keep the fat. Remove the sweeteners first. Modern-day fake sugars trap you with their sweet tastes. That sugary sensation triggers a memory. Longing for that familiar comfort starts when you tease your taste buds with the taste of sugar, even when no calories are there. Your brain is a sneaky little organ. Memories of that "feel good substance" awaken every time the sweet taste lands on your tongue. Relapse lurks in your future if you frost your tongue with that sweet memory. Taste buds sparkle with excitement. The signal travels from your tongue to your brain, igniting a craving for more. POW! Without warning or permission, your thoughts and body plead, scream, and squirm for more.

This signal needs to stop. Cravings will haunt you if you continue consuming sweetened drinks. The only way to suppress that memory is to stop adding sweet taste to your tongue. Abstinence! Your memory fades the longer sweetness stays away. Reset your brain with unsweetened drinks. No diet drinks. No sugar substitutes. No sweeteners, even if they naturally come from a honeybee. For the best results, stop all sweetened beverages.

In a perfect and advanced ketone world, drinks supporting keto-chemistry contain no calories and no sweeteners. That's right. They don't taste sweet. And no cream or oil swirls in them. That utopian drink is <u>not</u> for beginners.

Again, beginners start by first getting rid of the "devilish" sweet tastes in drinks. However, leave the fat, such as cream or MCT oil, in the drinks for now. Fat-filled drinks ensure a substantial shift in your chemistry. Adding heavy cream or butter to your coffee or tea pushes the amount of fat. This is critical when starting out. The more you take commanding charge to alter your chemistry using high fat, the easier and faster your transition.

Fix Chemistry before Calories

For decades, the medical establishment in the US has preached that calories matter. The truth? They don't matter when insulin reigns over your body. First, focus on reducing your insulin. Swallowing fat sparks minimal insulin to squeeze into your system. Beginners sail through the first weeks of keto when they eat an abundance of high-fat in the absence of carbs. *Follow this rule to lower your insulin.*

Only Fat

Don't focus on which type of fat. Confusion sets in when you start thinking about good fat, bad fat, seed-oil fat, animal fat, or dairy fat. Just focus on fat. Too many rules at first will overwhelm you. Eat and drink FAT. Period.

At first, some complain they don't like the taste of fat. An oil slick annoys their mouth and tongue. Stay the course. Once insulin drops, so many secretions change, thanks to keto-chemistry. One of those secretions is your saliva. Your teeth and tastebuds will praise the new chemistry in your mouth.

By 8 o'clock that night, David and his wife re-stocked their fridge with keto-friendly groceries. The temptation to snack on something sweet quivered through David's body. Irritability made itself known as he began to hunt for sugar. Salty macadamia nuts were the closest solution he could find. Down the hatch went four handfuls.

As the nuts descended into his gut, his mood settled. As his orneriness faded, he appreciated the importance of not having access to more carbs. He would have eaten them over those macadamia nuts for sure.

Bedtime was usually not for 2 more hours, but he felt strangely tired. Standing in the junction between the TV room and the hall towards his bedroom, he chose the latter. "Just go straight to bed," he told himself. Nearly 30 hours had passed since his last binge of carbs. Bed seemed like the least destructive option.

Go straight to bed.

Chapter 10

DAY 2: PINK PEETONES

David awoke the next morning after an unsettled night's sleep. That early bedtime wrinkled his routine, and unbalanced his rhythm. His mood changed when he peed on his Pee-Tone strip — Dark Purple! What did that mean? According to the bottle's instructions, that meant David had high ketones. His mood brightened; he stood a little taller, proud of his accomplishment. "I made ketones," he chuckled. "That was easy," he boasted as he headed to the kitchen to make some eggs.

If you peed ketones by day two, do a little dance and skip this chapter. If not, read about glycogen.

What is glycogen?

Thirty-eight hours had lapsed since David's last carb. Since that bite, he had burned the sugars circulating in his bloodstream. Poof! Pine needles crackled and snapped right through his mitochondria. When no more carbs entered his mouth, his system looked towards his stored sugar. Glycogen is stored sugar.

Glycogen had tucked into David's liver and muscle cells during his seasons of abundance dating back three decades. His sugars rose along with his insulin. Insulin commanded the excess glucose to quickly link arms and string together. Those strings of sugars wound into a vacuole or a bubble. Glycogen-bubbles had rapidly stored his unused, excess glucose in preparation for the expected drop in glucose and insulin. Once tucked away, glycogen sat there, just waiting, like a squirrel's nest of nuts in the Fall. David's thirty year supply of stored glucose overflowed thanks to his constant carb consumption. His squishy, plump, fresh glycogen bubbles had crystallized. Beyond his sleeping hours, he hadn't seen a 4-hour window without carbs in years. His constant carbs buttressed his level of insulin.

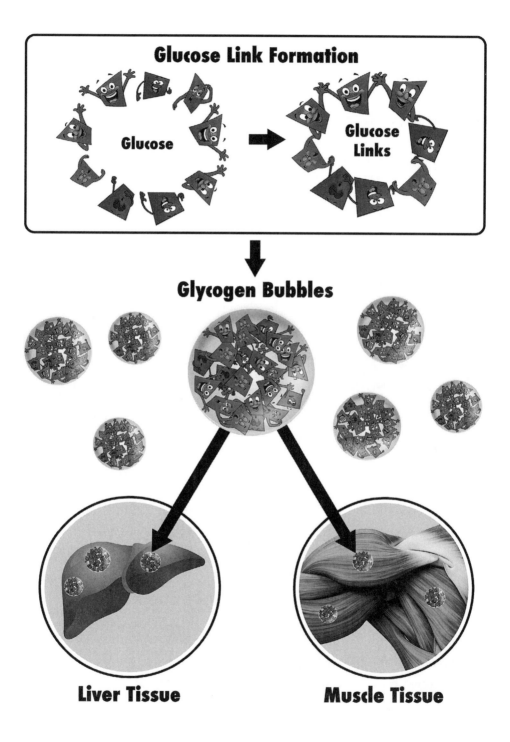

Glucose Link Formation

Glucose

Glucose Links

Glycogen Bubbles

Liver Tissue

Muscle Tissue

Nearly 40 hours ago, David slashed carbs. This dropped his insulin a bit, opening his access to years of stored glycogen.

How long does glycogen last?

Good question. Asked another way, "How long will it take to empty out all of David's glycogen-bubbles?"

The answer depended upon the amount of storage David had squirreled into his liver and muscle cells. He harbored the maximum number of cells that had stretched to full-capacity with glycogen-bubbles. After three decades of hoarding glucose, David's abundance would take quite some time to empty. The rate he depleted his stockpile depended upon how well he shifted his chemistry.

The more vigorous David's health practices veered towards keto-chemistry, the wider he opened his glycogen bin. Let's break that down further.

RATE of Glycogen Depletion:
How swiftly did you **shift your chemistry**?
How much **energy** did your mitochondria **use**?

MASS of Glycogen Present:
How many **muscle cells** do you have?
How many **liver cells** do you have?

Doc, how long will it take to empty my extra glycogen bubble?

$$\text{GLYCOGEN DEPLETION} = \frac{\text{TOTAL STORED GLYCOGEN}}{\text{RATE YOU BURN GLUCOSE}}$$

TOTAL STORED GLYCOGEN

Muscle Mass
Men Greater than Women

Liver Cell Mass
Size of liver is related to years
of alcohol or excess insulin.

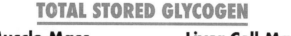

RATE YOU BURN GLUCOSE

**Energy Demand
of the Body:**
Exercise
Infection
Cancer
Injuries
Growth Spurt
Temperature
Baseline Functions

**Chemistry of
the Body:**
Insulin
Ketone production
Strict Low Carb
(<20 carbs Per day)
Eat only when the sun is up
Eat HIGH FAT until fat adapted
No sugar/sweet drinks

MITOCHONDRIA

Shift Your Chemistry:

David's strict adherence to cutting carbs dropped his insulin sharply in the first 24 hours. This blessed him with a wave of improved chemistry for burning stored glucose. If he would have denied that late-night temptation of macadamia nuts, it would have been even better.

Energy Used:

David spent most hours behind a desk and computer. His daily routine lacked a consistent exercise regimen; in short, he led a sedentary life. Thankfully, he wasn't fighting cancer or any types of infection. Medical issues such as those, as well as healing a broken bone, or repairing from an invasive surgical procedures, require extra fuel. David's body only asked for a minimum amount of energy to maintain his baseline functions. His mitochondria stayed in low gear, surviving on just a few ketones, or a few dozen glucose molecules per day.

Muscle Mass:

As a man, David stored more glycogen because of his higher number of muscle cells. However, his 63 inches held fewer muscle cells than someone a foot taller, but more than a woman of matched age and size. To further complicate things, those years of sedentary living estimated that one in three of his muscle cells actively burned fuel. The rest all but turned off their mitochondria from lack of use.

Liver Mass:

Finally, how large was David's liver? He'd never thought about that. Its size depended on how much he had stressed his liver over the years. He used to drink alcohol years ago, but never in excess. The chemical stressing David's liver was insulin.

The liver's response to insulin is to grow more liver cells. Yes! Insulin is a growth hormone. It instructs things to grow. Insulin grows liver cells along with skin cells, fat cells, cancer cells, and more. Insulin is not the only thing to spark new liver cell growth. Excess alcohol also triggers them to replicate. The growth of extra liver cells matches the amount of alcohol consumed. At autopsy, we can measure how many years of excess alcohol took place based on the liver's size. The same goes for excess insulin.

Extra carbohydrates stuffed David's liver cells with glycogen. When he ran out of storage space, his liver made more storage cells. His liver strained from the pressure of thirty years of extra carbs. His insulin worked overtime and always rang that alarm. David kept up with the carbohydrate onslaught by replicating liver cells as fast as he over-ate. When his liver failed to produced storage space for all the excess glucose, his blood sugars rose.

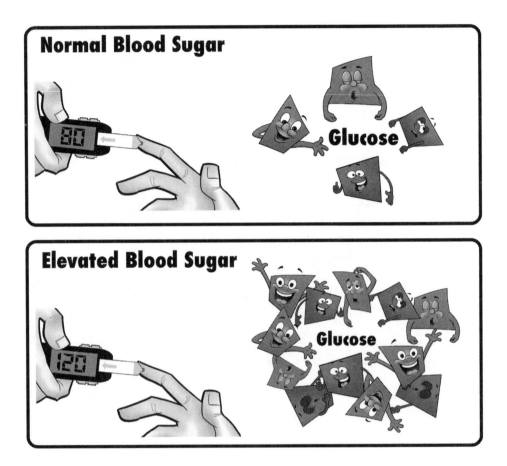

Did you empty your liver last night?

Let's check. After 12 hours with only water, prick your finger and check your fasting blood sugar.

Don't roll your eyes. You must know someone who has diabetes and checks their blood sugars. Borrow their glucose monitor for one day. No, they won't die if they don't check for a day.

If you burned through all your glycogen and emptied your storage, your fasting sugars will fall between 55-80 mg/dL. That's a surefire sign you have a normal-sized liver. However, if you've stretched and stuffed your liver with too many extra carbs, you won't burn through all the storage in 12 hours. It might take 20 hours to burn all those pine needles. Some overweight patients take a week. Others take up to a month. If your blood sugar first thing in the morning rises above 125 mg/dL, you HAVE DIABETES. No joke! That's the rule used to diagnose a diabetic.

David's morning blood sugars ranged in the 110-130. He did not know his glucose was that high. It would be weeks before he learned that. His body dripped with extra insulin and sugar. He drastically dropped carbs, lowered his insulin, and made his first ketones. He smashed those changes into his body in record time - under 36 hours. He wobbled into ketosis on a tightrope, unaware of all the shifting chemistry taking place behind the scenes.

Day 2 is the Toughest

David left his house with a belly full of eggs and cheese, sipping coffee with a generous dollop of heavy cream. He remarked that he didn't feel well. The universe seemed to have dialed up the gravitational pull. An invisible heaviness worked against him as he lifted his coffee for a sip. It seemed as if someone added lead weight to everything: His thoughts, movements, body sensations. He sank deeper into the car cushion as he drove. He pulled into the parking space at work, and just sat there for a few minutes. Something primal told him not to stand up.

David felt shaky, yet dense. He kept his butt in the driver's seat, thinking about, visualizing the stash of chocolate toffee he threw away. "Maybe it's still in the dumpster," he thought. An irrational craving for sugar made saliva leak out of his tongue.

Should David have pricked his finger at that moment, he would have seen his blood sugar at its lowest point in months. His "low" glucose would be considered average, compared to a healthy person. To David's body, this was "low." *His* body wanted — it begged for the missing glucose. His glucose had sunk so much that it triggered a craving.

The sight of his office door flashed pretzels and chocolate across his mind. He looked at his packed lunch of pepperoni, cheese, and nuts. Irritability wrinkled his forehead as he growled, "Don't want fat. I want carbs."

Where was that energy Grandma Rose had? He peed ketones! Wasn't that the point of this stupid diet? Why didn't he feel like she looked?

David pushed the car door open and stood, steadying himself. Something wasn't right. David never fainted before; but he was certain that what he was experiencing was the same as someone who's just about to pass out. The invisible lead weights pulled him back into the driver's seat. Moisture coated the back of his hand as he wiped it across his forehead.

"Is this a heart attack?" he worried. "Maybe this isn't the diet for me?" David took inventory. No chest pain. No left arm pain. His breathing seemed exaggerated. He just needed carbs — he was sure that was the answer.

With not a single carb within reach, time passed without David tracking it. When he notice that twenty minutes had lapsed, the sweating stopped, his breathing improved, and his weighted feet felt lighter again. He felt better. Whatever had temporarily overpowered him faded.

David cautiously walked into his office, steadying himself along the wall. He plopped into his chair, relieved to sit down. The phone rang. It was Kat, calling to tell him that she, too, felt crummy and was staying home. If she felt better she would come to the office. But for now bed rest seemed like the remedy she thought she needed. Hearing what his wife just said reassured David that he must have a bug. Kat never stayed home. She must have what he had. They both must've gotten a bug.

What if your PeeTone Strip is not Pink by Day 2?

If you're at the end of your second day and not turning your PeeTone strip pink, don't panic. You are not alone. Most Americans struggle with excessive insulin and livers stuffed with glycogen. Your insulin has been elevated, locking fat and glycogen bubbles into storage for the better part of a decade. They must fall to allow the purge that excess storage.

The ticket for folks who have not peed ketones by the end of Day Two is to eat more fat. Hold the carbs. Fat will also keep you feeling full. No matter how much fat you digest in the first several days of a keto diet, it will never stimulate as much insulin as the carbs that you used to consume. Eat fat! Stay the course! I cannot emphasize this enough. Do not pay attention to calories or grams of fat. Focus on swiftly switching your chemistry by cutting carbs and consuming fat.

SUGGESTION: Eat a burrito in a bowl: No tortilla — hold the rice, hold the beans. Order as much fatty meat as you like. Use guacamole. Include sour cream. Add as much cheese as you want. Hot sauce with a few roasted peppers and onions satisfy without too many carbs. Eat until you are stuffed.

Drink water, tea, or coffee. You will get there.

Chapter 11

THE PRICE OF FAT & NOT-SO-HAPPY

It's shameful to admit how quickly I sort people into two categories: Healthy and unhealthy. Decades of practicing the skill of sorting chronic illnesses from the healthy is now an unconscious habit for me. I just do it without thinking, not asking for permission. When I walked into the photoshoot with my mom, I automatically assessed David. A fifty-five-year-old man with a waistline thicker than his hips and a belt fastened in the final notch. His movements were just a milli-second too soon with a character of spasticity. Jerky; staccato. Something about his fleeting brain awakened anxiety in everyone in the room. David's body followed instructions from his fibrillating neurons as he jumped from topic to topic. His eyes bounced from one object to the next without quite enough time to focus. Words rapidly left his voice box without projection — like a partially connected micro-phone. His voice wasn't muffled, yet not crisp either.

His shirt buttons fastened with tension across the thickness swaddling his middle. Seventeen inches of collar cuffed his neck, and he left that top button un-fastened behind his tie. A seventeen-inch neck was three inches thicker than it should have been. The dark skin shadowing the back of his neck looked velvety. This darkness warned me of his years of high insulin.

Organ Analysis

I sorted through his organs one by one.

Lungs

David's belly wouldn't win the Santa Claus contest, but it stole real estate from his lungs. His stored carbohy-drates severely extended his waistline, while simulta-neously shoving his organs upward, squishing his lungs. What was the consequence? David's lungs failed to fully expand when he inhaled. The sound of restrict-ed airflow cut to my eardrums. I heard danger at the end of each breath — the end of his exhale was miss-ing. The pattern of breathing was unmistakable. On a medical chart, his diagnosis would be restrictive air-way disease due to a fat tummy.

Kat complained about the near-death episodes happening each night. For years David's snoring rattled the airwaves in their bedroom. His desperate gasps for air recently snapped her awake. David's breathing muscles naturally relaxed during the deepest phases of his sleep. Like many other overweight patients, his windpipe collapsed, and he suffocated every time he sunk into deep-sleep. Diagnosis: Sleep Apnea.

Those extra 20-30 pounds pushing on his abdomen made it impossible to pull in a complete breath. Without that full breath, his energy wilted.

Sleep Apnea robbed him of a good night's sleep. When David slept, each collapse of his windpipe rang alarm bells. Danger! Danger! Falling asleep threatened his life. Without air, his cells' oxygen fell - while his free-radicals rose. This deprived setting ping-ponged electrons and inflamed his tissue. Finally, in the dark of the night, a desperate rescue breath awoke Kat and pulled air into David's lungs. Oxygen billowed inward. David "slept" through all this unaware of the danger. His unsettled sleep and inefficient daytime breathing joined forces to deliver twenty-four hours of sheer cellular struggle.

David needed deep-sleep to heal, record his memories from the previous day, and strengthen his endocrine system. What was the price he paid for too much insulin and low oxygen? Brain cells. Sleep Apnea deteriorated his brain while the extra insulin sped up the destruction.

STATEMENT: If your neck measures 17 inches or more, get screened for sleep apnea. Nothing in this book will outrank the need for nightly oxygen. Your brain's health depends upon it. Address sleep apnea. Wear the Darth Vader mask. Using ketogenic nutrition, you will lose weight. Once that weight is off your body, ask your doctor if it's okay to sleep without your Darth Vader mask again.

Heart

For argument's sake, let's set aside David's history of elevated cholesterol. His fifty extra pounds pushed him into the obese category with a BMI of 30. Each pound of fat added seven miles to the hoses his heart pumped blood through every single heartbeat. David had three-hundred and fifty extra miles of arteries and veins. "Lub-dub, lub-dub, lub-dub," echoed through his tunnels. In between those two sounds hid a split-second of rest. That tiny, quiet moment predicted the longevity for David's heart. His heart squeezed harder because of those extra miles, and found no rest between heartbeats. He needed the increased pressure within his tubes to keep the flow moving through the extra miles. He needed his increased blood pressure.

Excess insulin burned through his veins and arteries leaving that grimy layer of inflammation coating the insides of his arteries — slowly decreasing the space for flowing blood. His heart muscle twisted and squeezed as hard as possible to push blood through his now thread-like pipes. Each added pound of fat decreased oxygen and nutrients delivered to the other tissues. Additionally, his mitochondria weakened because insulin remained high.

David's increased blood pressure mixed with low oxygen resulted in failure — Heart failure. Yes. That's correct. His heart failed to meet the demands of his body. When hearts fail, cells die. And some of David's heart-cells were dead. They had morphed into scars a couple of years ago. David knew none of this.

Liver

David celebrated five years alcohol-free on New Year's Eve. But unfortunately, his liver continued to harden even without the added stress from alcohol. Years of being overweight sparked a flame inside his body. Like lighter-fluid, insulin carried the flicker of fire throughout his body. The flame hid between his cells - all cells, but especially his liver cells. The spaces between David's cells slid further and further apart. This flame tunneled through out his body, burning and searing problems into his health. This was inflammation. The hottest fire camouflaged itself inside the strongest driver of metabolism: The liver. David's organ swelled with the build-up of grime. More lighter-fluid poured into the liver's spaces when his insulin rose. Insulin stuffed glucose into the storage bins throughout the organ's cells. Glycogen peppered his liver to the point of engorgement.

Years ago, David's liver cells switched tactics from storing energy as glucose to storing it as fat. Fat held more fuel-power than glycogen and packed into a smaller size. Layers of fat slithered between his sticky glycogen-filled cells. His fatty, sticky, flame-filled liver slowly hardened.

Tummy

David's paunch had embarrassed him, but it could have made him the runner up for being the next Santa Claus. In the upcoming months, keto-chemistry would melt away his paunch. As his waistline slimmed, David would feel healthier and would receive praise for the missing bulge around his middle. He would take pride in his shrinking mound of abdominal fat. Yet, although David looked better, it was his visceral fat that increased his chances of death.

That's correct. His visceral fat was the widow-maker. Visceral fat snaked in and around the gut's organs such as the kidneys, liver, pancreas, intestines, and adrenal glands. This serpentine slime increased his risk of heart disease, stroke, foggy brain, Alzheimer's, prostate cancer, and colon cancer. Ignited by insulin, his visceral fat subtracted months from his life.

Kidney

Thanks to excess insulin, David's kidneys filtered a high level of inflammatory enzymes. Cytokines, proteins, and inflammatory markers circulated in his blood. His overtaxed kidneys quietly worked overtime, straining to keep his blood clean. They declined each month in secret, without expressing any kind of symptoms. David didn't feel a thing.

Skeletal Muscle

David piped extra fat inside his muscle cells. How did the fat get there? You guessed it — via insulin. Insulin's authoritative voice commanded fat molecules to stay put inside his fat and muscle cells. The fat energy within his muscles just sat there inaccessible to David. That hidden power source could have helped David at the opportune moments whenever he felt tired, or his body needed energy. But insulin blocked that resource. His muscles, brain, and heart all could use fat for fuel if the chemistry was right. Instead, he used the inferior fuel — glucose. The slightest dip in his blood sugar, and he quivered, like a drug-addict, for more carbs. David was stuck. High insulin and carb-craving made it nearly impossible to shift gears to ketones. The symptoms that kept his butt sitting in his car on Day 2 had prevented his progress long enough. His obesity had cost him too much. For too long, he had sold his concentration, oxygenation, and energy. For David, this ended now.

No more!

	KETOSIS	STANDARD AMERICAN DIET
ENERGY PRODUCED (ATP PRODUCED FROM EQUAL-CARBON FUEL)	**2.6 X ATP**	**1 x ATP**
OXYGEN NEEDS	LOW	ELEVATED
VITAMIN NEEDS	LOW	HIGH
ANTI-OXIDANT NEEDS	LOW	HIGH
DIGESTIVE SECRETIONS	4000 - 5000 ml	8000 - 10000 ml
FOOD VOLUME NEEDED	350 - 450 g	1500 - 3000 g
WATER NEEDS	400 - 700 ml	1500 - 2500 ml
PROTEIN NEEDS (NITROGEN BALANCE)	~60 g	~55 g
CARB NEEDS	0g	UP TO > 600 g
ENERGY STORAGE NEEDS	NO	YES
INSULIN LEVEL	LOW	HIGH

ATP = adenosine triphosphate; ~ = approximately; > = greater than

Keto-Chemistry versus Standard Diet Chemistry

<u>The body functions better in ketosis</u>. The chart above unpacks the truth behind that statement. It compares the body's needs while in a state of ketosis to those associated with standard American eating. Let's work through that chart one row at a time.

Energy

David suffered from an energy mismatch. Fatigued, and run-down, he wanted more fuel chugging through his mitochondria. Despite copious amounts of unused glucose and fat stored in every possible corner of his body, he could not convert that to vitality. His insulin-soaked chemistry saved it for later. David joined thousands seeking a magical jumpstart into their power-circuits. He hungered for a secret ingredient to launch his revival. The answer: A ketone. The ketone fuel delivered the power he wanted, better than any prescription, remedy, or ritual. Carbon for carbon, twice as much energy flowed from furnaces that burned ketones versus carbs. When ketones processed through his mitochondria, the units of energy yielded over two and a half times as much power.

David's energy in the first few days didn't come from ketones. In fact, his energy was missing all around. Eating fewer than twenty carbs meant minimal glucose entering his body from the gut. Plummeting glucose dialed down his insulin. Padlocks restricting access to his storage slowly opened. At that moment, David was suffering from a mismatch. A trickle of glucose from unwinding glycogen-bubbles started to arrive in circulation - but not enough to make up for the previously swallowed carbs.

His liver cells had just begun to make ketones; yet, his cellular mechanics to burn ketones into energy were still hibernating from years of non-use. As that assembly line of keto-energy awoke, David needed to stay the course towards keto-chemistry. If he turned back now, his time, energy, and emotions invested would have been for nothing. His mitochondria were still several days away from furnish the superior, fat-driven energy.

Oxygen

Burning ketones requires less oxygen. Sliding ketones through his mitochondria instead of glucose delivered higher amounts of energy from fewer molecules of oxygen. This could help David on many levels. Nightly visits from the Grim Reaper occurred each time he held his breath while sleeping. His nightly breath-holds lowered his oxygen; this compounded his daytime fatigue.

The United States Navy Seals offer a no-nonsense lesson to demonstrate this keto-advantage. They tested their egos with breath-holding contests. Soldiers submerged into the water together, and the last one to surface won the bragging rights for the most-advanced-metabolism. Soldiers who practiced keto-chemistry for weeks before the contest outperformed those eating high-carbs. When carb-eating soldiers drank ketones-in-a-can for 2 days before the competition, they out-performed the carb-lovers who didn't supplement with exogenous ketones. Ketones increased the cell's efficiency to thread oxygen into its metabolic engine. If ketones were available to burn, soldiers held their breath longer thanks to improved oxygen efficiency.

Inside David's mitochondria energy came from the fusion of fuel, either ketones or glucose, with oxygen. David's energy depended upon how well oxygen got delivered to his tissues, along with the supply of fuel. In healthy cells, ample oxygen arrived at the tissue and lit the fuel into energy. Oxygen bound to hemoglobin, rode inside red blood cells to their destination. Upon arrival, oxygen joined with the available fuel inside the mitochondria to energize the cell.

David's paunch as well as his sleep apnea restricted his breathing at night, making it difficult for full oxygen intake. Compounding this was the fact that his red blood cells carrying that oxygen were sticky. Yes, sticky. Sadly, excess sugar had ruined his red blood cells. One out of every eight hemoglobin seats carrying oxygen throughout the body had been destroyed. Glucose had stuck to the hemoglobin — the place where oxygen should sit. That sugary mess acted like a pile of chewed gum filling the seat intended for oxygen. Once the gum stuck to hemoglobin, there was no fixing it. That red blood cell would live out the remainder of it's 100 days of life without the use of that seat. These lost seats added up. Less oxygen being delivered to the fires of the mitochondria, meant less fuel was made. Simply stated —sugar murdered his red blood cells.

David's body made pristine sugar-free red cells each day. However, his blood sugars ranging in the 110s and 120s spat glucose onto every eighth hemoglobin. His elevated sugars sabotaged his health. By reducing his blood sugars into the range of 60-80, his cells would keep the sticky gum out of the hemoglobin-seats intended for oxygen. But it would still take up to three months for David's body to rid itself of its sticky, corroded red blood cells. If he didn't want to wait that long to improve his oxygen performance, he had another option - switch the campfires from burning glucose to ketones. Less oxygen was needed for the ketone-fires.

Vitamins

When David started the ketogenic diet, his body hungered for deficient minerals and vitamins. Missing elements like magnesium, vitamin D, and vitamin K2, could have helped his body as it started to heal. The longer he stayed in keto-chemistry, the better his body would hang onto the needed nutrients and seal the defects in his leaking gut.

After months of keto-chemistry, David's gut stopped leeching valuable minerals and vitamins. Plugging the holes in his leaky gut replaced more vitamins than any supplement. My advanced, healed ketogenic patients maintain their health without vitamin supplements. NONE. Zero.

Anti-Oxidants

Take a stroll down your local drugstore's aisle that sells antioxidants. Each product promises to capture free-radicals bouncing around defective cells by absorbing the wild electrons destroying DNA, cell-walls, and mitotic-division. Free-radicals are free-floating electrons that have escaped the force field magnetizing them to their associated neutron. These wild whispers of electricity destroy cells from the inside out. Antioxidants capture those electrons and neutralize their energy. Once chemically neutral, they lose their ability to wreak havoc. Ketones nullify electrons, too, as they counteract these electrical puffs of destruction. Pour ketones into a free-radical storm and watch those little rascals disappear. Lastly, keto-chemistry prevents electrons from leaving their proper zone.

Compare keto-chemistry to a cart-full of antioxidant supplements, and ketones win every time. First, ketones start their quest already inside the circulation — flowing from the liver and swimming toward cells. Next, ketones naturally slip across the cells' membranes and into the mitochondria — where most free-radicals originate. Drugstore antics have several obstacles to overcome before they get anywhere near the campfires. Absorption, side-effects, and bio-availability place the supplements at quite a disadvantage. Add their costs and tolerance to the fact that most get gobbled up by the liver and never get a chance to penetrate the cell walls. In total, ketones win by a landslide.

STATEMENT: Ketones neutralize reactive oxidants as they absorb electrons. Ketosis further lowers the formation of reactive particles in the first place.

Digestive Enzymes & Food Volume

While in ketosis, David will need less digestive enzymes and less food. Every mouthful of ketogenic food equals 6-8 bites from a standard diet. Ketogenic menus deliver more absorbable vitamins, micronutrients, and essential proteins.

Poop gets dried out in the 2 feet right before your rectum. This section also houses the bacteria that ferment vitamins. The B vitamins, Vitamin K, and biotin spin out of the butts of bacteria living in your colon. These vitamins absorb into your blood along with water.

Patients in ketosis secrete half the volume of digestive enzymes to nourish their bodies. This matters a great deal to David and folks who've undergone weight loss surgery. David's enzymes fall short of emulsifying his standard diet. Most of his food slid down the tube of his intestines without a chance to nourish his body. Despite eating over five times the amount of food, it failed to enter his circulation. Instead, the excess flushed out his backside with a threat to clog his toilet.

Water Needs

Water enters your body from one opening: your mouth, and exits one of four ways: breath, pee, poop, and skin. Of these four, your bowel holds the most torque. Your colon can twist, squeeze, and wring your stools for every last drop of liquid. Poop gets dried out in the final two feet just before your rectum. This section also houses the bacteria that ferment vitamins. As the gut-bacteria gobble up nutrients in your stools, their waste products are our vitamins. The B vitamins, Vitamin K, and biotin spin out of the "butts" of bacteria living in your colon. They are then absorbed into your blood along with water. When life gets "messy" - the diaper kind of messy, it's an indicator that this section of your bowel doesn't work. When using keto-chemistry, the water stops filling up the ditches between cells and flows to the proper places within the body. This is how you stay hydrated instead of in-flamed.

WATER IN AND OUT OF YOUR BODY

IN: Water enters your body from one opening: your mouth.

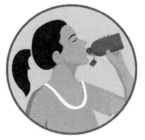

OUT: Water exits your body four ways: breath, pee, poop, and skin.

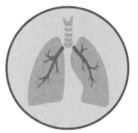

Through lungs as tiny droplets of water vapor.

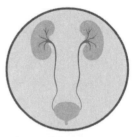

Through kidneys and blader as urine.

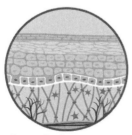

Through skin as sweat and water vapor.

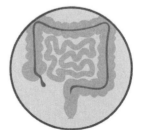

Through large intenstine and colon as poop.

Chapter 12

DAY 3 PRAY FOR PINK

On Day 3, David followed the same routine as yesterday. He began by peeing on a PeeTone strip.

Is your PeeTone strip pink? SUCCESS. You're making ketones.

Not pink? Hang in there. Keep carbs as close to zero as you can to swiftly switch your chemistry.

Glucose drops - first, followed by a decrease in insulin. *Both* need to reduce for a switch to occur. Once these two chemicals shift, ketones will flow.

Let me stress... Pink PeeTone strips matter. Without pink, your insulin churns too high to lose weight.

The trigger needed to empty glycogen starts with less insulin. How much less? Less than you had yesterday— it's a relative measurement.

The first three days of eating all fat popped open David's glycogen bubbles like wringing out a bubble wrap sheet. Pop! Pop! Pop! Next, thousands of glucose molecules swam into his bloodstream as glycogen emptied. These bubbles delivered a stable supply of glucose entering his circulation. Over the next several days his storage depleted, unwinding strings of glyco-gen as glucose trickled into the blood.

Failure to produce ketones by Day 3 means you haven't lowered the insulin enough to empty stored glucose into your bloodstream. You have not popped any glycogen bubbles. No stimulus to produce ketones occurs until both glucose and insulin have declined.

These sparkling crystals of stored sugar need to go! Hold the line. Keep eating fat without carbs.

Document Your Drop in Insulin

How? Pee on that stick.

The presence of ketones guarantees your insulin has lowered enough to instruct your liver to make ke-tones. Your liver swiftly responds when you remove all the carbs from your food. The length of time from your last carb to your first urine ketone predicts the size of your liver. Healthy livers transition quickly. The longer it takes to see pink, the larger and more damaged your liver. So keep track of how long it takes your liver to produce the first ketone.

But stubborn livers beware! Overworked, stretched out, engorged livers take days. Carb junkies or full-blown diabetics have even longer before Pee-Tones turn positive.

Your liver produces ketones the moment your sugar-dependent system smokes away the circulating pine needles. Some cells rapidly throw those logs into their mitochondria, while others resist the transition. Fat and muscle cells quickly adapt to burning ketones for fuel; while brain cells are the last. But when the brain cells finally convert — Euphoria. It feels good. SO GOOD!

Follow these steps for the smoothest transition — when your cupboards are empty, and your initial pages of the workbook are complete: Eat your last meal in the evening before starting ketogenic nutrition. Avoid alcohol. The fewer carbs you consume in this meal, the better. Allow your meal to digest for several hours, and then go to bed. When you awaken, you'll be nearly ten hours into your transition. Within the next 12 hours, your liver should empty a hardy section of your stored sugar.

Eat a HIGH FAT BREAKFAST - Even if you are not hungry. Do this! The first two weeks of keto are all about SHIFTING YOUR CHEMISTRY. You are not diet-ing. You are chemistry shifting. Eat HIGH FAT for BREAKFAST. Don't mess with this. Don't argue, "I don't eat breakfast." Just follow this rule for two weeks.

Also, document exactly when your liver pumps out its first ketone by checking your urine ketone strips several times per day. Put 4 more strips in your pocket. Each time you pee, check your PeeTones. We are hacking your chemistry.

Breakfast

- Start your day with heavy whipping cream, or butter, or MCT C8:C10 oil in your coffee.

- Drink water.

- Eat all the eggs you desire for breakfast. Cook them in butter.

- Add cheese.

- Add sausage or pepperoni.

- Eat until you feel full —to satiety. This correlates with your chemistry.

Lunch

- Eat a couple of sausage patties or bacon. Dip the meat in mayonnaise with hot sauce.

- Eat hamburger meat soaked in butter. Spread a layer of sour cream on this patty; add a salty pickle, and/or green olives.

- Take a can of sardines as your lunch. Add mustard, a squirt of lemon juice, and ¼ cup of diced onion.

Snack

- Bring to work some high-fat cheese with slices of pepperoni or beef salami. If habit or hunger strikes your brain to eat, eat them. It's ideal to keep a supply of these at work, too.

- Stop agonizing over the type of fat in these snacks. Or contemplating whether these snacks are "processed, canned meat" versus "grass-fed beef.". Those details don't matter when compared to excess insulin. <u>Focus on converting your chemistry.</u> Initially, every food choice depends on flavor, number of carbs, and high amounts of fat.

PeeTone Strips Prevent Frustration

Before I insisted that patients rigorously check their PeeTone strips, several who needed this lifestyle change the most, sadly gave up. Their failure to produce results led to frustration. They asked for help; yet, the answer hid deep inside their body's chemistry. Insulin and glucose needed to drop to produce ketones. Sneaky carbs lurking in gum, toothpaste, cough drops, and sauces kept their urine free from ketones. Their casual selection of carb-heavy foods such as mayonnaise or soup also blocked success.

Negative PeeTone strips served several purposes: They communicated the need to further lower their carb intake. They needed fewer carbs — yes. But they needed know they needed fewer carbs. PeeTone strips told them. Negative PeeTone strips also helped patients to identify and fix hidden habits and mistakes. This monitoring strategy also instilled tenacity into my patients, motivating them to stay the course.

Monitoring PeeTone strips offered a tangible way for patients to see their progress. Pink strips left them tingling with delight — mentally and physically.

Do any of these statements sound like you?

'Doctor, I have tried every diet. None of them worked. I can't lose weight.'

'Doctor, I look pregnant. I am a dude. Can we fix this?'

'Doc, I had a gastric bypass and lost a bunch of weight... but I gained most of it back.'

Some of these patients had gastric bypass, gastric banding, or balloons placed to restrict foods from entering into their stomachs and still failed to achieve lasting weight loss. Others used speed pills, anti-depressants, injected hormones, underwent hypnosis, participated in group therapy, and counted calories with obsessive accuracy, all to no avail. Hidden high insulin with abundant glycogen storages resulted in zero to minimal weight loss after 5 years. How can you tell if you suffer from this? Perform any of these tests: A liver or muscle biopsy. It will show your stored glycogen. Or an expensive, carefully timed, five-hour-long test to measure your blood insulin after drinking a bunch of carbs.

Save your money, time, and blood — pee on a strip.

Keto Flu

David, sluggish and crabby, barely made it through the second day of his keto-diet. Kat felt ill, too, expressing symptoms of headache, nausea, sleepiness and lightheadedness. They struggled to identify where they contracted the sickness. Why? They had no known infections. So why are they having these symptoms? What in the world is going on? - KETO FLU!

Yes. Keto Flu. The KETO FLU got its name because flu-like symptoms manifest when transitioning from glucose to ketones. Dropping carbs changes the chemistry causing symptoms that feel exactly like the flu. David was a prime candidate for Keto Flu.

These symptoms felt exactly the same as the last time David contracted the flu. A virus had invaded his body, set up an illegal residence, and then went about wreaking havoc inside his system. Those invaders stole his water, drank his salts, and devoured his sugar. David's body provided the ideal living conditions for that infection to occur. The critters replicated quickly, draining his energy and causing his tummy to ache. Flu symptoms spread throughout his body with a headache, loss of appetite, and an irritable mood. As the community of bugs conquered more of the real estate in his gut, he struggled to stand up. Dizziness and a racing heart prevented him from standing every time he tried. His symptoms came from dehydration.

Dehydration occurred when David vigorously flipped from sugar to fat. Dehydration caused the keto flu symptoms by rapidly dropping in his blood pressure. What's so dehydrating about producing ketones? Ketones weren't the cause. Instead, the sudden drop of those glucose molecules put a strain on David's body. These vast, monster-sized glucose molecules flowed and tumbled through David's veins, soaking up, holding onto, and trapping any nearby water molecules.

Eating nearly zero carbs dropped David's blood glucose level, which meant fewer water molecules circulated in his system. His body expelled the excess water through his kidneys. Over the first week, David lost nine pounds. Some of my patients have lost as much as 20 pounds - that's nearly three-gallons of extra water.

David's 'flu' or dehydration symptoms appeared because he was unprepared in mind and body for ketosis. With little forewarning, he got a headache and felt tired. After his short office commute, David stood up. Sudden dizziness and a pounding heart caught him off-guard. The water loss lowered his blood pressure enough to create an unsafe and unsteady feeling. Perspiration and a massive sense of fatigue stemmed from his newly suppressed blood pressure.

In the long game, the extra water David lugged around in his system needed to go. Like lighter fluid, the excess fluid irritated David's body down to a microscopic level. Removing extra water, reducing his blood pressure, and decreasing his glucose were the right answers. But removing them too quickly shocked his system, causing keto flu.

Salt, Salty Water, & Speed

Salt

Yes, I mean salt. Like the white stuff in the shaker on your table. Pink, mineralized salt offers a better range of important elements, but ordinary table salt will do. Salt, like fat, has been overly demonized.

Fat and salt are essential to keto-chemistry. David feared salt almost as much as he feared fat. He avoided doctors, but could not escape the decades-old message from the American Heart Association that, "Low salt was good for your heart." Adding salt to his meals felt counter-intuitive, so David sprinkled a stingy amount, in secret, onto his food.

On Day 3, David needed to replace the fluid he'd lost. His kidneys had flushed salt along with that tidal wave of fluid. Had David known that keto transition sucked salt and water from his body, he could've prevented the flu. Replacing the salt as fast as he lost it could have diminished his suffering.

Drink Salty Water

By adding salt to his food and drinks, David would have quickly reversed the symptoms of dehydration. Instead, he tried drinking plain water. This satisfied his thirst — for a few minutes — but his kidneys naturally flushed it out. Unsalted water failed to fix his flu-like symptoms. In fact, his ad-hoc remedy further upset his salt/water imbalance and complicated matters. The more water he drank, the worse he felt. David needed salt to retain the replacement water in his circulation. Only then would he have corrected his troubles.

Drink salty broth to keep the keto flu away!

Speed

Finally, David needed to slow down. His rotten mood, nausea, and fatigue signaled that something was wrong. These symptoms prompted him to take life slower for a few days. That was a good idea.

200 CLUB: Let's Start Again

David belonged to the The 200 Club — he ate more than 200 grams of carbs a day before starting keto. Because he never counted carbs prior to starting, he was unaware of his membership in this club. From somewhere north of 300 grams per day, David slammed his carbs under 20 putting him at increased risk for KETO FLU. He could have prevented this with these tips:

1) Drink Ketones-In-A-Can.

Ketones-In-A-Can prepares the body for the up-coming transition. The 200 Club gains the most bene-fit from sipping on ready-made ketones for 10 days be-fore starting. The healthier you are when you begin the change, the less you need this assistance. However, in several of my young, carb-eating athletes, I have used this intervention to prepare their bodies for the transi-tion. Much like adding powdered sugar with elec-trolytes to water, ketones come in a powdered form, too. Drinking powdered ketones awaken the cellular parts of the body that use them. Add ketones into cir-culation by drinking the ready-made versions. **Then** take away carbs. Buffer the change by sipping ketones before you start.

2) No Carbs in Drinks.

If you are in The 200 Club, cut the sweetness out of your drinks — Zero calories, zero carbs, and zero sweeteners in your drinks. Yep. The goal is zero calories, zero carbs, and zero sweeteners in your drinks. However, I make this exception with Ketones-In-A-Can because... frankly - it works. Someday all the sweeteners should go, too. For now, ketone-supplement-drinks offer a perfect trade-off.

Ketones enter your circulation and deliver more than just fuel. Ketones signal your cells to change the way they work. That advantage matters greatly to folks in The 200 Club. Add fat such as heavy whipping cream, coconut cream, or MCT C8:C10 to that ketone drink. Added fat improves the absorption of the ketone salts along with enhancing the taste.

Be prepared for your tongue and taste buds to go on strike when you omit sweetness and carbs from your drinks. Your palate has grown used to those addictive substances. Don't advance to the next step until you reset your taste buds away from sweeteners.

Much like the lima-bean-guy, your system will adapt. Give it a chance.

3) No White Stuff.

If you are still in The 200 Club after cleaning up your drinks, add the following restriction: No white stuff.

- No bread.

- No rice.

- No potatoes.

- No pasta.

- No pastries.

Keep that rule for seven consecutive days — that means seven days in a row. No cheating. This gives your brain and body the ideal time and space needed to gently shift chemistry. Your neurochemistry gets a chance to adapt ahead of time. This also prevents keto flu and the crabbiness on the second and third days.

And finally, this schedule also gives you time to clean out your cupboards. ALL OF YOUR CUP-BOARDS.

High Blood Pressure Medications

If you are on blood pressure medication and want to get off of them, this lifestyle is the answer. Thanks to keto-chemistry, helping patients get off blood pressure medication has never been more successful. However, the transition can be dangerous. Prepare.

My patients taking high blood pressure meds must check their own blood pressure at home. Your body's blood volume drops in the absence of those large glucose molecules dripping with excess water. It takes far less medication to control blood pressure when all that water is gone.

Here are the rules I tell my patients:

1) You must use a home blood pressure monitor. Blood pressure is impacted differently for each person. After years of trying to predict who will have the worst or easiest time with blood pressure, I fail.

Monitoring pressures at home saves lives. Get a monitor. Take a pro-active stance for this.

2) Check your blood pressure two-three times per day when transitioning. Your blood pressure will advertise any problem that presents. Don't be surprised when your blood pressure numbers vary during the transition. Blood pressure fluctuates every time your heart beats. Your readings can range 10-15 points from one check to the next. That does not mean your blood pressure cuff isn't working. It means your system is transitioning. As you remove carbs from your diet, your blood pressure will quickly fall. So be careful.

3) Ask your doctor to rank your blood pressure medications from most important to least important. Use your doctor's advice to help you remove those blood pressure medicines as quickly as your body adjusts. Again, you will know this by checking your blood pressure.

4) Ask your doctor what pressure is the right number to start lowering medications. I use 100-110s/60-80s as a guide. If my patients have pressures in that range for several checks, it's time to reduce medications.

Stop the carbs, and you will lose water. Less water means a lower blood pressure. It's that simple. If you expel a gallon of water via urine and sweat, your blood pressure math equation has just changed. For example, if your blood pressure medication lowered your blood pressure by 15 points, pre-keto diet, then it also lowered it that much after starting the keto diet, too.

Take note: It is ill-advised to simultaneously lower your blood pressure from both meds and keto-chemistry at once. You'll end up on the floor. And when you awaken, you'll learn that you passed out. You'll most likely discover a bump on your head as well from hitting the floor.

Prevent This.

Let me repeat: Study your blood pressures. Check pressures several times a day. Know them before you begin and during the transition into keto-chemistry.

In a matter of five days, I removed five blood pressure meds from a patient! The only way we kept him out of the emergency department was through careful monitoring of his blood pressure as we walked through the first seven days of his keto transition.

Day 3 marks a significant transition in keto-chemistry. Pink PeeTone strips will guide you to improved health. Stay the course if your PeeTone strips aren't pink yet. Soon you will improve your health one ketone at a time.

Chapter 13

DAY 4   OH POOP!

On the forth morning since ditching carbs, David awoke, feeling rested. Normally, he felt tired upon arousal, as if not sleeping at all. But last night was different. He slept for nine deep peaceful hours. That hadn't happened in years. If eating keto caused this, he was definitely on board; the keto lifestyle now commanded his attention. Even though yesterday's flu symptoms, the racing heart when standing, his pounding headache, and heavy feeling, lurked in the back in his mind, David went about his morning routine. He rechecked his PeeTones. The dark pink color on the strip awarded him an exciting success.

The aroma of coffee led him to the kitchen where he fried two eggs in leftover bacon fat and added salt. Bacon-greased-eggs delivered on taste and not carbs. A smile slid across his face, "Salty eggs fried in bacon grease! Is this even legal?"

He accelerated the car down the street. A sharp pain caught his breath as he pushed on the pedal. Deep in his stomach, on his left side, just north of his pelvis, a twisting, heavy cramp siphoned all of his attention. It had been four days since his last poop. Worrying thoughts about constipation flickered across his mind.

Poop Problems

Fat coated David's gut lining for the first time in years. From lips to anus, a layer of slime lubricated his tubular food-tract. But he worried when symptoms of change writhed through his abdomen. For what he was feeling, seeing and experiencing were new to him. Like most patients, David cared about his poop. Changing the way his body expelled waste was frightening. A change in poop can ignite panic in folks. Pooping matters. From the first day of life, to the last— it matters.

Bowels: TOO HARD [Constipation]

Constipation and hard bowel movements natural-ly and commonly occur in the first days of ketosis. This is part of the keto transition. In the first couple of weeks, patients struggle with what to eat. They load up on fatty, greasy meat. Too many carbs sweep roughage, or high-fiber foods, off of their new keto-menus. The volume of food decreases because of that missing fiber. As ketones begin to flow, constipation often stops their momentum.

To help understand why, a brief review of how stool moves from top to bottom sets the stage. Let's begin at your stomach.

Chewed food mixes with slimy enzymes to form a ball, or a bolus of food. This glob leaves the stomach with a strong push into the top section of the 'hose.' The bolus stretches this section of your intestines. Ex-panding the tube triggers wave-like muscle contrac-tions, called peristalsis. One nerve zaps the neighbor-ing nerve. Muscles within the wall of the intestines squeeze and shuffle the message downstream.

If you've ever watched a group of people per-form the wave at a stadium filled with a cheering crowd, a leader shouts, "Let's do the wave." Someone stimulates the action. The movement of bowels acts similarly. It begins with a spark. The arrival of that ball of food stretches the tube and sparks action—the more massive the food, the greater the wave.

When eating smaller amounts of food, waste collects into one area creating a 'pile of trash.' As it accumulates, each tablespoon of food stretches the bowel further. Eventually, enough collects to trigger another wave of contractions within the bowel-muscles.

On a ketogenic diet, the stretch response is weaker in comparison. This is due to the decreased volume of food taking place by eliminating carbs and high-fiber foods from the diet. This requirement is mandatory for ketogenic chemistry. For years, processed foods overflowed from the standard American diet. Strong bowel movements came from stretching their intestine with a high volume of food. Eating high-fat, low-carb cuts the quantity of food. Keto-eating is nourishment without the bulk.

Instead of a mound of food zapping muscles to contract, little pings of pulses instructs the muscle to squeeze. Much like the human wave in that stadium, when only a few people participate, the message dwindles quickly. Without a dominant message from neighbors, the bowel stays in rest mode. The first two weeks of a ketogenic diet reset your system to infrequently move stool. Prepare for this constipation challenge.

Four days of no movements and David hurt from the inside out. Cramp! Sharp, rising pain stole his breath as he drove to work. His stool collected in the last section of his bowel. The low volume trickled in and slowly stretched his tube. That gradual expanse allowed a pile of poop to acquire *before* his muscles contracted. This part of the intestine, called the distal colon, or the descending colon, draws water from the debris and recycles that water throughout the body. When this section of the bowel fails, deadly consequences related to dehydration occur. David collected four days of leftover food in his descending colon. This poop was so dry it could be mistaken for cement. Hours into his workday, he was sure he knew what labor pains felt like. His bowel squeezed and cramped, trying to inch the bolus to the exit. The waves of pain grew unbearable. Each pain weakened his resolve. "Maybe this diet isn't for me," he complained.

Before giving up, take my advice: milk of magnesia and chia seeds.

Chia Seeds to the Rescue

Chia seeds work like magic when constipation attempts to impede your keto-transition. Here's how to demonstrate their power: Add one-tablespoon of chia-seeds to one-half cup of salty water. Over the next minutes, watch them expand into little gelatinous globes. This happens inside your intestines when you ingest chia seeds with salt water.

If constipation strikes, drink one tablespoon of dry chia-seeds with a glass of salt water every hour — you can use a timer to remind you. These seeds have little to no taste and do not trigger an insulin response. Dry chia seeds don't raise blood sugar. You can swallow them whole, or chew them before washing them down. Keep drinking this chia-seeds / salt water mixture until you have a bowel movement.

Keep track of how many tablespoons you've swallowed before your first bowel movement occurs. Ideally you should have a bowel movement within eight-hours of starting this protocol. Keep this 'eight-hour window' in mind. If it's bedtime, and you still haven't produced a bowel movement, — stop! Wait until morning, and start again. Count the first tablespoon of seeds as your ninth one. Keep going until you have a bowel movement. The total needed to stretch your intestines into motion determines your chia-seed dosage for the next few days. For example, if you swallowed 12 tablespoons of chia-seeds before your bowels finally responded, take 12 spoonfuls per day for the next three days.

Instead of portioning out your dosage hourly, take 1/2 the dose first thing in the morning and the other half at noon. In our example, swallow six tablespoons in the morning and the other six at noon. With that large dose, instead of chewing them dry, try mixing them into the saltwater and washing them down quickly before they expand in the container. After three days, decrease by one tablespoon. In our example above, that would be eleven per day. Continue tapering the tablespoon dosage by one serving every other day.

This resets the trigger inside the gut, and reactivates the natural stretch-factor the intestines had before the ketogenic diet. With the stretch-factor properly functioning the muscles will now contract to move things along. Once bowels move, step down slowly. Decreased seeds decrease the stretch.

David wanted to solve his constipation with laxatives or high fiber supplements. However, both options fight the forward progress of ketogenic chemistry. His laxatives delivered cathartic results but failed to fix the underlying issue to re-train his bowels. On top of this, fiber supplements combine carbs that claim to stay inside the intestines. Their claims of non-absorption ring untrue when blood sugar spikes after each dose. This spike halts the ketone production.

Healthy bowels don't need fiber. Diseased and inflamed intestines do. Bowel biopsies from folks eating high-fiber diets show unhealthy slime coating the intestinal walls. They also show tiny gaps that opened between cells. The tight-junctions sealing their cells together, wiggled apart due to chronic inflammation. These microscopic changes often go unnoticed, yet they significantly impact the function of the bowel. In diseased intestines, we trick the muscle into contracting by stretching it. Healthy colons should contract without the exaggerated stretch stimulus. Salty water with chia-seeds expands without adding carbs.

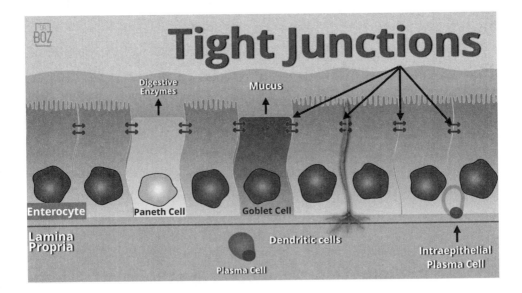

Life without fiber is possible. Keto chemistry will resolve your poop problems.

Try Milk of Magnesia

If constipation hits as intensely as with David, add Milk of Magnesia (MOM.) This over-the-counter medication delivers the perfect short-term antidote. In the first weeks of keto, the most commonly deficient mineral is magnesium. This magnesium-filled liquid helps replenish missing magnesium while boosting stools to flush along. David solved his bowel trouble using Chia seeds and a few doses of Milk of Magnesia. The MOM rescued him quickly.

David also swallowed Ketones-In-A-Can when he felt any possible intestinal problem about to return. Adding Ketones-In-A-Can boosted the salt intake and helped his keto chemistry not slip out of ketosis.

Bowels: TOO LEAKY [Diarrhea]

Two decades of practicing internal medicine sorted the most difficult cases. The easy cases got better; the difficult ones taught me how unhealthy a body can get. The most difficult cases presented with severe malnourishment and chronic inflammation. Initially, neither the patient nor I knew these problems harbored deep inside their cells. Crohn's disease or ulcerative colitis demonstrated the devastating price paid when the gut was compromised.

Colitis, also called leaky gut, starts with microscopic defects in the barrier between food and human. These tiny gaps progress to ulcerated wounds bleeding inside the bowel. Leaky gut refers to the error that allows particles to traverse back and forth across this barrier. Healthy intestines inspect every particle that enters and exits through this security system. When items come and go as they please, without permission — health declines.

A highly choreographed policing synchronizes which particles of food get absorbed and which ones pass by. The gut regulates which vitamins, minerals, or essential proteins to flush out of the body when they aren't needed. A body low on iron should never allow it to slip into the waste headed for the toilet and should grab every element of iron hidden in food. Inflammation promotes a leaky environment. When the gut 'leaks,' depleted nutrients accidentally flush away, while unwanted particles sneak in. The most advanced medical treatments fail to compensate for all that is lost when the gut leaks.

Malnutrition starves the body in phases. See *Appendix I* explaining the 4 phases of leaky-gut malabsorption.

Small Bowel Overgrowth

Did you know your small bowel or small intestines are supposed to be sterile? Yes! Sterile-as in no bacteria. Your large intestines are packed with bacteria, but your small has none. The small intestines pull in nourishment and swiftly move the food to the large intestines. Anxiety, stress, and chronic illness cause dysfunction within the waves of the bowels. Instead of a well-paced forward movement from top to your bottom, cramps from the bowel muscles shuffle the food back and forth. This mixes everything up.

Bacteria commonly found in the large intestines wiggled into the upper real estate of your digestive tract. These critters trekked into the small intestine; and there they flourished, reproducing with little to no resistance. This massive proliferation and bacterial overgrowth lined — or even haunted — the interior of the small bowel. This is known as: Small Bowel Overgrowth (SBO.) These overgrown colonies of bugs block the absorption of fat-based nutrients in that small intestine. When patients with SBO eat high-fat, they can't absorb the fat, and severe symptoms blast out their backside. Their muscles cramp with misery, and uncontrolled diarrhea derails their progress. They soon declare, "This is NOT the diet for me!"

Those with SBO may be unaware of their diagnosis, but they all share the same history. They have avoided eating fat for years because according to their predictable verbal utterance, "It always gives me diarrhea." Oily eruptions grease their toilet after each fat-filled meal, causing them to flush the toilet two to three times before the stools disappear down the drain.

I rid my mind of any doubt about their diagnosis by checking their Vitamin D blood test. Vitamin D is one of the fat-based vitamins—one of the four vitamins built from fat. Thanks to their strict avoidance of fat, their lab results hover at the dismal number of 20. Healthy levels of Vitamin D soar above 50.

"Doc, prescribe me a pill for that."

Patients with low vitamin D limp along with minimal fat entering their bodies. Unfortunately, current medications have proven almost useless when the flaw originates at the site of absorption for this fat-built nutrient. The consequences are awful. Patients suffering from a leaking gut have left me sleepless over the years. Silent symptoms lead to extreme suffering, and their souls melted away with their nutrients. Their spirit died.

Attempts to seal the gaps have included probiotics, prebiotics, colostrum (yes — drinking breast milk!), fecal transplantation (yep — putting someone else's poop into their bowels!), FODMAP diet (Fermentable Oligosaccharides, Disaccharides, Monosaccharides, and Polyols), and the Paleo Diet. What's worse is that the trend in prescribing mega high-doses of Vitamin D prescriptions of 50,000 units per pill, only moved the needle slightly after weeks of replacement. Then we added expensive medications that targeted an overactive immune system. All failed to reverse the damage until the ketogenic diet.

If diarrhea splatters your throne after going keto, you need this anti-inflammatory, nutrient-dense way of eating more than most. Allow your body the time needed to adjust. Don't give up! The flare from high fat is more than just an annoyance. The staples sealing your gut have wiggled apart. Go see a gastro specialist and share that your poop floats and your vitamin D is low. Those clues will start the correct workup.

Teaching your gut to absorb fats again is a slow process. Jumping into high-fat eating can send greasy-poopers racing back to the high-carb world for relief. If you struggle to absorb fat, we must fix this for the long-term health of your body and brain. I cannot overemphasize this enough. Reversing the extreme intestinal inflammation takes weeks. Years of this hidden problem led to the chronic swelling of your bowels' inner lining. Time spent in ketogenic chemistry will mend that chronic wound inside your gut.

While you work with your gastro doctor, get ketones into your circulation.

Ketones-In-A-Can, also called exogenous BHB, offers a beginning step. The only advantage to a leaky, swollen gut might be the quick absorption of ketone supplements. Adding ketones begins the process of ketogenic chemistry. When in circulation they tell your body that "Fuel is changing. Make more ketones." Supplemental ketones only stay in circulation for a couple of hours. Still, that short time in blood flow is usually enough to flicker on the chemistry for beginners.

Lick the Spoon with MCT C8:C10 Oil.

This tasteless, super-fat absorbs directly into your circulation instead of going through the lymph digestion process. Instead of waiting hours to find recently consumed fat in circulating, MCT C8:C10 can be found within minutes. Start with one soft-gel filled with this oil. Bite it open. This tiny dose of fat should not send you trotting to the toilet. If it does, *stay* the course of treatment until it fades. Then increase your soft-gel intake to two. The cells designated with the task of absorbing fats have hibernated from lack of use. Awaken them slowly, and you will find diarrhea subsides. Give your gut time. Once these cells return to their functional state, their neighboring cells awaken. Unlike Ketones-In-A-Can, MCT C8:C10 elevates blood ketones for several hours. This unique fat zips into your liver's mitochondria to spit out ready-made ketones. Within weeks you will tolerate a tablespoon or four - six soft-gels of MCT oil. That's a success!

Other tips to tide you over as the diarrhea settles down include:

Loperamide: This over-the-counter medication curtails bowel movements. Most people cannot put their life on hold to deal with intense diarrhea. It takes time to fix this problem. In the meantime, don't take all this suffering lying down. Control your symptoms. Take Loperamide. This will settle the unpleasant symptoms while you work through the problem. The medication is safe to use. Take a single dose after each bowel movement until the moments slow to a tolerable rate. As your gut lining heals, taper off the medication.

Chia Seeds: Yep. Those little seeds I have already spoken about. Do the same protocol. Add one-tablespoon of dry seeds every hour for eight hours, or until you feel relief. As stated earlier, when you get the chia-seeds dosage properly measured, you can slowly reduce the number of tablespoons. I suggest decreasing by one tablespoon every three-four days until done.

Kombucha Tea: This ancient drink is a bubbly, fermented beverage that contains healthy live bacteria. Many of my diarrhea patients reversed their bowel problems when they re-populated their gut bacteria with 'good'-bacteria, and spending thousands of dollars on this process. Save your money. Drink 1/4 of a cup of this per day until the diarrhea is resolved. Notice that I said ONE-FOURTH-of A-CUP. Too much of that type bacteria is often not tolerated by those struggling with bowel problems. Also, many store-bought Kombucha teas contain a large amount of carbohydrates. Read labels for guidance or consider making your own drink. If you home-brew your kombucha, titrate the tea to a pH of less than 3.2.

The F word

Finally, the surefire antidote that transitions patients through the roughest part can be an unsettling word: Fasting. The F word. The term for NO EATING. Fasting of any kind sounds like a strange idea. But diarrhea caused by eating fat often means an injury inside your gut exists. The intestinal lining needs to heal. How? Rest. In other words - *intermittent fasting*.

Fasting is a universal remedy for many medical problems. When I suggest this to patients, they often resist due to fear of going without food. To persuade my patients to consider the option, I remind them that animals instinctively fast when they are ill. Rest your gut for healing. Stop eating. No snacking. No nibbling.

Complete rest for your intestinal system for 20-hours each day. With the sun's rise, your bowel enzymes churn inside that dark tunnel. Your circadian rhythm can't stop those hormones from firing. They follow the rising and setting of the sun. Fast with water and salt for 20-hours of the day. Then use the remaining four-hours, following sunrise, to consume all your calories. That's the remedy for an injured gut. The grave lessons from severely malnourished patients prompt me to share this rule. It is not easy to follow; but it saves lives when fiery inflammation burns in the lining of your gut.

A note: Once you produce ketones, your appetite decreases. So don't be surprised when you uncon-sciously begin to eat smaller food portions.

The ancient Greek physician, Hippocrates, re-garded as the father of medicine, said this about fast-ing, *"Everyone has a doctor in him; we just have to help him in his work. The natural healing force within each one of us is the greatest force in getting well. To eat when you are sick is to feed your sickness."*

Chapter 14

PULL THIS CHORD IF YOU NEED HELP

More hurdles lie ahead for David. Grandma Rose attracted him to the ketogenic diet like a moth to a bug zapper. He tumbled into ketosis, ill-prepared. Oblivious to his undiagnosed diabetes and elevated blood pressure, he struggled with headaches, pounding heartbeat, muscle cramps, plummeting blood sugar, constipation, and low energy. If you're having as much trouble as David, or still have gray PeeTone strips on Day 4, take a different path. Within 100 hours of starting, you should be through the most challenging chemistry changes. Keto-chemistry delivers more than just weight loss. It offers life's best health; but it begins with a change in chemistry.

Why No PeeTones by Day 4?

1) Your PeeTone strips are bad.

Double-check your PeeTone strips. Are they bad? If you bought them a month or two ago, and are just starting the keto diet, they might be deactivated. Fresh air and time deactivate the sponge at the tip of the PeeTone strip. If the top of the bottle leaked a bit of air into the canister, the strips would undoubtedly be compromised. You could pour a bucket of ketones onto those strips, and they wouldn't turn pink.

ANSWER: Get new strips.

2) You're eating more than 20 carbohydrates.

You started this process expecting a smooth transition, but each person has their individual "keto path" to walk, so to speak. There's no need to beat yourself up if you have failed to keep your total carb-count under 20. This is an arduous challenge for some. Carbs are addictive. Most don't realize how loudly they scream to be eaten until they stop them. This realization slaps the truth into Day 4.

ANSWER: Get the Cronometer App. Invest in this resource. Hidden carbs or inaccurate measuring tools have left patients without pink PeeTone strips for days. Measure accurately with Cronometer.

3) You're drinking too much alcohol.

Alcohol burns as fuel inside your mitochondria. When alcohol is present, you stop burning ketones and glucose. This means you're going to struggle to maintain ketosis when alcohol is present. Place all three fuel options (glucose, ketones, and alcohol) in front of hungry mitochondria and alcohol burns first, followed by ketones, and then carbs. Alcohol stops ketones from burning, and from being produced. That's double trouble. Besides, you tend to eat more carbs than you normally would when with booze on the menu — your ability to resist temptations decreases.

ANSWER: If you have not peed ketones by Day 4, the best answer is to abstain from alcohol for six-weeks. Ideally, stop consuming alcohol first before stopping carbs. Letting go of both chemicals at the same time proves difficult. Not impossible — but pretty tricky. Your brain and body chemistry need time to reset after removing these substances. If eliminating booze seems unlikely at this stage of your life, shift to no-carb alcohol. Use distilled alcohol, and stay away from most wine and all beer. Distilled spirits drip out of a distillery from six fermenting options as Brandy, Gin, Rum, Tequila, Vodka, and Whiskey.

I've had patients mix distilled alcohol with BHB ketones. Not my idea ... but it worked. When they felt the need for alcohol, ketones added to distilled drinks seemed to be the least derailing option.

4) You are a type-1 diabetic and your average blood sugar ranges above 150.

Translation: You have a liver filled with stored glucose thanks to years of injected insulin. You have muscle cells crammed full of stored glucose from that prescription. Do not be discouraged, this will get better. We must apply twenty-first century chemistry to help you. Hang in there.

5) You are a type-2 diabetic and your average blood sugar soars above 150.

You have that same liver condition mentioned in #4, but your insulin came from your pancreas. Their insulin came from a prescription.

6) You have insulin resistance or undiagnosed diabetes.

David had this. He didn't know he was insulin resistant, nor that his blood sugars sky rocketed so high. His story wouldn't reveal this for several weeks. Even with this hidden problem, he successfully peed ketones within hours of giving up carbs. David's early production of urine ketones assured me that he was early in his metabolic troubles with insulin resistance.

How will you know if this is you? I just told you: You fail to see PeeTones by Day 4. David's keto-transition occurred rather swiftly, albeit a rocky road. David's side effects within the first few days revealed his hidden insulin resistance. Thankfully, David arrived just in time on the side of ketone-production. At this point, his best and wise solution was to stay the course. The more robust and longer David produced ketones, the further he defeated insulin resistance.

Twenty carbs or less will push every person into ketosis within four days unless you fall into category 4, 5, or 6 above. Like David, insulin-resistant students need keto-chemistry the MOST. Ketones will reprogram your insulin resistant system, but the transition will be rough. Let me help you with a different plan.

BIOHACK

The word biohack refers to the clever, often unconventional, use of science to make your body function at its peak. The methods used in biohacking are the same in most scientific processes: Measure a problem. Begin the plan to fix it. Re-measure to see how it worked.

A biohack fix can be a change in diet, behavior, adding supplements, or medication. The biohack for smoothing the keto-transition in insulin-resistant patients is a supplement.

Beta-Hydroxybutyrate

Shortened, this is BHB—also called exogenous ketones. My favorite term for this is *"ketones-in-a-can."*

I coined the term ketones-in-a-can because it's fun to say, and it delivers the message, "Ketones you can swallow." Most often, ketones-in-a-can are sold in powder form. Mix them with a liquid and drink your keto-chemistry. Just swallow it.

In the 1960s, chemists manufactured ketones in their lab. These ketones were bound to salts. If you tasted these powders in the raw form, you would understand why their popularity has remained dismal. However, in recent years, sugar substitutes have softened the bitterness to improve the taste, thus helping to popularize this powerful chemical.

Ketone supplements used turned me off before I understood the research. Hypocritically, I wanted my patients to do this "all-natural." Yet, I ordered "unnatural" prescription medication for blood pressure, depression, water retention, and vitamin deficiency.

BE KETO - Use Ketosis Chemistry.

Ketogenic chemistry means adding ketones into your circulation. Improved health from ketones takes place only when ketones are present. Like David, those with chronic inflammation will benefit the most. The transition into ketosis is the critical step. A rugged shift repels those who need it the most. Let me help you. Outsmart or "biohack" that chemistry with supplemental BHB. Ketones-in-a-can radically changed the success of insulin-resistant patients' arrival at ketosis. This biohack won't be needed forever. But powdered ketones bridge the transition, and help if you fall off the wagon. The healthier you become, the less you will need these supplements.

Start by lowering your total carb intake as much as you can. I acknowledge that this is easier said than done. But, once you identify your weaknesses — those carbs that keep tempting you —the reality of learning this skill will seem as if you've just been kicked in the buttocks. Let Ketones-In-A-Can carry you to this destination.

For folks like David or those who have grey Pee-Tone strips on Day 4, I place them on a twice-daily Beta-HydroxyButyrate regimen, where they mix ketones into a drink and ingest it several times an hour by sipping on the drink. The goal is to consume at least 16-grams of ketones during the daylight hours. Drinking Ketones-In-A-Can saturates the blood with ketones for two to four hours after swallowing, so be careful not to guzzle the drink. Before you think about chugging ketones-in-a-can, remember, these are salts. Sip slowly. Adding a bunch of salt to your gut produces diarrhea! If your gut rumbles when sipping BHB, try adding fat such as heavy whipping cream to your drink. This improves the taste, slows down the rumbles, and increases the amount of BHB absorbed.

For two-weeks, drink the 16-grams of ketones throughout each day. During this two-week period, lower your carb intake to as close to 20 as possible.

Keep checking your PeeTones. The science behind the hack starts with circulating ketones. When first adding ketones to your circulation by way of supplements or by stopping carbohydrates, you can't use all of them. What hasn't been used by your body will show up in your urine.

"Wait! I pay money for ketones only to flush them down the toilet?"

Yes. Don't stress about that. Your PeeTone strip will be positive not because you're making ketones, but instead, you've been drinking them. You must expose your cells to ketones to transition the chemistry. When first adding ketones to your circulation by way of supplements or by stopping carbs, you can't use all the ketones. Your cells are not ready. Transition begins with exposing the cells to excess ketones.

Our goal is to raise ketones while lowering glucose. Ketones-In-A-Can adds those ketones. You reduce the carbs.

Stevia Sweetens BHB

Stevia: The most common *fake-suga*r added to BHB. Stevia naturally comes from the leaves of a plant in the ragweed family. Many allergic to ragweed also 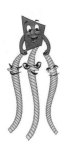 react to Stevia. If you are allergic to Stevia, use one of these three: MCT C8:C10, Ketones-In-A-Capsule, or straight beta-hydroxybutyric acid. Capsules filled with BHB salts hide the taste, but you need quite a few pills to get 16 grams per day. Straight BHB acid is a liquid and has the best bioavailability. If you can pucker past the sour taste, it guarantees ketones in circulation within minutes. A better answer might be MCT C8:C10.

MCT C8:C10

MCT stands for medium-chain triglycerides. Triglycerides are fats in your blood. Every time you see the word 'triglyceride', think fat. Triglycerides are named based on the length of their chains. Short triglyceride chains have 4-6 links in them. Long-chain fats have 12 or more links. Medium-chain triglycerides, MCTs, have eight to ten. Much like Goldilocks, MCTs are not too short, not too long — they are just right.

Just the right size for what? For slipping through a special nutrient trapdoor hidden in the first part of your small intestine. This trapdoor dumps into your portal vein. Direct absorption of certain select nutrients happens here. Typically, nutrients filter through your lymph system as a safety check. Food particles trickle through, getting sorted, screened, and shuffled before entering into your bloodstream. For your survival, this slower lymph network protects against the entrance of any toxins, poisons, or bacteria attempting to enter.

FAT UNZIPPING INTO KETONES

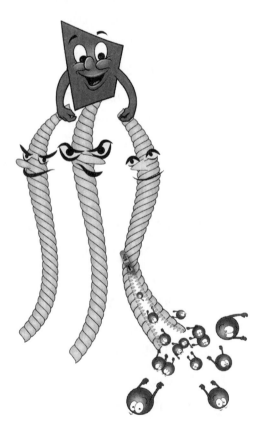

Valuable foods gain direct entry to your blood through a unique trapdoor. These select foods bypass all the sorting and shuffling processes taking place in your lymph system. Instead, these coveted nutrients drop through the trapdoor and into your portal vein, where they head straight into your liver.

MCTs are one category of nutrients allowed through this special entrance. In fact, all fats with 10 links or less fit through the trapdoor, port over to the liver, and rapidly unravel into ketones. Unlike other fats, these VIP morsels cut to the front of the line and shave hours off the trip. All other fats use the standard digestion process trickling through your lymph system for 2-3 hours before entering your circulation.

Length of Fat Chains

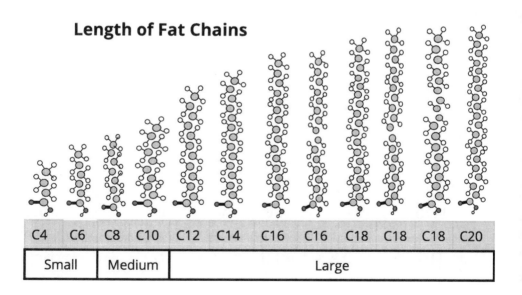

C4	C6	C8	C10	C12	C14	C16	C16	C18	C18	C18	C20
Small		Medium		Large							

MCT C8:C10 comes in supplements of liquid oil or soft-gels. These VIP super-fats work ideally to train your bowel to absorb fats again. As outlined previously, the key is to start small, "Lick the spoon," or bite open one soft-gel. Once that dose glides through without causing your gut to rumble, increase the dosage. This biohack heals the gut while increasing circulating ketones. Be sure to check PeeTone strips each day. You will know your gut started to absorb the oil and transform it into ketones by watching those strips. Expect it to turn pink sometime during the first two-weeks.

Biohack Your Brain Chemistry

A persistently negative PeeTone strips on Day 4 discourages the greatest of intentions. Sadly, grey PeeTone strips mean you have farther to go before your brain feels better. Your mental fuel currently tosses glucose in 100% of those campfires. This means your brain's transition has yet to start. Ironically as vital as this organ is, it is the last to transition from glucose to ketones. This ornery organ protests producing a myriad of symptoms before eventually surrendering, adapting to, and then using the new fuel. A little bio-hack-tweak softens the blow and reduces the struggle.

The new brain-fuel transition starts by getting ketones into the sac that holds and protects the brain from toxins and other dangers through a screening process. When it comes to fuel, the brain is really picky. It carefully screens the fuel it uses-not once, but twice! Before you can burn a single molecule of glucose, you must lift the glucose into the brain. The same rule applies to ketones. Individual transporters lift glucose from the blood and deliver them to your brain. In contrast, different transporters carry ketones over that same blood-brain barrier. Only after glucose and ketones are lifted across this barrier can they supply the brain with energy.

The transport of ketones slowly takes place when adding ketones into your circulation for the first time. Like other cells, the brain hardly remembers or even knows what to do with a ketone in the beginning. But slowly the mitochondria within the brain adapt. And over time, glial cells will prefer ketones over glucose.

In a perfect world, we would pump ketones inside the sac holding your brain and force the transition to begin. There are several flaws in that daydream. Instead, the closest option is to fill your blood with a high volume of ketones. This will instruct your brain to begin the process of scooping them up and transport them across the blood-brain barrier. Once inside, a few ketones percolate into the brain cells and through the mitochondria. The brain's mitochondria will rapidly prefer and adapt to this reliable, stable ketogenic fuel over the flash-flame of sugar-energy. The secret to the biohack is to offer ketones as a constant option. How do you do this?

Ketones-In-A-Can or MCT C8:C10 start the shift.

Nearly every brain cell in patients suffering from Alzheimer's used glucose for decades before their symptoms appeared. But it's now clear from the latest cutting-edge brain research that their brains significantly show improvement when they switch fuels, from glucose to ketones. When I think of an Alzheimer's patient's brain cells, I imagine their mitochondria with soot and holes burned through the sides. Hot flames of pine-needles flashed and flickered through their furnaces for thirty years, on and off. Adding glucose every few hours to meet the brain's volatile energy demands, fried the interior of their mitochondria, causing severe memory problems, the kind that seems insignificant to the patient in the early stages; then and without mercy hijacks their entire brain.

Sipping on ketones awakened the hibernating brain-ketone transporters in Alzheimer's patients', and in persons suffering from brain-fog, lethargic thinking, and depression. Brain cells, specifically astrocytes, might not have seen ketones since the early days of breast-milk dependency. But once the transporters were back in action, ketones became a powerful ally in the mental and physical wellbeing of the individual, with patients showing signs of improvement within ten days. The steady supply of ketones offered a superior fuel that didn't ebb and flow so much. They faded cravings and increased mental performance. This constant source of energy awoke sluggish astrocytes in patients with memory problems, anxiety, mood swings, attention lapses, and Parkinson's disease.

If you're struggling by Day 4, biohack. Supplement your blood with ketones. Drink down BHB salts or swallow MCT C8:C10 to switch energy. Keep supplementing and checking PeeTones for fourteen days. Wake up your transporters that lift ketones across the blood-brain barrier. Bridge your body and brain to a new fuel.

Chapter 15

DAY 5,6,7 MAGNESIUM

Friday morning, David fastened his belt into a new notch; a notch indicating he was losing weight. He stepped on the scale— 9 pounds missing since Monday. On top of this, the past three nights delivered progressively better sleep than each night before.

There's more: Yesterday, he, as if by magic, arrived to work ahead of schedule. That's never happened. Usually, his scattered thoughts lead him through a checklist that didn't fit into the allotted time. But yesterday, his mind focused. Period. This mental happiness seemed dreamlike.

Standing alone in the kitchen, David smiled, staring at his coffee. This mental happiness seemed dreamlike.

PeeTone strip positive= ✅ CHECK

Coffee with heavy cream = ✅ CHECK

Eggs and Sausage for Breakfast= ✅ CHECK

David's morning sped by as he raced to meet a deadline for several high school seniors. He submitted their graduation portraits by noon, an hour ahead of schedule. Next, he loaded his vehicle with the equipment for the afternoon shoot. David carefully reviewed his gear and studied his checklist. He looked forward to the winter outdoor photoshoot for one of his oldest accounts. Distracted by the importance of this situation, David forgot to grab his packed lunch. Cold, South Dakota air cut through his layers as he shivered for most of the shoot. Despite the intensity and windchill, his brain kept up. A week ago, a hyper-scheduled day with several hours spent in the cold, without lunch, would have resulted in failure. That was the formula for a grumpy mood and disregard for the details needed to produce what his client wanted. Remarkably, he snapped frame after frame from the sweet-zone. Perfect performance.

Satisfied, he returned to the studio late in the afternoon, put his gear away, and called it a week. He ate a few bites of his packed lunch as he reflected the difference a week had made. This Friday afternoon seemed a lifetime away from last Friday.

His son, Joshua, enjoyed cooking, and affectionately identified himself as the family chef. Joshua used Friday night for a standing invitation to gather the family around food. David's praise of keto over the past week led Joshua to make keto-chili. Joshua's version of keto-chili recipe contained no kidney-beans and corn-chips. It used tomato paste and bone broth instead of his usual canned tomatoes. He topped each bowl with sour cream, cheese, and a sprinkle of green onions. Joshua worried that his parents would drop dead from all the fat. Over the past week, he'd looked into keto-cooking. Every recipe blubbered with fat.

"You've got your will and testimony in place, right? This meal could kill you." The fatty meal drew praise from everyone, including the chef. Filling. Tasty and satisfying. Respecting the diet, Joshua served no sweets or carbs. David and his wife tucked into bed with stretched, satiated bellies.

Saturday morning should have marked another perfect day, but, once again, David felt off his rhythm. A headache pounded him out of sleep at the break of dawn. David squinted his eyes to reduce the morning light as he waddled towards the bathroom. "Kat, help me!" he suddenly yelled, while clutching the dresser to prevent himself from collapsing. David managed to steady his gait and continue towards the bathroom. Pain from his left leg-muscle forced him to tip-toe and limp to the toilet as the sound of his heavy, pounding heartbeat filled the room.

Kat rushed over and assisted David. "Take it easy. You're okay," she said. He tried to convince himself, of what Kat was saying, as he slowly inhaled, and then let it out. A couple of breath-cycles later settled his heartbeat. David, rubbing his left leg muscle, remembered his middle-of-the night awakening. Pain had shot through his foot and into his calf muscle, causing a sudden bolt out of bed. While still partially awake and asleep at the same time, David danced around in the darkness, in the hopes of making the pain go away, and wishing it would just stop on his command. "A Charlie Horse?" David thought.

He sat on the toilet, wondering how he was going to manage his day with a gimp leg and a pounding head. Minutes passed. His hands involuntarily began to massage the fullness in his belly. His night-shirt stretched over his rounded paunch. A full, tight drum pushed his belly-button out. Too much chili?

No. He felt bloated. Distended. His bowels had barely moved since Monday. Constipated?

David showed all of the following signs:

- A grumpy mood.
- Muscle cramps.
- Sluggish bowels.
- A headache.
- A thumping heartbeat when he stood.

Symptoms of Low Magnesium

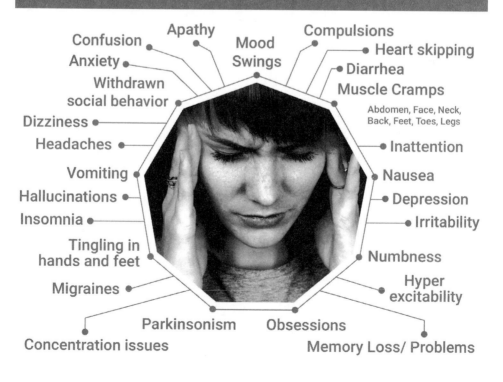

Confusion — Apathy — Mood Swings — Compulsions — Heart skipping

Anxiety — Diarrhea

Withdrawn social behavior — Muscle Cramps

Abdomen, Face, Neck, Back, Feet, Toes, Legs

Dizziness

Headaches — Inattention

Vomiting — Nausea

Hallucinations — Depression

Insomnia — Irritability

Tingling in hands and feet — Numbness

Migraines — Hyper excitability

Parkinsonism — Obsessions

Concentration issues — Memory Loss/ Problems

His hidden health problems haunted him again. To compound worsening matters, an irritable mood, low energy, and a pounding heart swept him out of "keto euphoria." This was hours after his body had flushed away several pounds. Add a startling muscle cramp that jerked him out of slumber to clinch the deal: His magnesium was low.

MAGNESIUM

Most reading this book hover on the precipice of low magnesium. Almost every patient I see suffers from low magnesium. The symptoms usually go unnoticed until keto-chemistry tips them over the borderline-from low to deficient.

Magnesium

- Sparks muscle contraction,
- Regulates blood pressure,
- Lassos insulin metabolism,
- Tames the excitability of your heart muscle,
- Relaxes the tone of the muscles lining your blood vessels,
- Sets the proper pace for nerve transmission,
- Harmonizes the messages between nerves and muscles.

Magnesium (Mg++), a required body salt, reigns as one of the most important nutrients. It activates 300 enzymes, stabilizes cellular structure, and instructs many cell proteins to do their job. "Magnesium is da' bomb!"

You feel like dying when it slips too low. And WITHOUT it — you die! Period. Low magnesium triggers headaches, dizziness, confusion, mental cloudiness, nervousness, and tingling in your hands and feet. Have a foggy brain? Blame magnesium. In some way, you'll be right. When Mg++ falls below the needed threshold, muscle cramping tops the list of complaints. The lower the magnesium, the more muscles spasm into a cramp. One muscle affected is your heart. Changes in magnesium can interrupt your heart rhythm, causing your heart to - to skip a beat. This is serious stuff.

David's magnesium level hit a tipping point just five days into keto. He had earlier warning signs before his muscles squeezed him out of bed. David failed to recognize the warning signs and attribute them to low magnesium. Like most, he didn't take them seriously. These early signs of low magnesium teased David with general weakness, low concentration, constipation, and an unsettled stomach. Muscle cramps, such as his "charlie-horse" or the crick in his neck, rang the second alarm of low magnesium. His squeezing muscles around his head caused a headache, and the muscles lining his bladder cramped to cause deep tummy pain. David complained of low back pain, twitching eyes, and ringing ears—all from muscle cramps.

David's most devastating symptom on Day 5 was a wake-up-call for him. It wasn't the headache, nor his sensitivity to light, either. It was his lowered brainpower! Down went his magnesium, followed by his energy, his cognition, and his newly adopted belief in ketones. David chalked up his irritable mood and grumpiness to the imposters that typically caused those symptoms. He even blamed the chili from the night before, and naively concluded that his rotten sleep was the result of yesterday's shivering photo-shoot. And he scolded his bowels, "My constipation must have caused this bloating."

That entire Saturday slumped by without improvement. The next morning David left the house with weighted feet. On his way to Sunday mass, David's boots clobbered down three wooden steps and into the garage. Kat turned around to find the cause of the sound. Sadness passed from David's face to hers. The radiant joy she'd seen in his eyes this past week — was gone, - again.

"David, are you okay?"

"Ya. ... Why?"... David replied in a slow, monotone voice. "I think that bug from the other day came back. I don't feel good."

David moved towards the car with downward cast eyes. He slid behind the wheel and put the car in reverse.

"STOP!" Kat yelled. "Open the garage door first. Do you want me to drive?"

"No. No. I'm fine. I just wasn't thinking."

David tried to fake joyfulness at church. But he abruptly stopped participating during the second verse of the first hymn. The force of the cloud of gloom was stronger. And it won. He sat heavily in the pew, pushed inward by this returning fog that possessed his mind, body and soul. He felt like he was inside a tunnel yet distracted by every movement. Zoned, yet worried. "I thought keto made it better, but it didn't last," he pouted to himself.

Low magnesium swallows you inside a cloud and traps you there. You may have felt the effects of plummeting magnesium the last time you had diarrhea, and you flushed this vital salt down the toilet. Magnesium poured out of your body with the loose stools. In quick succession, severe fatigue, irritability, and depression took over. Similarly, when you shift your body chemistry from standard eating to keto-genic, your magnesium washes away.

A few days into ketosis and David dropped half a stone. His belt slid tighter, and his scale read lighter. What could be wrong with that?

Answer: Low Magnesium.

Without correction, David will give up and blame keto for all those symptoms caused by low magne-sium. Proper guidance is needed ASAP.

Measurement

Magnesium deficiency is not easy to measure in the laboratory. Trust your symptoms. Not the laborato-ry. It's a rare day when I ditch checking a lab value and trust the patient's symptoms. I am an internist known for ordering a test for each and every one of your symptoms. But NOT this time! When it comes to as-sessing magnesium, *symptoms* matter most.

Magnesium blood tests fail to show who is truly low in magnesium, and who is not. Don't waste your money on the lab test. The results will confuse and dis-tract you.

The standard blood test for magnesium mea-sures the minerals floating in the liquid part of your blood— the serum— called *serum magnesium*. Our kidneys keep a close check on serum magnesium, and rarely let it dip below the normal range. The slightest shift from normal sends your body to mine the massive magnesium deposit stored in our bones. Magnesium robbed from your bone-storage keeps the level in the blood out of the danger range—but just enough to prevent your ticker from skipping heartbeats.

Advanced researchers measure magnesium by collecting urine for 24 hours and tallying the total magnesium in the jugs of urine. This concluded number gets compared to the amount of magnesium the patient consumes. Subtract what comes out from what goes in, and you have the numbers to figure out the rest. That is hard to do, expensive, and takes a lot of time and effort from the patient.

Magnesium inside red blood cells can also be measured. This number is slower to change and more accurate. For a nominal amount (example $50.00 in 2021), you can order this test, but I don't recommend any of them. The best way to measure your magnesium is through symptoms.

Replacement

The science of magnesium replacement is complicated. Type "How to replace magnesium" into any search engine on the internet and hundreds of answers populate your screen. Not just one. Hundreds. Why?

Shouldn't the answer be: Take magnesium? If it was that easy, the search engine would show a few high ranking answers. Instead, you have every marketer who sells magnesium paying for that top click.

Many advisors bluff their way through, with half-truths about magnesium replacement. They teach a tiny segment of this meticulous equation and leave out the pitfalls. Most "students" buy their solution.

ANSWER: Replace magnesium slowly and steadily.

Slow & Steady

So many things influence how you absorb magnesium that textbooks on this subject still leave you wondering what's best. The factors impacting your gut's magnesium absorption stretch beyond my attention span — and I love this stuff.

The ability to absorb magnesium is influenced by so many factors it could be likened to the changing wind from the north. Swallow your magnesium with some MCT oil and increase the amount that gets into your blood. Add some apple cider vinegar, and you'll poop all of it out. Stir in any form of fake sugar, and you nearly halt all absorption of magnesium.

Change when you eat, what you eat, your age, your last bowel movement, your supplements, or your body temperature and magnesium absorption changes. Plop your magnesium into some water. Does it make the water fizz? That seems to help absorption — especially if you take it on the second Sunday before Easter. (Just kidding about that last part.)

If you think your magnesium is low, you should replace it. Sounds simple enough, right? Telling you to eat high magnesium foods should be good advice. But this also falls short.

When the lowest link on the food-chain breaks, the rest of food-chain suffers. Magnesium enters into the food-chain from nutritious plants — unless you eat plants grown from the 21st-century soil. Today's food should be bursting with magnesium. Roots should have sucked magnesium from the ground into the plants we eat. In reality, our food fails because the soil lacks magnesium too. The marked decline in soil-magnesium plagues the whole globe. This vital mineral dwindles in plants and the animals that eat those plants.

Your system gets caught off guard when you expel large amounts of magnesium from the body at once. The results can be dangerous. Rarely, too low of magnesium can be a medical emergency from irregular heart rhythms. Long before that crisis, patients suffer from warning symptoms, much like David. The body cautions the patient that something is wrong.

In an emergency, I can write an order to drip a magnesium solution into a patient's veins. Obstetricians prescribe this same antidote to a uterus muscle that won't stop cramping. The protocol for preterm labor often reads, "Intravenous magnesium drip. Titrate to contractions." If an unborn baby threatens to enter the world too soon due to pre-term labor, one solution is to flood the mother's blood with magnesium. That magnesium settles down twitchy muscles and stops contractions. One or two grams of magnesium and preterm labor disappears. If excess magnesium circulates, your bones will reabsorb some, and your kidneys will eliminate what's not needed.

Instead of always playing catch-up with magnesium, fix the root cause. The origin of low magnesium begins with the gut lining. A swollen gut lining allows precious magnesium to slip away unchecked. Without fixing that leaking gut, expect to fight low magnesium symptoms.

Adding a big dose of magnesium to anyone's gut shocks the system and causes diarrhea. One gulp of milk of magnesia (magnesium hydroxide 500 mg in a tablespoon) will flush away the constipation. It also increases your serum magnesium. With hopes of avoiding the side effects of loose stools, vitamin suppliers have a history of adding only a stingy amount of magnesium to their supplements. But these tricksters have a tough time fooling educated consumers. If the magnesium supplement you're taking does not cause your tummy to rumble, it's probably a minor quantity of magnesium. The rumbles of your bowels subside when you lower the dose or slow the speed. Slowly add magnesium to your gut with a tiny amount of magnesium in each swallow. This allows it to get absorbed instead of squirting out your backside. Slow and steady wins the magnesium race.

ANSWER: Replace magnesium, track your symptoms, and stay keto. Use the chart in the workbook to guide you.

Pick one or both of these options

Take a Supplement

Magnesium supplements include magnesium citrate, magnesium carbonate, magnesium chloride, magnesium hydroxylate, and magnesium glycinate. Of these, magnesium glycinate and Slow-Mag (a slow-digesting form of magnesium chloride) prove least likely to cause loose stools or other digestive problems.

Early in my medical career, I used to care about all this. But time spent practicing medicine has taught me to care less about the type of magnesium, and more about getting some magnesium into the bodies of patients. Just pick one. Go with Milk of Magnesia. Find it in every gas station across the globe. It's in the laxative section.

I guarantee it has magnesium in it. Take a big swig. Thirty minutes later, the gurgles in your tummy followed by diarrhea prove you chugged magnesium. Flushing most of it down the toilet isn't the plan. Instead of a gulp, add a tablespoon to the water you drink. Using the unflavored Milk Of Magnesia works well. Sip magnesium-spiked water all day long. This will undoubtedly increase the magnesium in your body. It is cheap, easy to find, and safe.

Use Your Skin

Yes, that's right. Use _your body's largest organ_ to absorb magnesium: Your skin.

Add six to eight cups of magnesium salt to hot bathwater. Sink into the warm water up to your armpits and soak for at least 40 minutes. Ideally you'd soak for an hour, but 40 minutes is a minimum requirement. Twice weekly baths are a good goal. This delivers magnesium to your circulation while adding relaxation time to your schedule. Epsom Salt, magnesium sulfate, can be found in every drug store. Magnesium Chloride salt offers another option.

Don't be stingy on the amount of salt you put into the bath. The only way the magnesium gets into your circulation is through the layers of skin cells. Too little salt or too short of time in the tub, and you don't get much magnesium.

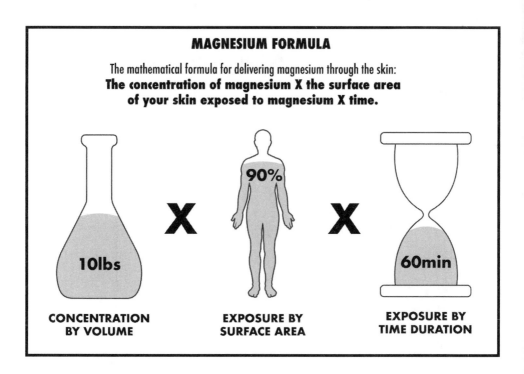

MAGNESIUM FORMULA

The mathematical formula for delivering magnesium through the skin:
The concentration of magnesium X the surface area of your skin exposed to magnesium X time.

10lbs **X** 90% **X** 60min

CONCENTRATION BY VOLUME   EXPOSURE BY SURFACE AREA   EXPOSURE BY TIME DURATION

Float Therapy:

Floatation tanks add 1500 pounds of Epsom salt to a single-person pod. This is a maximum Epsom salt bath. Much like the Dead Sea, the salinity of the water is so high, you can't sink. Enter into your private pod wearing your birthday suit. My favorite experience, close the cover to your pod for a vacation wrapped inside an hour. Time-out. No light. No sound. Ignoring the passage of time. Just floating in warm water. Suspended without touch, light, or noise, all sensory input stops. Your mind drifts into a vacation.

The mathematical formula for delivering magnesium through the skin looks like this:

Concentration of Salt **X** Exposure of Skin **X** Time

Let me break that down.

Epsom Foot Soak:

Pour two five-pound bags (12 cups) of Epsom salt into your foot basin filled with hot water. Mix. Place feet in water for 60 min.

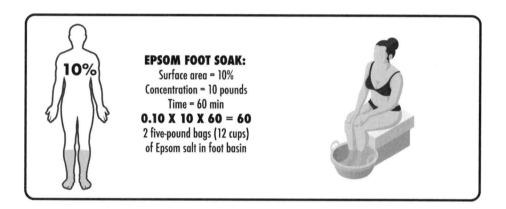

EPSOM FOOT SOAK:
Surface area = 10%
Concentration = 10 pounds
Time = 60 min
0.10 X 10 X 60 = 60
2 five-pound bags (12 cups)
of Epsom salt in foot basin

Epsom Salt Bath:

Pour one five-pound bag (6 cups) into the bathtub. Suspend your body towards your armpits. Relax for an hour.

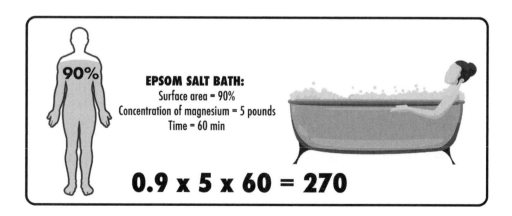

EPSOM SALT BATH:
Surface area = 90%
Concentration of magnesium = 5 pounds
Time = 60 min

$$0.9 \times 5 \times 60 = 270$$

If you throw two bags of salt in the tub, the number would be 540.

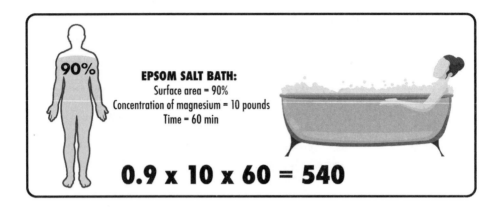

EPSOM SALT BATH:
Surface area = 90%
Concentration of magnesium = 10 pounds
Time = 60 min

0.9 x 10 x 60 = 540

Float Spa: There is no comparison.

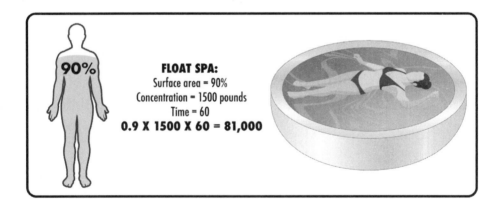

FLOAT SPA:
Surface area = 90%
Concentration = 1500 pounds
Time = 60
0.9 X 1500 X 60 = 81,000

Patients ask about rubbing magnesium spray onto their skin. This falls short, too. These sprays are a combination of magnesium salt and oil, making the total amount of concentrated magnesium variable, and sometimes falling short of the required amount for your body to fully benefit.

Too much magnesium crystallizes and turns your spray-oil into a salt scrub. The first few times someone adds the oil to their legs or arms, they may cover 25-30% of the skin. But as time passes this percentage of skin coverage lessens to just a few inches. Minimal sustained improvements happen with the oil spray.

The fastest reversal of low-magnesium happens when I drip the magnesium into their veins by I.V. during an emergency. The next best option I recommend to my patients is to float five hours in the floatation. Spread those five hours over seven days.

No matter which magnesium you chose, remember that absorption increases with the dose. So if you only soak in magnesium once a month, not much changes. If you only take magnesium supplements 3 times a week, that, too, will do little to reverse symptoms. Rubbing magnesium oil into your skin twice a week doesn't move the needle much either.

Stay Keto

Pouring magnesium into your blood only fixes things short term. All that magnesium wiggles out of circulation if inflammation whispers through your system allowing it to leak out the gut. Stop those precious minerals from sliding out your swollen gut-lining. Seal your intestinal wounds by steadily peeing ketones.

Keto chemistry reduces inflammation - stay keto to fix your magnesium.

Take notice of the list of medical problems linked to low magnesium — and this is only the severe conditions. The complete list would take pages.

On Tuesday, David acquired some of this knowledge about low magnesium. Deficient magnesium twitched his tiny eye muscles, slowed his bowel movements, and twisted his larger muscles into cramps. His somber mood teetered on the edge of giving up. Education and encouragement to replace this mysterious mineral helped him stay the course. He longed for the blissfulness from his previous week. When he learned that a silly crystal stole his mojo, he identified his enemy. He loaded his car with bags of magnesium bath-salts, several bottles of Milk of Magnesia, and enough supplement pills for the whole block.

He made every mistake I warned against. He swallowed a half dozen supplement pills the first day. This did little for his low magnesium, but it corrected his constipation. His bowels educated him far better than my lecture could have.

Conditions that "leak" magnesium

Alcoholism

Diabetes

Malabsorption

    Crohn's disease
    Ulcerative colitis
    Celiac disease
    Short bowel syndrome
    Small Bowel Overgrowth
    Whipple's disease

Endocrine causes

    Aldosteronism
    Hyperparathyroidism
    Hyperthyroidism

Kidney disease

    Chronic renal failure
    Dialysis
    Gitelman's syndrome

Medications

    A variety of antibiotics
    Chemotherapeutic agents
    Diuretics (pee pills)
    Proton pump inhibitors (stomach acid pills)

His eagerness to re-capture his early keto feelings motivated him to fill his bathtub with bags of salt. Ten pounds at a time. He soaked in a half-dozen home baths before he grew tired of buying, carrying, and pouring salt. He finally conceded to trying the local floatation spa.

Desperate, he prayed for happiness to return. Four days of swallowing, soaking, and rubbing magnesium into his body, and the grayness began to fade. It took nearly two weeks before the sun shone with full brightness in his life.

Longterm Replacement:

David replaced magnesium daily for eight months. At first, he used up the magnesium pills he'd bought. He keenly, and rightfully, connected his symptoms of low magnesium: erratic muscle twitches, distracted thoughts, and sully mood to low magnesium. All bowel problems, he blamed low magnesium.

David added unflavored Milk of Magnesia (MOM) from the gas station to all of his water. One capful of MOM per water bottle. He kept a bottle of MOM at work, in the car, at home, and in his travel bag. He even tried adding it to his coffee. (I did not recommend that!) Every sip inched him closer to a restored level of magnesium. He suspended his deficient body in the float spa a half dozen times over the next month. And as predicted, the improvements with the floats helped him the most.

As ketones healed his body from the inside, his magnesium requirements decreased. Deep within the cells of his gut, the chronic, hidden injuries repaired thanks to ketogenic chemistry. Circulating ketones delivered more than weight loss. They strengthened his immune system, organized his thoughts, tightened his connective tissue, and repelled swelling. David improved his health one ketone at a time.

Chapter 16

DAY **8, 9, 10** CRAVING PITFALLS

David struggled with depression in the past, haunting him for months at a time, sometimes years. Originally the sadness gradually appeared, the symptoms imperceptibly snuck up on him, making them hard to recognize. "Did the weight-gain come first, or the low energy?" he wondered. David got used to soothing his mood with carbs, affectionately called "comfort food" or "therapy food," for almost six decades. Feeding on carbs fostered the symptoms of depression. The more he ate, the higher the symptoms stacked — feeling down, no joy, difficulty sleeping, fatigue, scattered thoughts, and thoughts that death would just be easier. All of them at once. He recalled his darkest days. David understood why people gave up and threw in the towel.

Those shadowed days scared him. But never again. Magnesium, carefully tailored for David, allowed him to feel hopeful again. His recent extra magnesium swept away his clouded thoughts.

His first week of keto circulated ketones and reminded him of life before his depression. Not a perfect life, but compared to the recent months of darkness, the first week of ketosis saved his life. And then it switched off. Seven great days of steadily climbing out of a dreary mist, only to be engulfed in it again. But blaming magnesium helped David to fight; it gave him the pathway to victory. Sometimes you just need an enemy to work against.

Craving Pitfalls

Modern-day sweeteners line our grocery shelves. Brilliant chemists delivered numerous substances that mimic the look, feel, smell, taste, and the power of sugar. Place these creative combinations on your tongue, and your brain will think sugar. Your soul will feel the satisfaction of sugar.

Is it real sugar? Is it fake sugar? Your brain doesn't really care. Once the chemical lands on your tongue, dopamine relieves the craving. If you didn't believe this before starting the ketogenic diet, Day 10 offers an excellent opportunity to test this theory. Most people miss the feeling of sugar by this time.

David's brain and body weren't an exception. He responded to sweets the same as every human. His carbs got burned or stored when he abundantly and regularly ate them. His metabolism acclimated and used pine needles as full-time fuel. His worst cravings for carbs were in the evenings. Against better advice, he stocked up on "healthy keto snacks" and then placed them where his comfort foods used to be. The packages marketed him with slogans of, "No net carbs." "Only two carbs." "No carbs." Macadamia nuts were his kryptonite. The label read "four carbs in 10 nuts, two-grams of fiber," and boasted "24-grams of fat." Every keto chart ranked them at the top of the list for the best, fat-filled nuts. He found a massive bag of roasted, salted macadamia nuts for $30.00. A month's supply? Nope. It was gone in under a week. How? David ate them all - Mindlessly.

The reach inside the cupboard for a handful happened without thought. It was as if unconscious hand-levitation took over. Just like the words of an addict, David admitted, "I don't know how it happened." Over the past decades his dwindling metabolism created gnarly brain-wiring that sparked his cravings. David's addicted brain needed rewired.

Protocols that work on healing addiction start with proximity. Proximity matters — it's the first rule toward eliminating temptations. David needed to remove the nuts from his house. Just like any addiction, the first phase began with the removal of his tempting, over-used vices. The cleaned-cupboard exercise at the onset of keto was not an accident. This cleansed environment waxed the first steps for success.

Rules of addiction begin with proximity. So do other protocols used to heal from addiction.

ABSTINENCE vs HARM REDUCTION

Management of addiction battles between two camps: abstinence versus harm reduction. While abstinence completely removes the addicted substance, harm reduction offers clean IV needles to heroin addicts. Harm reduction saves lives, decreases diseases, and provides a beginning to many stuck in the depths of addictive behavior. Abstinence heals a brain. Harm reduction offers hope to those who did not think it was possible. This method applies to sugar.

The Best Answer Is Abstinence

The best answer is - NO SWEETS. Period.

On a ketogenic diet, sugar cravings decrease. Your taste buds will reset once you stop putting sweetness onto them. Rip the bandage off quickly by stopping all sweet consumption. Reminding your brain of those deviant tastes is akin to alcohol to an alcoholic; you are flirting with danger. When sugar-addicts hear this strict rule, these questions arise:

"What about honey?"

"How about fruits — they have sugar?"

"What about fake sugar?"

Questions such as these are a last ditch attempt at holding onto a semblance of the addictive substance in question, to keep your addiction alive. The answer is NO! We must change the way your brain responds to sweetness. Treat sugar and sweet tastes like poison, especially during the first six months of your addiction recovery ... I mean your ketogenic diet.

If you can follow that no-sweets-rule 100% of the time, avoiding any games or tricks, you can skip the next chapter. You're good. The rest of us will reduce harm with our 'clean-IV-needle' program.

Harm Reduction

I find teaching the rules of harm reduction allows folks to fail upwards. Harm reduction slowly pulls off the bandage. It begins with a dramatic decrease in the drug dosage —in this case, CARBS. Start with 20 grams of carbs per day. Period. That rule needs to stand. If you were part of that 200 Club, set your course with a slower decline to 20, but the number to reach is still 20. Don't be deceived that the gradual re-duction means you stop at a higher number of carbs.

Next, fructose remains on the forbidden list, along with a few others. Fructose processes through your liver exactly as booze does. The two chemicals responsible for fatty livers hardening into cirrhosis are: Fructose or alcohol. Both poison the liver when consumed in excess. A damaged liver only has a chance of healing if you dial the total grams of carbs back to 20 or less.

Fructose commonly hides on labels disguised as

high fructose corn syrup,

fruit juice from concentrate, or

agave syrup.

All of these should be called "super sugars." Banish them along with honey, molasses, and any fruit sugar from your menu. No. None.

HARM REDUCTION sweeteners include allulose, stevia, and monk fruit.

Let's go through these.

#1: Allulose

Allulose (also known as D-Psicose) identified in the 1940s, is an ultra low-calorie sugar found naturally in wheat, figs, raisins, and jackfruit. Recently, chemists have found an enzymatic way to transform the fructose in corn to allulose, thus enabling the mass-production of allulose. With corn as the source of sugar, the cost remains reasonable. Gram for gram, allulose has one-tenth the calories of sugar. Hopefully, we process less corn into evil high-fructose corn syrup and more into allulose.

Allulose absorbs readily into the body, but very little gets burned in your campfires as fuel. Most of it is excreted via urine. Allulose, studied in insulin-resistant diabetics, caused negligible increases to their blood sugar or insulin. That is remarkable! Other studies show less tooth decay and increased fat loss when allulose was consumed.

When you see it on a label's Nutrition Facts, you will notice that the Federal Drug administrators have allowed allulose to be excluded from the total and added sugars. Strangely, despite having no effect on blood sugar or insulin and minor amounts metabolized for energy, the FDA requires allulose to be included in 'total carbohydrates' on the label. I tell my patients to not count those carbs.

Add another point for the clean taste of allulose without a cooling effect like xylitol. Artificial sweeteners like sucralose and aspartame are hundreds of times sweeter than sugar. This high-intensity sweetness leaves an aftertaste in the mouth because of how those chemicals fit into the tastebuds. Allulose is different. In the eyes of a chemist, it looks and acts like sugar. It's a chemical sibling to cane sugar, with about 70% of the sweetness; yet, a tenth of the calories. It depresses the freezing point of foods, and caramelizes when exposed to heats similar to sugar. It is highly soluble and works well with monk fruit and stevia. Allulose wins for minimal processing, natural origin, abundant resources, and cost.

#2: Monk Fruit

This incredibly sweet fruit from Southeast Asia was first consumed by 13th century monks, hence its name - monk fruit. Today, you'll find it in every Chinese medicine market. Drying and extracting the molecule from this fruit has been taking place for centuries, which requires minimal processing. It only takes a few flakes of dried monk fruit to sense optimum sweetness. Think of the specs of monk fruit as diamonds. Crystals. Powerful.

Monk fruit wins on taste, minimal processing, and limited troubles with digestion. In the grocery stores, it's frequently mixed with stevia or erythritol, so read the labels carefully. After seeing the cost of pure dried monk fruit, which will shock you, you'll know why I equate the tiny specks of monk fruit to diamonds.

#3: Stevia

Of all the sugar-demons consumers live with, Stevia is a lessor evil. You just can't ignore this sweetener. "Stevia's too big to fail," and has an excellent marketing team. On the package of most stevia products, you will find a vibrant, wholesome green leaf that connects your brain to the words NATURAL or HEALTHY. Stevia is derived from a South-American plant. Indeed, that part is natural. But buyer beware! Do not be deceived with photos of a stunning Brazilian woman holding a green leaf. The majority of stevia comes from China. Chemists process the leaf into powder through bleaching, de-coloring, and chemical transformations. Before it hits your tongue, more than forty steps of chemistry have been applied to create this substance. There are no carbs; no calories either. But nobody told that to your brain - or your pancreas.

Stevia's sweetness soars 200 to 350 times sweeter than cane sugar. Sprinkle a tiny bit onto your tongue and watch your brain crackle, spark, and light up with dopamine. Simultaneously, as the pleasure centers of your brain are being distracted and hijacked by the sweetness, your pancreas will squirt insulin.

Don't believe me? Do a home experiment. Check your blood sugars. Sprinkle ONLY stevia on your tongue. Wait 20 minutes. <u>During those twenty minutes, keep track of how many sweet foods circle through your thoughts.</u> Addicts beware! Recheck your blood sugars, and you will find that it should not rise. You read that correctly. NOT RISE. When using stevia, the studies show the blood sugars stay stable. What no one talks about is <u>the sudden rise in cravings associated with stevia.</u> The other detail left out of those trials was the audience in the studies. Stevia did not spike blood glucose in lean, healthy people. I have pages of insulin-resistant patients who show a rise in glucose after a sprinkle of stevia.

Stevia doesn't taste exactly like sugar. That's a downfall. Also, stevia comes from the same family of plants as ragweed. If you're allergic to ragweed, watch out, sometimes the allergies cross-react. The allergic reaction to stevia often manifests as loose stools. When Gastro doctors snapped pictures of a susceptible patient's gut lining after swallowing stevia, it looked like hives. Their gut swelled and reacted to the chemical exactly the same way their sinuses responded to ragweed.

So that's it. No sweetness is best, but if you're going to minimize the damage with sweet relief, use allulose, monk fruit, or stevia. Those are the three harm-reducing sweeteners I recommend.

Beware of Other Sweeteners

When you ferment corn, you make corn-sugar-alcohol. Another name for this chemical is erythritol. I don't recommend erythritol, with the exception of its use in sugar-free-gum. Sprinkle this sweetener onto your tongue, and a cooling sensation accompanies the sweet taste. Only a tiny amount gets absorbed by the body when sweetening foods with it — the rest slides into the toilet. Swallow a spoonful and you'll have an "explosive date" with the porcelain god. Just like stevia, erythritol contains no carbs or calories. Your blood sugar, once again, should not rise. But tiny amounts do pass into your urine after being absorbed into the circulation. Scientists are not quite sure what the long-term consequences on kidney-health will be. Research is still pending.

Xylitol is also on the naughty list. If you've ever chewed sugar-free gum, then you've tasted xylitol. If you've used a sweet, mouthwash product, then you've also tasted it. These aforementioned products aren't meant to be swallowed. The best advantage to xylitol comes from the substantial evidence that it suppresses the growth of oral bacteria. Much like erythritol, only a minimal amount of xylitol gets absorbed into your circulation. Your blood sugars do rise in response to this sweetener. WARNING: This sweetener is extremely deadly to animals. Even a small lick can be deadly.

Maltitol also failed to make the nice-list. Maltitol is used in medicine as a potent laxative. Just saying. Guess what happens when you swallow it? Yep, a bowel cleanse.

** Note: The expensive types of sugar-free gum use erythritol as an ingredient. Cheap sugar-free gum uses xylitol.

Zero Calorie Artificial Sweeteners

Be aware of things that look too good to be true. Zero calories are not actually zero calories, especially for products such as Stevia In The Raw, Equal, Sweet n' Low, and Splenda. The literature gets messy and nebulous when you search for scientific answers about fake sugars. Short-term studies linked certain artificial sugars to weight loss in the first year. Questionably, nearly all of those studies were funded by The American Beverage Association — the folks who make diet-sodas.

Here's the skinny on "zero" calories. The Federal Drug Administration (FDA) allows manufacturers to round down to zero for carb servings under one gram or fewer than four calories. In the bigger scheme of things, this sounds like a reasonable rule. Manufacturers and marketers border on unethical while wiggling around this rule. They package sweeteners right under the cutoff. Instead of a serving size of one gram of carbs, their serving size tops at 0.9 grams. Similarly, they have a sweetener with 3.6 calories, sneaking under the 4.0 edge. They legally round down to zero. Don't be tricked. Those carbs add up. You'll be outside your 20 grams of carbs with several servings per day. More noticeably, your brain gnaws at you with cravings.

Observational studies have retrospectively re-examined a decade's worth of using sugar substitutes. These studies contained many flaws. For example, asking people to remember what they ate yesterday is problematic. Think about this: Imagine reporting what you had to drink for the last 10 years. That's how this information was collected. For what it's worth, these observational studies showed higher risks of obesity, hypertension, metabolic syndrome, type 2 diabetes, stroke, and cardiovascular events in the group that used fake sugars.

Reading the scientific literature on sugar substitutes guarantees frustration. Skip that.

The best approach to artificial sweeteners remains LESS IS BETTER.

David used sweet temptations to satisfy his cravings. This sparked an increase in his desire for treats. Only when he ceased eating all sweet tastes for several days did it improve.

RECOMMENDATION: Pull the bandage off.

PART TWO

ketoCONTINUUM		WHO DOES THE WORK?	TEST	
BEGINNER	1. I EAT EVERY 2-4 HOURS	CHEMISTRY CARRIES YOU	NONE	4-6 WEEKS
	2. LESS THAN 20 TOTAL CARBS. I EAT EVERY 6-8 HOURS.		URINE PEETONE STRIPS	
	3. I "ACCIDENTALLY" MISSED A MEAL. [KETO-ADAPTED]			
BASELINE METABOLISM	4. EAT 2 MEALS PER DAY.	YOU DO THE WORK. DISCIPLINE NEEDED FOR EACH NEW STEP.		LIVE HERE
	5. 16:8			
	6. ADVANCED 16:8			
	7. 23:1 OMAD: ALL IN 1 HOUR.			
STRESSING METABOLISM	8. ADVANCED 23:1/OMAD	PSYCHOLOGY. USE TRIBE FOR BEST RESULTS.	BLOOD KETONE STRIPS	USE INTERMITTENTLY
	9. 36 HOUR FAST			
	10. 36 HOUR FAST WITHOUT CELEBRATION MEAL			
	11. 48 HOUR FAST			
	12. 72 Hour Fast			

GUIDELINES	NEXT STEPS
Fueled on glucose. Must refuel often. Never fueled by ketones.	
Eat <20 total carbs per day. Ketosis begins. Fat-based hormones rise. Eating happens less frequently.	Be sure to eat high fat with low carbs. Your body uses the fat to restore your fat built hormones. Elevated insulin within your body prevents you from using the stored fat. You must eat the fat.
Fat supplies the resources needed to make fat-built hormones. Fat based hormones approach healthy levels. Appetite decreases according to body's chemistry.	Sometimes it takes 10 weeks before this moment happens. Don't look at the scale. Listen for the absence of hunger.
Choose to eat only 2 meals per day.	Succeed 7 days in a row before advancing.
Eat ALL food, snacks, and supplements in an 8-hour window. No eating, snacking, or chewing for 16 hours.	That means no gum during fasting hours. Suck on salt if you need a substitute. Keep your coffee filled with fat.
Clean up your morning drink. Remove all calories and sweeteners. Morning drink = no fat, no MCT, no butter, no sweeteners, no calories. The 16 hours = only salt, water, black coffee, or tea.	Don't remove the fat from your morning drink before this phase. You needed it to get here. Now it's time to let it go.
ALL calories & sweeteners in one hour. 23 hours = Only salt, water, tea, or coffee.	Begin checking blood numbers right before you eat.
Move eating-hour within 11 hours following sunrise to match your circadian rhythm.	Record the Dr Boz Ratio first thing in the morning. Repeat before eating.
Fast for 36 hours. No calories. No sweeteners Start in evening as to use 2 cycles of sleep during the 36 hours.	Begin fast after evening meal. DANGER: If on blood pressure meds or blood sugar lowering meds. ASK YOUR DOCTOR
After 36 hour fast, return to your normal pattern of eating without a splurge meal.	Offer a group fasting routine to others in your tribe. Fast together.
Fast for 48 hours. No calories. No sweeteners.	Safe to try twice a week. Unlike the 36-hour fast, this option keeps meals at the same time each day.
Fast for 72 hours. No calories. No sweeteners.	When the timing is right, stress your metabolism with 8 weeks of a 72-hour fast. The rest of the week, return to your BASELINE METABOLISM. The best transitions happen through this challenge.

Chapter 17

KETO**CONTINUUM**

To change behavior, you need motivation, clear instructions to get started, and a roadmap. You proclaimed your motivation not only to the world, but to yourself, when you articulated your WHY. Eating 20 carbs or less offered clear initial instructions. ketoCONTINUUM maps where you're going.

Let's Recap

Weeks ago, glucose saturated David's brain, insulin inflamed his body, and he limped through his daily tasks. Grandma Rose, a 72-year old cancer survivor, inspired David after she adopted the ketogenic diet. He threw out the carbs and joined her in slurping down fat. Despite David's missed steps, he persisted with this newly adopted eating lifestyle.

Brazilian Mama

While parked in the line of cars to pick up my middle schooler, a jolly-sized Brazilian woman knocked on my frosted car window. Her eyes betrayed her desperation. 'Had we met before?' I tried remembering, but to no avail. The winter froze my window from opening, so I motioned her into my front seat. "I need your help. You wrote dis book?" she asked, showing me a copy of ANYWAY YOU CAN. I nodded and forced my brain to process her thick Brazilian accent. "You need to teach more people dis! I just got out of hospital for they removed my colon cancer. Do you know what they fed me in hospital?" Before I could answer, she sped forward, "PUDDING!!" Over the next 15 minutes, Brazilian Mama did her best to talk me into adding her to my clinic-roster as a new patient. I refused, "You don't need a new doctor to do the ketogenic diet. Your healthcare has several good doctors. I know your doctors. They are not telling you anything medically that I would not tell you. You need to follow the instructions in that book and eat a ketogenic diet. That does not require a new doctor.

She did not like that answer.

Brazilian Mama persisted. In an attempt to dissuade her, I layered on the complication that her insurance would not pay for "keto-coaching," even if it saved her life. No diagnostic code matched — not to mention the amount of time needed to teach the nutritional approach toward consistent keto-chemistry.

By now, our kids watched two first-born females, Brazilian Mama, powered by her desperation for help, and me, a doctor and first-time author, battle with words, wits, and tenacity. A wave of patients like Brazilian Mama, needed hours of education to satisfy their hunger for improved healthcare. She, along with countless others had reached out to our clinic in hopes to help them succeed like Grandma Rose had. Traditional medicine had abandoned these patients — those starved for intimate, high-quality care.

Unbeknownst to either of us, my car threw disorder into the middle school parent-pickup line where parents grew frustrated by the blocked flow of traffic. Honking parents with bushy eyebrows glared and maneuvered around our argument. In the stress of this circus, Brazilian Mama proposed a solution without thinking. "Lead a class for keto students. I'll be your first student." The simplicity of her compromise rang true as I impulsively accepted her proposal.

The following week "class" started in the basement of my office building. This birthed the ketoCONTINUUM support group. Cold folding chairs and minimal heat traced the edge of our first classroom. A handful of people came to that first meeting. David attended the following week and rarely missed one since.

Brazilian Mama's hare-brained idea, combined with my acceptance of the idea and commitment to it, gave birth to the ketoCONTINUUM support group. Renowned mythologist, Joseph Campbell famously said, "When you are on the right path, you will find invisible hands helping you along the way!"

ketoCONTINUUM Support Group

The effort to host the gathering was minimal. No cost; no food; no gossip and no suffocation. The attraction grew slowly at first, but then dynamically. Soon, that hour became my weekly favorite. People came and shared their keto-journey. We created a community of folks trying to improve their health. Lives changed each week.

The support group evolved with just enough structure to be functional, but informal enough to attract beginners. The secret code that got you into our meeting was to know what a ketone was. Most attendees had a basic education about ketosis from reading ANYWAY YOU CAN. But years of leading small groups helped me set the expectations for an impactful process. Each meeting started with the announcement that this is not a substitute for your doctor.

Using the industries best practices for addiction-recovery meetings, I grew a nurturing environment with a few simple guidelines:

- Share your own thoughts and feelings with focus on your personal issues. Limit advice to others by sharing your experiences.

- No cross-talk. A separate conversation with your neighbor limits the sharing. Bring forth your comments in a way that all can hear and participate.

- Anonymity and confidentiality are basic requirements. Share the education you learn in ketoCONTINUUM without sharing identities.

- Veterans check-in first. Newbies wait to introduce yourself until you've seen several examples of how it works.

Human beings, by default, are constantly learning. This innate ability never stops. It is one of the ways we survive and thrive as individuals. Observing others is foundational for the succession of skills into the next generation. One of the biologically built-in strategies we use in order to learn is simply watching others - "look, watch, and learn." On the surface, it seems like individuals are simply "looking on" during a support group meeting, yet a deeper set of mental processes are taking place. Neurons are at work — firing, rewiring, and establishing new neural connections. The neurons in charge are called mirror-neurons. What are they? Mirror neurons help us imitate, or "mirror," new behavior. Mirror-neurons capture information not seen before. Successful meetings educate through mirror neurons. Watch group members struggle. Watch them succeed. Observe them encouraging one another. Mirror neurons capture all of these moments and tuck them into the grey matter.

Some folks attend for a season, and then disappear for months. Others might return when they need encouragement. Students watch others cycle in and out of the group without shame or guilt. Newbies watch the veterans share their WHYs. The established members demonstrate honesty, vulnerability, and acceptance of your strengths and fears stimulating the mirror neurons of newbies.

We gathered weekly for an hour to share our journey along the ketoCONTINUUM. The ketoCONTINUUM maps the pattern I've seen in patients. As numbers rise from one through twelve along the map,

ketoCONTINUUM		
BEGINNER	1. I EAT EVERY 2-4 HOURS	**4-6 WEEKS**
	2. LESS THAN 20 TOTAL CARBS. I EAT EVERY 6-8 HOURS.	
	3. I "ACCIDENTALLY" MISSED A MEAL. [KETO-ADAPTED]	
	4. EAT 2 MEALS PER DAY.	
BASELINE METABOLISM	5. 16:8	**LIVE HERE**
	6. ADVANCED 16:8	
	7. 23:1 OMAD: ALL IN 1 HOUR.	
	8. ADVANCED 23:1/OMAD	
STRESSING METABOLISM	9. 36 HOUR FAST	**USE INTERMITTENTLY**
	10. 36 HOUR FAST WITHOUT CELEBRATION MEAL	
	11. 48 HOUR FAST	
	12. 72 Hour Fast	

so does metabolic strength. Each number marks a learned skill. Practice one skill before advancing on the continuum. The goal is health, not reaching the highest number on the ketoCONTINUUM. Once health improves, stay at that number. Each level on the continuum stresses cellular metabolism higher than the previous one. We encourage advancement only when they want it and feel ready for the next step.

Like David, most folks needed a nudge to achieve better health. He had dropped the ketogenic way of eating into his life like a bomb. After the dust settled, he was lost without a roadmap. David used the support group to find and then stay the course.

Roadmap

ketoCONTINUUM divides 12 stages of metabolism into three sections: Beginners, Baseline Metabolism, and Stressing Metabolism.

Beginners eating a standard-American, high-carbohydrate diet start at ketoCONTINUUM #1 and often take 4-6 weeks to progress through the rest of the beginners' phases.

ketoCONTINUUMs #5 through #8 represent the four metabolic options to stay healthy with consistent ketosis. These lifetime options are called the Baseline Metabolisms and have the potential to sustain ketosis for life.

	ketoCONTINUUM	WHO DOES THE WORK?	TEST	GUIDELINES	NEXT STEP
BEGINNER	#1. I eat every 2-4 hours	CHEMISTRY	NONE	Fueled on glucose. Must refuel often. Never fueled by ketones.	
BEGINNER	#2. LESS THAN 20 total carbs. I eat every 6-8 hours.	CHEMISTRY	URINE STRIPS	Eat <20 total carbs per day. Ketosis begins. Fat-based hormones rise. Eating happens less frequently.	Be sure to eat high fat with low carbs. Your body uses the fat to restore your fat built hormones. Elevated insulin within your body prevents you from using the stored fat. You must eat the fat.
BEGINNER	#3. I "accidentally" missed a meal. [Keto-adapted]	CHEMISTRY	URINE STRIPS	Fat supplies the resources needed to make fat-built hormones. Fat based hormones approach healthy levels. Appetite decreases according to body's chemistry.	Sometimes it takes 10 weeks before this moment happens. Don't look at the scale. Listen for the absence of hunger.

The final section offers four ways to stress your metabolism. Adding one of these stressors to the baseline metabolisms strengthens the cellular performance each time it's applied. Categorize ketoCONTINUUMs #9 through #12 as workouts for your mitochondria. Stressing Metabolisms are not recommended until you've practiced life at one of the baseline levels for a season. Strategically stressing one's metabolism will push the efficiency and strength of cells. When the loss of weight has plateaued or stalled, stress the metabolism to push through that stall. Similarly, cells' highest performance is required to combat against cancer or auto-immune problems. Stressing Metabolisms strengthens cells to their peak performance with hopes of reversing chronic metabolic illness.

Find the ketoCONTINUUM number where you spent the most time during the previous week.

Find your number.

1. I eat every 2-4 hours
2. LESS THAN 20 total carbs. I eat every 6-8 hours.
3. I "accidentally" missed a meal. [Keto-adapted]
4. Eat 2 meals per day.
5. 16:8 All food, snacks, and supplements in an 8-hour window.
6. Advanced 16:8 Clean up morning drink. No calories or sweetener in A.M. drink.
7. 23:1 OMAD: One Meal A Day. All calories & sweeteners in one hour. 23 hours = nothing.
8. Advanced 23:1/OMAD Move eating hour within the 11 hours following sunrise.
9. 36 Hour Fast
10. 36 Hour Fast without Celebration Meal
11. 48 Hour Fast
12. 72 Hour Fast

ketoCONTINUUM #1 through #3

Eating 20 carbs per day for 10 days stretched the hours David went without food. Instead of adding pine needles to his metabolism every 2-3 hours, he ate closer to every eight hours. He was not expecting the chemistry shift to occur so quickly; in fact, weeks later, when looking at the ketoCONTINUUM roadmap, that was when he realized that the chemistry shift occurred, automatically — and outside his awareness.

Within days of starting the ketogenic diet, David's high-fat breakfast powered him until 2 PM. Hunger slowly signaled him to eat his packed lunch of hard salami and cheese. His previous warning to refuel twisted his mood into grouchy Mr. Grump. Any delay in feeding him escalated his irritability and dropped his energy. He never missed a meal when fueled with carbs for fear of those symptoms overpowering him. Now, the sensation of eating whispered subtly, "It might be time to eat, David."

During the second week, David's hunger pains passed quickly. With barely a notice, he brushed them off and promised to eat as soon as he finished editing the photos. When he looked up at the wall clock, it read 5:10 PM. Bewildered, he realized he had missed a meal! That *never* happened before keto.

When beginners study the ketoCONTINUUM they naturally lock their eyes onto the transition from keto-CONTINUUM #2 to #3. This step marks keto-adaption. Keto-adaption, also called *fat-adaption*, refers to the ability to quickly shift from burning pine needles to logs. David transitioned rather quickly. Though he took a beating from the unexpected symptoms of lost magnesium and low blood pressure, his mitochondria gracefully converted ketones into energy. Not everyone is that fortunate. But David was blessed.

The time it takes to hit ketoCONTINUUM #3 depends upon two things:

1) The amount of fat-based hormones at the start.

2) The level of compliance with eating high-fat during ketoCONTINUUM #2.

David's fat-based hormones, like everyone's, are made from the fat called *cholesterol*. Before keto, his elevated insulin locked the fat molecules away from his body's hormone-factories. The longer his cells remained saturated with insulin, the lower his fat-based hormones. On a scale from one to ten, with ten being abundant fatty hormones, and one being none, I'd rank him at a four.

Low-fat and high-carb eating had depleted David's fat-based hormones. But a robust keto-chemistry fixed all that, and produced far less insulin. Eating multiple servings of high-fat meals per day permitted his body to quickly transition to keto-fuel. By avoiding carbs, David created a small window of time when the recently ingested fat turned into ketones. The only fat David's insulin-soaked body had access to during the early days of ketoCONTINUUM was the fat he ate — his stored fat swaddling his mid-section. If David had failed to eat abundant amounts of fat in the first days, keto-chemistry would only have trickled ketones into his body, versus the vast internal keto-transition his body underwent.

Eating globs of fat produced far less insulin than when he ate carbs. Lowered insulin started David's cascade of change. Even the slightest reduction in insulin allowed fat to flow throughout his system instead of staying locked up. Flowing fat led to higher fat-based-hormones.

Those fatty hormones satiated David right through that afternoon, and because of that, he missed a meal. That history of "accidentally missing a meal" signals the transition from ketoCONTINUUM #2 into ketoCONTINUUM #3.

ketoCONTINUUM #4

	ketoCONTINUUM	WHO DOES THE WORK?	TEST	GUIDELINES	NEXT STEP
BEGINNER	#4. Eat 2 meals per day.	YOU - DISCIPLINE NEEDED.	URINE STRIPS	Choose to eat only 2 meals per day.	Succeed 7 days in a row before advancing.

Keto-adapted chemistry carried David into keto-CONTINUUM # 3. Keto-chemistry did most of the work curtailing his eating pattern from multiple times per day down to three to four. After "accidentally" missing a few meals, David needed to make a decision about progressing to ketoCONTINUUM #4: Choose to eat two meals per day.

Moving from #3 to #4, required a conscious choice on David's part. At ketoCONTINUUM #3, David's chemistry lubricated his body with fat. He greased up his dusty mitochondria. Eating fat improved his thinking, honed in his immune system, greased his dusty mitochondria, and delivered a teenage-libido-like energy. David, by all observance, felt great. Alive. His spirit crackled. He surely had no desire to quit keto now. But for the life of him, he couldn't think of a single reason to push further. Without advancing to the next level, his health improvements would stall.

David discovered many keto-friendly snacks after the newness of keto-eating faded. He first swapped out his mid-morning pretzels for some cheese and meat. It wasn't long before he found keto-friendly bars to munch on. David also added back mixed nuts to the office under the disguise of "snacks for the client." He rationalized the snack by calling it his "handful of keto-healthy." These habits felt comfortable; and "I like the variety," he said to defend his keto snacks.

His weight loss had stalled after several weeks at ketoCONTINUUM #3. At one of the weekly keto-support groups, he heard others talking about giving up the snacks he enjoyed munching on throughout the day.

He recounted his carbs to find he had inched back up to 45 carbs per day. Most came from healthy, but sneaky, snacks. When David shared this setback with the support group, he truthfully shared, "I have to stop buying them." Indeed, this pattern of eating had stopped his metabolic health improvements. Observing others within the group encouraged him to move from ketoCONTINUUM #3 to #4.

Cutting down to two meals a day did not happen by accident. David made that choice — and followed through. Riding that initial wave of ketosis delivered a graceful transition. This next step, however, did not feel so lovely. David felt deprived the first few days he limited his meals to two. His heavily creamed coffee in the morning became a lifeline. He traded his usual cup for a bigger version. Despite this, he nursed his fatty-coffee throughout the morning with visions of salty nuts and fat-bomb-snacks. His mood grumbled midway through the morning, teasing him to give up. Removing snacks was definitely a challenge.

Setbacks of ketoCONTINUUM

Let's face some facts: Setbacks will occur on the ketoCONTINUUM. Everybody has them. Instead of focusing on your stumble, reflect on what happened. Critically analyze why the setback occurred, where it started, and how can you try again.

Flipping your metabolism from sugar-fueled to fat-fueled is easy … at first. It's the unseen potholes along the path that disrupt progress. After you've flipped from carbs to fat, the real struggle begins—foods from fat overflow with satiety and savory flavors.

However, when compared to carbs, the variety of flavors is boring. The abundant world of carbs tempted David every waking moment, even haunting him in his sleep. His brain remembered the comforts of his favorite carbs, and seduced him with not just images, but also by deluging his body with dopamine, yes, that "feel good" chemical. Every memorable carb linked to a feeling, sound, smell, and taste that added dopamine to his brain.

David succeeded because he didn't struggle alone. He unpacked his setback with others. With who? Anyone who would listen. David used his relationships from the group. He also shared Grandma Rose's story with hundreds of others.

I walked hand in hand with my mom as she crawled through a profound, dark chapter filled with cancer. The threat of death honed our focus. Do or die. No guarantees. We did not know if the change in her metabolism would do any good. Grandma Rose did great for the first six weeks, improving mental focus, and restoring much of her immune system. But over the next six months, despite feeling great, she, too, had her setbacks. It felt like driving into a ditch.

Ditch driving has some rules. The moment your car veers off the road determines how bad this trip through the ditch will be. It happens in seconds. The first tire hits the grassy shoulder, and then the entire car slants towards the bottom. This critical moment separates minor from major ditch driving. Factor in your speed, the shape of the ditch, and the mud's consistency to determine how deep into the ditch you'll find yourself. If you can steer along the bank of the ditch, many times, you can drive right out. No harm. No foul. The same calculations apply to staying consistently keto.

Speed: The speed at which you implement new behaviors predicts success. When behavioral changes take place at a snail's pace, the old, established patterns dominate before the new ones ever settle in. David made the opposite mistake. He changed nearly everything in one day. He reduced 250 carbs to less than 20 in an afternoon. By the grace of God, and plagued with many bumps in the road, he sustained that change. Often dramatic changes like his can't find the brakes when that front tire touches the grass. Just a single bite of their familiar carb-filled foods, floods their brain with the desire for more.

Steep Ditch: If carbs jump back up to 250 in one fell swoop, even a slow-moving car rolls side-over-side to the bottom of the ditch. Add alcohol to those carbs, and the image of driving off of a cliff fits best. In contrast, repeated handfuls of macadamia nuts fails in a different pattern. Too many keto-snacks sneak you into the bottom of the ditch. You can ride the shoulder with two tires in the grass and convince yourself you're safe. Bite by bite, inch by inch, the car slides down the ditch with cravings pulling you down.

Mud: If you drive into a spring South Dakota ditch, you will need a tractor to pull you out. The thick, sopping, sticky mud sucks you into the goo up to your hubcaps. If you are the only one you know doing keto, it's easy to get stuck—support matters.

STATEMENT: When in the keto ditch, be kind to yourself. Change is hard. Pressures around you to conform with the "normal" way of eating will pull you in like the mud in the ditch. Stuck. Again - support matters!

Take a deep breath. We have a plan after a setback.

If you've had a setback or stalled in your weight loss, follow these steps:

1. Read your WHY

The first part of this book instructed you to write down your WHY. Re-read that statement. We did that exercise for moments like these.

2. Call a Tow Truck

Support groups are tow trucks. They get people out of the ditch. There's no better time to start a support group than after a fall off the keto-wagon. Humility runs high and attracts the right kind of people. Find others trying to improve their health. Join forces. You're not the only one struggling. Look around. Waistlines everywhere have stretched to their limits.

Get out of your cubicles, homes, and comfort zones. Take some time away from social media or virtual meet-up-groups, and start a group that meets in-person ... where humans actually meet each other and interact. We are social creatures. It's in our DNA. I guarantee you that others in your community want to do this, too. So be brave. Announce what you are doing. Post the sign-up sheet in the workbook. Begin again.

Changing behavior is hard. Inspiration grows in support groups. Setback or stall — be brave enough to try again. Get into the habit of forgiving yourself. Give yourself the gentle grace you need.

Use this outline for a meeting:

Arrive a few minutes early. Set up the room to promote eye-contact between attendees by placing the chairs in a circle or around a table. Think of a specific check-in to share with the group. In the spirit of triggering mirror neurons, I offer my example for the first check-in. Following my case, I encourage those who have attended previous meetings to check-in next.

I don't allow food at our support group. I also remind attendees to stay focused on their own experiences and choices. Sharing struggles and successes with one another connects a group. Offering too much advice between attendees divides a group.

Examples of check-ins include the following:

• Share your KETO WHY

• Share your place on the ketoCONTINUUM.

• Set a goal for the upcoming week.

• Identify coping skills you are working on.

• Share a personal tactic on how to avoid carbs.

• "How do you say, NO?"

• HI/LO check-in.

HI: Share the best keto-success of your week.

LO: Share a keto disappointment from the week.

• Click Play Together

Go to YouTube. Find the Dr. Boz Channel. Focus on the playlist for beginners called <u>BEGINNERS: All</u>

<u>Things Keto</u>. This playlist in a mini-tutorial that takes you from the beginning of the keto process all the way through to adopting keto nutrition. Some of the videos last as little as four minutes. The videos are free, and they're there to help you. Don't carry this alone. Let experts help you with education.

Click play at the beginning of the meeting and watch it together if the video is short. Another approach is to assign the videos as the pre-group preparation. Watching the video before the group provides an excellent foundation for discussion.

If no one shows up, just push play. Know that the persistence of a meeting will attract people. Stay the course, don't give up.

3. Grab those urine ketone sticks.

Testing PeeTones sounds goofy. But it works, because it offers personal accountability. Use PeeTones as a plus or minus at this stage of the game. Did you produce ketones? Yes, or No? Keep those ketone strips in your pocket. Use them two or three times a day after a setback. Check! I can't over-emphasize this enough: ***Ketosis is not a diet; it's chemistry flowing through your veins.*** Prove to yourself that your chemistry is ketosis.

4. Listen to <u>ANYWAY YOU CAN</u>

If you've experienced personal setbacks, encountered stumbling blocks, and temptations during your keto journey, I urge you to listen to the audiobook, *Anyway You Can*. This is the first book I wrote. It is truly a gift from God. I shared a story about my mom and the lessons that I wrote down for her. Those lessons rescued her during this critical phase of her life. The story reminds the listener of how many ways ketones help and revivify an old chemistry set. The compassionate story helps you root for the underdog, Grandma Rose. You will finish the book inspired and willing to try again.

5. Return to Cronometer

Go back. Remember the app I asked you to download at the beginning. Find that. Start over. Take an honest count of your carbs again. Be real. Don't round down.

Instead of suddenly slamming your total carbs from over 200 to under 20, let's step down a bit slower. Cut your carbs by 'some.' Use your tracking tool to see if you kept the number steady for five straight, uninterrupted days. Then cut the number again.

Stay there for a week. This shift isn't as dramatic to your system. It allows time. Time to assess your relationship with different carbs. That sounds weird, "Relationship with food." During these steps, pay attention which foods trigger you the most. Which carbs do you "make room" for? What food seduces desires and stimulates your taste buds? Track to see if you stayed out of the ditch for an entire week with your newly reduced carbs. With this success, you can set another minor, yet, measurable goal and be proud of yourself. "A journey of a thousand miles begins with a single step." - Lao Tzu.

6. Biohack with BHB.

Biohack yourself. If you fell off the wagon and you dread the effort of transitioning again, HACK IT. This time, let me help you, chemically. Do the 14 Day BHB Challenge. For 14 days, sip on ketones-in-a-can. Let ketones percolate around your bloodstream for most of the waking hours in a day.

Carbohydrates won your first round. Temptation conquered your brain. This time around, we'll fight those carbohydrates with a little more chemistry and a slower transition. Work to reduce those carbs while drinking ketones.

When folks get stuck in a season of temptation, a bottle of ketones-in-a-can rescues them. When snacking derails the afternoon or evening, sip on BHB to suppress hunger and satisfy cravings. This delivers a safeguard and bridges through a struggle. Increase your circulating ketones and let chemistry lead the way. As ketones circulate in your veins, it gets easier each day—Supplement for 14 days. Use BHB to boost you out of the ditch.

Ketones also increase GABA, a 'feel-good' hormone inside our brain. Stay the course. Don't give up. The greatest struggle with a behavioral change starts with our mind. Keto chemistry reverses depression. Ketones lift your mood, settle anxiety, and slow down racing thoughts. Add ketones to your brain. Use BHB or MCT C8:C10 to boost you out of the ditch. Deliver the chemistry, and your mind will follow.

Chapter 18

CALORIES SCHMALORIES

O ver a decade ago, David joined his son's quest for weight loss. Both men shoveled their money into a program that idolized protein and packaged food. The program started out on the right path with two weeks of ketogenic chemistry. Sadly, they shifted lanes to calorie counting. The initial two weeks of ketosis unlocked fat cells with a drop of insulin and a shift in chemistry. Both men shed weight dramatically. The watershed of insulin, ketones, and inflammation lifted a cloud of fog from their sensorium. Had they stayed with keto-based weight loss, David and his son would have fully restored their metabolic health. Instead, this in-fashion, trendy program switched tactics by restricting calories using processed, packaged food. The program measured success through weekly weigh-ins, and dispensed the following week's worth of packaged food rations based on their results. The scale led the program. If no weight loss over the past week, no problem. The program simply packaged them less food. And if they lost weight, they kept the same calories of packaged-food as the previous week.

Fourteen days of keto-chemistry flushed out inflammation and reduced their insulin. Each day after that, their chemistry slid further away from ideal to lose weight. By the end of that year, David lost 50 pounds, most of which happened in the first few weeks. David and his son ended the year lighter, but they were grumpier, hungrier, and depressed. Their metabolisms had all but shut down.

The mistake this fad program made originated inside the mitochondria. The hormones that signaled their metabolism came from fat. Surging those hormones kept their mitochondria humming along with steady energy. If the program had reduced calories while protecting their metabolism, the company might still be thriving. Instead, they made zombies out of their paying customers. The program abandoned the science after the second week and measured success solely on weight loss. When their clients failed to lose weight, they reduced calories instead of surging their fatty metabolic hormones.

In the decade that followed, both men regained the weight. The saddest part happened to their brains and mitochondria. They shut down. WAY DOWN. As calories slid down, so did the gears of metabolism. Less energy led to fewer mitochondria, while the fat supply for neuroendocrine hormones all but stopped. These hormones faded as insulin circulated. This chemistry kept them overweight, depressed, and aging faster than the clock.

CALORIE BASED WEIGHT LOSS

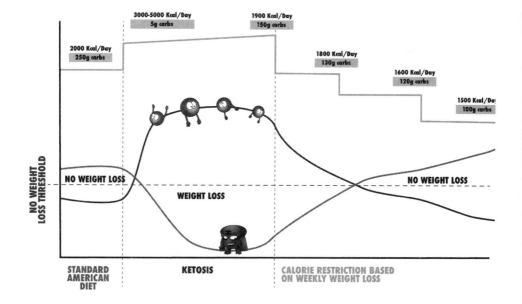

David and Joshua wanted to awaken their dreary, zombie metabolisms. Reigniting it required lots of fuel. Both bodies needed an infusion of energy. The measuring unit for the energy found in food is called a *kilocalorie*, commonly shortened to *calorie*. They needed to mine lots of calories without raising insulin. Their broken metabolic engines needed high energy-food. REALLY HIGH. Bite for bite, fat delivered the top performance. Due to their chronic inflammation, they needed to do this without raising their insulin. Eating high fat without carbs added fuel to their smoldering fire. One little spark would excite the explosion required for a comeback.

Nothing quiets a pessimist like success.

David and Kat followed instructions from ANYWAY YOU CAN, filling their cupboards with fatty-ketogenic foods, eating whenever they felt hungry, and adding salt to every bite. But Joshua watched with skepticism. At first, David and Kat shared their enthusiasm with him. Joshua, astounded by the concept of high fat and heavy salt, looked for the problems with this type of eating. He scolded his parents, even shamed them, for consuming so much fat and salt, and for thinking fat could do anything but shove them into their graves. Joshua had already witnessed his parents flirt with fad-dieting—only to give up weeks later. So

Joshua played along and prepared a few keto meals knowing the novelty would fade soon.

By the end of the second week, Kat had lost 10 pounds, and David was down nine. More importantly, they had energy. They danced circles around their son. No one spoke about it, yet the message rang clearly. Something healthy had taken over the ones eating fat.

Why count calories when your body doesn't?

I took a poll of over 50 middle and high school health teachers asking, "Does the body keep track of calories?" Forty-seven of the fifty teachers answered YES.

These teachers, influencers of young minds, taught their health students that our bodies have a sort of ticker tape located at the bottom of our esophagus that counts calories. That propagation didn't stop with the teachers. Nearly all of my patients failed this quiz too.

Let's set the record straight. There is no such ticker tape, no cell, hormone, or magical green troll measuring calories. Every time a morsel of nutrients slips into the stomach, no counter tallies up the calories.

TALLY TROLLS

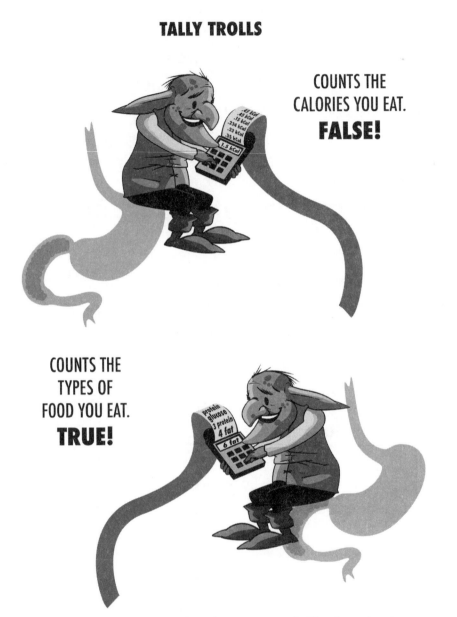

COUNTS THE
CALORIES YOU EAT.
FALSE!

COUNTS THE
TYPES OF
FOOD YOU EAT.
TRUE!

My entire medical career drilled calorie-counting into ideal weight loss advice. How is it that we've spent decades focused on the number of calories? We screwed this up - for generations. It's wrong. Calories do not top the list for losing weight. If you want to lose weight, think as your body does.

How does the body think?

Our body measures what we eat. It detects different types of food, <u>not</u> the quantity. Food drains out of the stomach and into the first part of the intestines — called the duodenum. As food parades by, millions of receptors await listening for specific contents. Different nutrients fit into matching receptors and spark action. Fatty foods trigger absorption while spiking their endocrine hormones to surge. Carb-based food, at the other end of the hierarchy of absorption, causes insulin to spike. Our ancestors survived through this critical distinction.

Evolutionarily, survival depended upon a person's ability to store and preserve carbs. Our gut used the receptors found in the duodenum to signal the storage of this quick energy source. Times of scarcity emptied the excess carbs, while seasons of harvest refilled it. Our ancestors consumed seasonal nature-made carbs. Fruit trees bore sweets a few weeks out of the year. Similarly, grains of wheat, corn, or rice provided a harvest-feast. Our ancestors celebrated eating those carbs with this refrain in mind: "Eat all you can before it spoils." Some seasonal items traveled with the tribes, but most were eaten.

Modern-day food distribution offers different problems. Foods once available for a few weeks now sit on shelves for years. But the millions of receptors in the first section of your gut did not change; they stayed the same. Carb consumption still triggers storage, while scarcity of food signals the body to empty stored energy.

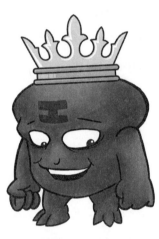

Top Weight Loss Secret: Do Not Store Food

Stop instructing your body to store fat. This is the obvious "secret!" to weight loss. The chemistry to make this happen oozes from your duodenal cells nestled in the first inches of your intestines. It's in the chemistry, folks! What did David eat? Well, millions of his receptors awaited the answer. When David tickled his receptors to life with carbs mixed with vitamins and minerals, his chemistry responded, snatching the precious commodities passing by, like iron and potassium. But the loudest signal from that bolus of food came from carbs triggering his insulin.

Carbs passed over David's receptors. The higher the carbs the higher his insulin rose telling his body to "STORE THE FOOD!" This caused David to gain weight. Though our current habits and attitudes about food consumption have changed, how the body responds to food has not. This weight gain is evolution's way of protecting the individual from the possible future nutrient scarcities.

This biological survival imperative is often abused by today's food consumers. David's gluttony of carbs led to increased blood sugars which led to a steady, unhealthy rise of his insulin, day and night, for years.

In order for David to turn off his spigot of insulin, the signal triggered by his duodenal receptors had to change. To stop that message, he needed to switch the instructions by switching his food to fat. David exchanged carbs for fat and flipped his chemistry from storing to emptying. He swallowed fat, and millions of receptors changed their tune.

The adage that says "You fight fire with fire," is misleading—you fight fire with water. But every fire-fighter knows there is truth in the statement. Regarding weight loss, replace the word "fire" with fat! "You fight fat with fat!"

Increase your Cholecystokinin

One of the receptors awaiting the arrival of ingested fat is linked to cholecystokinin. Cholecystokinin, like insulin, is a hormone that responds to food sliding past the receptors in the first inches of the intestines. It listens for fat and is built out of fat. When fat cuddled into David's duodenal receptors, cholecystokinin oozed out of those cells. The hormone, cholecystokinin, sent two powerful messages throughout his body:

1) Stop eating.

2) Add slimy bile to the fatty food in the gut.

1) Shut Down the Appetite

Particles of fat sent cholecystokinin slithering to David's brain with a single message, "Stop eating." Before switching to ketogenic eating, David made little to no cholecystokinin. His body rarely called for it to be made during his years of carb-feasting. The resources to construct cholecystokinin came from fat. David didn't have much of that available. Due to his high carb consumption, his fat was locked away imprisoned inside his cells.

David began to awaken and liberate those cells at the start of high-fat eating. The resources required to build cholecystokinin were now finally available. Over the first five weeks, his complex intestinal universe practiced sending that message from the cells listening for fat. Over the previous years, David's supply of fat-built hormones had fallen way below empty—that included cholecystokinin. However, the restored and liberated allocation of fat revived his ability to make hormones built from fat—like cholecystokinin as well as testosterone, cortisol, norepinephrine, and growth hormone. Hormone supplies throughout his body began filling their reserves.

David felt an abundance of cholecystokinin one night during his fifth week of keto. At a yearly board meeting, he entered the boardroom feeling famished. Hunger gnawed at him as he scanned the appetizers for fatty-food. The chef answered his prayers with bacon-wrapped cheese and deviled eggs. He ate four … of each. The main dish offered a choice of prime rib with a healthy rind of fat, or greasy pulled-pork with a sour-cream sauce. He ate both.

Somewhere after the prime rib was devoured, but before David finished the pulled pork, a wave of nausea stopped his fork on the way to his mouth. He felt sick. He just couldn't take another bite. Cholecystokinin created the sensation of nausea and fullness. Every cell capable of making cholecystokinin emptied their load into his endocrine system. That mountain of fat had just hit his listening cells, and they delivered.

When abundant cholecystokinin lay in waiting, fat triggered its delivery. The message from this fatty-hormone said, "Stop eating." And so, David stopped. The signal echoed so loudly throughout his body, he couldn't hear the speaker with the microphone. There David sat, in that room of board members, just listened to his hormones.

The discomforting fullness faded over the next half an hour, just in time for the sugar cookies being delivered to each table. Despite the recent repulsion of eating another bite, the cookies tempted David. Strange. How could he possibly think about eating after that?

Had David taken one bite of that sugar cookie, he wouldn't have added more cholecystokinin. He could have stuffed one half-dozen sugar-cookies down his gullet without a drop of that hormone. Why? Because that hormone was never linked to carbs. Only fat.

Fat triggered the message to the brain, "Shut off the eating." Carbs said, "Insulate."

2) Add Slimy Bile to Fatty Food

Fats require emulsion in bile for them to be engulfed by the digestive lining. Cholecystokinin told David's gallbladder and liver to produce bile, that oily, slimy substance.

David and Joshua entered their weight loss program wanting to lose excess fat. The first 2 weeks used ketosis to unlock their fat stores. Then their program cut the fat, squelching the production of fat-hormones. They were no longer fighting fat with fat. Their levels dwindled the longer they ate mostly carbs-filled menus.

To restore their weight-losing chemistry, David and Joshua needed to eat fat without carbs. To spark their metabolism and fat-based hormones, they needed to fill their bellies with fat.

David made several mistakes when he started the ketogenic diet, but he did one thing correctly: he ate abundant fat starting on day one. The most significant error in the first weeks of a ketogenic diet comes from eating too little fat. Those who make this mistake only add small amounts of fuel-energy to their wilted metabolism. They feel fatigued, tired, and crabby. David avoided this by weeks of eating high fat.

Mommies, don't let your babies grow up to be fat.

Moms, I give you permission to take back your role and establish the rules about snacking between meals. I grew up on a farm where no one snacked between meals. No after school snack. No mid-morning snack. No snack before bed. Kids ate three squares. Period. The adults on the farm ate twice a day. No one on the farm struggled with a weight problem ... until our family adopted the snack mentality that swept the country.

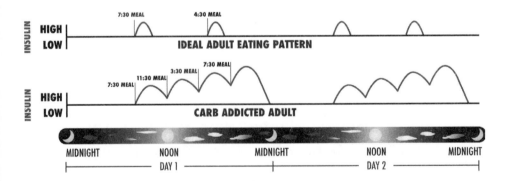

The chart shows the insulin response in adults who ate two meals per day versus those who snacked several times throughout the day. Each time food entered their system, insulin followed. The higher the carb count, the greater the amount of insulin. After their morning meal, insulin never returned to baseline again. Only after they slept for several hours did it slide back down to normal. Insulin resistance correlates to an insulin level that never returns to normal, even during their sleep. Their insulin spigot delivers so much insulin that it takes days of consuming salt and water - only - before it returns to baseline.

Look around a first-grade classroom today. Schools coordinate a mid-morning snack and a mid-afternoon snack. Guess the first thing parents offer their child after school? Yep, more food. That's five or six feedings a day. That makes sense for a baby. Not for a first-grader. Each time they eat, their listening receptors signal *'store food,' 'store food,' 'store food.'*

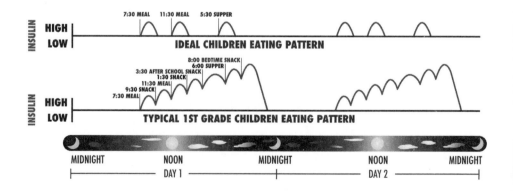

Notice in the image above what happens to insulin as children eat carb-laden foods five to six times per day. The time between carb-feedings doesn't allow for insulin to return to baseline. Only during their overnight hours of sleep does it sink to normal. Insulin levels in children soar at a record high level. This is not necessary. In fact, it damages their body, slows their brain development, and programs them to be overweight.

"But Doc, my kid is hungry every 2-3 hours."

Yes, they are. Your kid makes a wimpy amount of cholecystokinin, Peptide YY, and leptin. Like David, when kids lower their insulin, these appetite suppressing hormones rise. Reducing the number of feedings per day cuts down insulin significantly. Start there.

'No' is a complete sentence.

Eat only when hungry. When children want food outside of mealtime, use these two letters: N. O.

That's it. NO.

This clear message helps them understand, "No." Remove the processed-carb temptations from the cupboard, ...for you, for the kids, for the grandkids, and for the pets, too. NO!

Food pacifies the stress or boredom in children the same as adults. Carbs surge their dopamine to inundate their bodies. Adding that dopamine squirt of happiness creates an addiction to carbs. Before you know it, the whole bag of carbs tickles through their intestines. Recognize these habits. Remember the word, NO. Stop the carbs and fill their backpacks with pepperoni and cheese WITHOUT JUICE OR CRACKERS. NO CARBS.

High-fat food without carbs signals their hormones. Start signaling and watch what happens. Don't expect perfection on the first feeding. Hundreds of high-carb feedings allowed their cholecystokinin and Peptide YY to get lazy. The first time they skip the carbs and eat fat, only a trickle of these enzymes drip out. A few meals of practicing and their digestive enzymes will rally in response to fat.

It took David over a month to see his hormones successfully suppress his appetite. Kids course-correct much faster. Within two to three days, their hormones flood into circulation, and hunger disappears for hours.

Chapter 19

DAVID'S TRIBE

Joshua

Joshua, David's 30-year-old son, had seen his parents try every diet possible, from the All-Banana-diet, the Cabbage-Soup-diet, Eat-Right-for-your-Blood-Type-diet, all the way to the South Beach Diet. Each culinary adventure repeated the pattern where they ended back at their same old habits with very little to show. He'd joined his dad years ago in a quest to lose weight. Sixty pounds lost - only to have it all return and then some.

Joshua knew his dad had avoided the doctor for at least a dozen years. David's last cholesterol results from a health fair scared the daylights out of him. Joshua knew eating all that fat was dangerous. But somehow ... at the end of two months of keto, his parents looked fine. He noticed that they also had reservoirs of higher energy. Joshua had never witnessed this energy expression from his parents before. And every conversation with them was better than the last.

Even though Joshua held on to his skepticism about his parent's new way of eating, despite evidence to the contrary, he valued the return of his father's cheerful, upbeat spirit that had blessed their family for years. Everyone who'd missed it, definitely noticed its return.

John & Darlene

Joshua poked fun at his parents and their crazy fat-feasting-friends, John and Darlene. They were like second parents. John had as much problem with his weight as Joshua. They weren't father and son, but they carried the same shape. John dominated the room with his rotund 350 pounds. On more than one occasion, John's heart problems sent family rushing him to the hospital. It didn't take a medical doctor to see the troubles. If you sat next to John, you could hear the rattle in his breath. He sighed frequently, and when he drew in those deep breaths, the sound of gurgling water cracked the air. Everyone in earshot shifted their eyes when it happened. That sound surely meant danger.

John vetted a myriad of methods to shed the pounds — fad diets, exercise programs, and weight loss procedures had all been adequately vetted. The collective effort to help John always roped the rest of the gang into his plan. John's pattern of recruitment started with his wife, Darlene. She needed little assistance with her weight and joined her husband, "to help him." Next, John and Darlene would convince David and Kat to pledge loyalty to the latest attempt to lose weight. As soon as the parents acquiesced, John recruited the next generation to join him. Not this time. Joshua, had seen this scenario too many times. Everyone would swoop into the newest diet with obnoxious enthusiasm. Then fall off the rails.

No thanks. Joshua would wait. Watch. And cook.

Joshua gave credit to the fantastic tastes in this weight loss gimmick. As the guy in the kitchen, he loved the way fat delivered on flavor. Pride would keep him from admitting this to his parents, but these recipes made the cook look great.

Aunt Know-It-All

Each February, Dad's family celebrated Aunt Know-It-All's birthday. Like most family traditions, some parts attracted Joshua, and others repelled him.

Joshua entered the restaurant, and the reality of his genetics slapped him. Every single person in the room was fat. Like a sloth of bears, the family all looked the part. The least overweight people in the room were his parents, but they still layered the insulation into every part of their body. Joshua's reflection in the window told him he was not adopted. He definitely fit the mold.

Aunt Know-It-All announced her presence when she entered. She topped the family in her size and authority. The family designated her as their medical expert--more accurately, she designated herself. Her medical expertise came from being bossy. Her first-born female pedigree awarded her a master's degree in telling people what to do, especially if she was related to you. She had spent twenty years as a medical technician dispensing medications to patients. Her career gave her proximity to every doctor in town. Aunt Know-It-All had cultivated relationships with all of them, even having them on speed dial. If you asked Aunt Know-It-All a question, or challenged her advice, she readily took advantage of the latticework of doctors just a text away, who promptly answered her. You can poke fun at her medical expertise, but don't tell Aunt Know-It-All. She found it her personal mission to make sure that everyone in the family knew her advice and opinion on "all things" health. She maximized her social capital and used that knowledge to be the top

Mama Bear. Honestly, her education wasn't half bad. She repeated what the doctors told her and often knew the sources of the information. When she really wanted to flex her authority, she reminded you that she raised a child to become a doctor.

Joshua watched from across the room, as the family praised David for his recent weight loss. It took Aunt Know-It-All seconds to notice David's weight loss. Joshua prayed silently for his dad as Aunt Know-It-All moved in for her attack. He hoped his dad could find the words to outsmart her or stand his ground against her. This wouldn't be the first family event she'd used as an intervention. She was just so extra.

And there she went. The top blew, "HIGH FAT!! You're going to die. Keto is fad science." She squawked with condescension as only a big sister can. Every little brother in the room shrunk as she consumed all the energy with her supercilious scold.

David's sister towered over him by a solid seven inches. When you add the mass difference to the height, she had at least 100 pounds on him. Her berating, authoritative tone made everyone cringe and root for the underdog. Who cared that they were both over 60 years old, they'd regressed to teenagers battling over the keto diet.

Soon the whole family extended heartstrings to David in hopes of empowering him. They all felt Aunt Know-It-All's wrath. She destroyed her opponents. The world would stop turning if she was ever wrong. She continued to lambast until the last whisper of courage squelched out of her target. Most looked away, afraid to watch the final blow. But out of the ashes arose an articulate, strong, confident younger brother. Precise words pelted his sister onto her heels. No stuttering. His freedom from doubt grew along with his height. In less than 30 seconds, he conquered her with his argument about ketones and health. He spat words like mitochondria, autophagy, and ATP. The room witnessed David shed his 'exoskeleton' that had protected him against Sister Know-It-All. He won.

Could that be the diet?

As the evening closed, David shared a peace-offering to his sister. "Read this," he said as he handed her a copy of ANYWAY YOU CAN.

Aunt Know-It-All wrinkled her nose and tilted her head, looking down at the book. As if the information were contagious, she took it between her thumb and first finger, not allowing it to touch the rest of her.

Joshua couldn't stand to see his father flogged by this obese, obnoxious, arrogant woman. He didn't say a word, but at that moment, he proclaimed, "Yes" to keto. Joshua was in.

Sometimes spite motivated more than love.

Chapter 20

WEEK 6: DAVID'S TIPPING POINT

By week 6, David had a rhythm. His fat hormones had measured near zero at the start. But after weeks of feasting on fat, growth hormone, testosterone, cortisol, and other vital hormones slowly replenished. David lost weight - 20 pounds, and counting. The creative part of his brain returned. And it rose to the occasion to outsmart his older sister. He converted the skeptic hiding in his son, inspired his three pinochle players, and shared Grandma Rose's story with dozens of customers. David's work-performance hit record highs. But most importantly, he just felt wonderful deep inside. Within the folds of his brain, fewer drips of murky fluid submerged his glial cells. He was on ketoCONTINUUM #4, eating two meals a day without trouble.

David and his band of fat-feasting friends walked in step. His wife was down over a dozen pounds and also feeling great. His son proudly wore the badge of a keto convert and officially joined the tribe. The original four friends succeeded on many levels, weight loss, increased energy, lowered blood pressure.

David felt he could eat this way for the rest of his life. That's a win!

Aunt Know-It-All returned the book after a week with the spine barely cracked. But that didn't slow David's momentum. He couldn't stop talking about how amazing his 60-year-old body felt, which was way better than it did ten years prior. Like a walking advertisement, David reflected the energy he saw in Grandma Rose.

He attended the weekly keto-support group, even giving credit to his mirror neurons for spouting the information he acquired from attending previous meetings back at his sister. He witnessed other group members tackle the same bad habits he had. In addition to copying their behavior, he slowly appreciated how much stress and boredom influenced his desire to eat.

Week Six

In the sixth week, John and Darlene attended the group with him. He introduced them during his check-in and then reported no further weight loss the past two weeks. Twenty lost pounds in four weeks, but nothing since then. He enjoyed hours of productive time without the distraction of food. His tasks fit into the allotted time better each week. His brain performance improved. Steady. Enjoyable. No more carb-grazing. No Friday afternoon slump or naps with his head on the desk.

After several check-ins, I asked the group, "Who checks their blood sugar?" Some nodded. But David sat quietly, his eyes scanning the room, as if the question didn't pertain to him. David had never checked his glucose. I slid my chair closer to David, and said, "May I check your blood sugar?" David looked bewildered. His eyes honed in on the lancet in my hand. His pupils dilated, and cheeks flushed. "ME?"

The phobic fear of a needle stared back at me. David's apprehension riveted the room. I backed away from his anxiety by saying, "I will check mine first. Watch. It's okay."

"The word ketogenic does not refer to what you eat. It's a state of chemistry. You will know if you are keto by checking your chemistry." I said as I readied the kit and pricked my finger.

David could go hours without feeling hungry. His body had shifted from using glucose to using ketones without much notice. His mitochondria had improved and adapted to using ketones regularly. This improvement is called *keto-adaption.* Once keto-adapted, he needed to level up! He was ready to measure his chemistry and plot his progress.

David's instinct to flee from the meeting passed, and he offered his finger for a check of his sugar. He had drunk black coffee that morning because the heavy cream at home was empty. We pricked his finger at 8:30 A.M. His blood sugar came back at 115 mg/dL.

David looked at the meter, then back at me as if it was normal. His blank expression showed he had no reference range for blood glucose. I seized the teachable moment by asking him, "What do you think it should be?"

He looked at the monitor and said, "115?" The room chuckled.

"Nope. What time did you swallow your last bit of supper last night?"

He thought for a minute, "5:40 P.M."

"Any snacking after that?"

"Nope."

With fifteen hours since his last calorie, his blood sugar should have dropped well under 100.

Snacking in the evening used to be David's staple. A predictable pattern every night for years left him grazing throughout the close of the day. I cautiously double-checked, "Not a single bit of food since supper?"

"Not one bit. I followed the rules last night, Doc."

"Do you still check for PeeTones?"

"Not recently. I ran out of strips, and I can tell when I'm in ketosis. I can smell it on my breath," he replied.

David's blood sugar of 115 signaled danger. His elevated blood sugar foreshadowed the work that lay ahead. It also told me that David hovered on the edge of diabetes. I praised David for losing 20 pounds of fat off his body. Eating high fat improved his metabolism and health dramatically. However, David was diabetic before he lost those 20 pounds.

Diabetes is defined by the excess glucose circulating in his system, 12 hours after eating. David had clocked 15 hours since the last snitch of food, and he teetered on the threshold for the diagnosis. If we rewound time and peaked at his morning fasting glucose before the ketogenic diet, David would have been above 125 mg/dl of glucose. That's diabetes.

David didn't care for doctors. He navigated his healthcare without stepping foot into a doctor's office. Thoughts of a bossy older sister easily shape-shifted the doctor into Aunt Know-It-All. He did not want to change that part of his identity. I insisted David get a home glucose monitor, "David, you've graduated from PeeTone sticks." I asked him to spend a bit extra and purchase the meter that checks both ketones and glucose. A glucose-strip detects glucose in the drop of blood. Another strip slides into the same meter, but measures ketones in the blood.

David shared his most significant improvements in the last two months since going keto. He stated, "My brain. The cobwebs are gone. I can think. My focus and energy improved. I don't feel depressed." He paused for a moment, "And I don't have to go to the bathroom as often."

"David, lift your foot onto my lap. I want to look at your shin," I said. David pulled up one leg of his pants as I slid down the top part of his sock. I found his shinbone and pressed my thumb into the area right over the bone.

"Ow!" David remarked as I pushed firmly. I didn't lift my thumb for 30 seconds. When I released it, I left behind a crater.

Everyone watching drew their breath inward. Seeing the indentation sent a message to the room, "Something was wrong."

When teaching new doctors the art of examining the human body, we show them how to measure the extracellular fluid. Students learn quite a bit from an example like David. The shin bone offers one of the places in the human body that does not acquire fat. That bone should have a layer of fascia and skin over it —nothing else. If you press firmly on the shin bone for 30 seconds, nothing should happen.

David had struck out with all three 'P's.

A **P**lateaued weight, a **P**oke to the finger showing high glucose, and a thumb **P**rint on his shin. It's time to take action.

David's new assignment: Check morning fasting blood sugars for the next week. As soon as he awoke, I asked David to prick his finger and write down his morning fasting blood glucose. We were going to look inside David's liver. While David gathered his data, I asked him to get a screening of his coronary arteries called a **Coronary Artery Calcium Score**.

Chapter 21

DAVID & DR. STENT

The first week David checked his morning fasting sugars as instructed. He hoped to find all his sugars in order and chalk the experience up to mistaken identity, or a faulty meter. However, not one stinkin' blood sugar measured less than 100.

"Am I doing this right?" he asked his wife. She checked her sugar, 75.

David found the removal of his food in the evening the most challenging. Even though the best of intentions filled his thoughts, he oftentimes found his hand, filled with food, moving towards his mouth. The muscles in his arm had a memory of their own. They did things without asking his brain. Munching his way through the evening had been hardwired into him.

Those nuts were keto, and eating the whole bag wasn't his plan. Yet the bag lay empty the next morning. This nasty habit caused his morning fasting glucose to rise way past his target.

Over the next week, he managed to sneak ONE of his morning fasting blood sugar results under 100. Only after he skipped supper the previous night did that happen. Nearly 16 hours without food before he cleared the hurdle of a morning blood glucose under 100.

With this success on his mind, David called to schedule an appointment for the screening of his coronary arteries.

The scheduler on the phone said, "Along with that calcium screening, we check your cholesterol and a few blood tests. You can add an ultrasound of the arteries in your neck too. Would you like to be screened for a stroke?"

"How much more does that cost?" David asked with a thick tone of incredulity.

"An additional twenty-five dollars."

"Wow. That's pretty cheap. Ok, I'll do it."

David fasted for 18 hours in preparation for his heart screen. On the morning of the test, he entered a mobile van where they drew his blood. The nurse asked a few questions while checking his blood pressure: 128/76. He entered the CT scan and was finished with the test in a few minutes.

As he left the test, David sat on the bench, hunched over, tying his shoes. Nurse Fright rushed in, "David, ... you okay?"

"Oh, ya. I was just tying my..." he tried to answer.

"Please stay sitting," she blurted. "You need to see the cardiologist right away. Stay put while I call the doctor." She swung his feet up onto the bench and firmly guided his head down.

David asked the nurse, "Are my results back already?"

"Your coronary calcium tests won't be ready until later today," the nurse replied. "Your cholesterol tests are back and they are very concerning. You need to see the doctor immediately. How do you feel?"

"Well, now that you're rushing around acting like I might die, my heart seems to be pounding a bit," David said sarcastically.

"When is the last time you had your cholesterol checked?" she asked, looking over the top of her glasses.

"When I got life insurance. About ten years ago." David answered. "It was high then; but they insured me. And in case you missed the obvious, I'm still alive. This bench is stiff. Can I sit up?" David protested. This interaction with Nurse Fright was squelching his budding attraction to doctors.

She spoke into the phone pinched between her shoulder and ear, "His total cholesterol is over 400. He doesn't have a primary care doctor. He came in for a screening. No. No—he said no chest pain, but he reported palpitations recently. No, his scans aren't back yet. Okay, thanks for fitting him into your schedule, Doctor." She hung up the phone and spoke directly to David. "Dr. Stent has generously shuffled his schedule to see you immediately. Your appointment is in two hours." She turned on her heel and spoke over her shoulder, "I'll be right back."

	GOAL	Keto Month 3	Keto Month 15	Keto Month 25
Total Cholesterol	**<200**	440	293	336
LDL-C	**<130**	353	221	239
Triglycerides	**<150**	128	84	91
HDL	**>40**	61	55	79
Total Cholesterol /HDL	**<3.5**	7.2	5.3	4.3
hs-CRP	**<1.0**	2.0	1.5	0.5
HG A1C	**<4.6**	5.4	5.5	5.3

Twenty minutes later, Nurse Fright reviewed David's lab results with him. The nurse chirped, "The only nice thing I can say about your labs is that you're not dead ... yet. The amount of fat floating around your veins verges on an emergency. Are you sure you are not having any chest pain?"

David then said the most dangerous words, "Well, I have been on a ketogenic diet for a few months, and I feel great! I've lost 25 pounds and ..."

Nurse Fright morphed into David's older sister as she scolded, "That diet will kill you! Your labs prove it. Your total cholesterol should never be higher than 200. Yours is over 400. Your bad cholesterol is over 350. It needs to be less than 130!" The high-pitched chatter continued on, but David closed his eyes and mentally hit the mute button. He wished to be any-where else other than trapped in the mobile van with this nosey, overbearing nurse.

Three hours later, Dr. Stent covered the same topic pleading David to stop eating all that fat. In addi-tion to the labs, Dr. Stent shared David's coronary artery calcium score. "Well, thankfully it came back at ZERO. That's excellent news. This means we caught you in time. No calcium has hardened into your coro-nary arteries yet. It's a good thing you came in when you did."

David walked away from the mobile screening lab eight hours later with the prescription medication to lower his cholesterol: A statin.

What is CAC? A coronary artery calcium scan screens people who show no symptoms of heart dis-ease, but may be at risk for getting it. The test uses a small amount of radiation with computed tomography (CT) to check for calcium buildup in the coronary ar-teries. The coronary arteries wrap around the heart and supply it with blood and oxygen. The higher the coronary calcium score, the greater the amount of hardened plaque in the artery walls. And, the higher the score, the higher the risk of a heart attack. A zero calcium score all but guarantees protection from a heart attack for the next few years. A high calcium score sends a warning flare that your coronary arteries are up to no good.

Chapter 22

DAVID'S CHOLESTEROL

Keto diet and cholesterol. It's one of those topics that overwhelm the best of students ... and teachers alike. Before we begin, take a deep breath. Inhale - slowly. Exhale - even slower.

Now let's begin.

"Doctor, will my cholesterol rise when I'm on the ketogenic diet?"

Answer: Yes.

Don't panic. Keep reading. This chapter helps you get past the good, bad, and sticky realities of cholesterol. My first advice regarding the ketogenic diet and

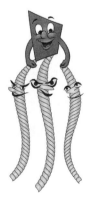

blood cholesterol is to NOT LOOK for six months. Yep. Temporarily IGNORE your cholesterol numbers. Prove to yourself that keto-chemistry coaxes your health in the right direction by confirming ketones in your urine or blood for six months. If you're worried about heart disease, or your longevity, ketogenic chemistry offers tremendous advantages. Go keto! But don't play around! To reap keto advantages, you must step into ketosis and stay there.

Inflammation is the cause of heart disease. Keto-chemistry is the opposite of inflammation. It will reverse the inflamed aspects of heart disease.

Start keto. Stay keto. And measure. MEASURE! To reap keto advantages, you must stay in ketosis. If you go keto and remove that inflammation, only to have it return because you failed to stay consistently keto, you aren't winning health awards. If you fall off the keto-wagon in those first months, push "reset." Use the strategies in Chapter 14 to do so. Get out of the ditch, and stay the course. Six consecutive months of keto protects your heart. It may take you a year to remain consistently keto for an uninterrupted six months straight. Measure it and time it. Track your progress. Measure. MEASURE! Then, and only then, after you've have produced ketones for six months would I approve measuring your cholesterol numbers. That means out of the 180 days, most days your PeeTone strips were pink.

For beginners on the keto diet, that first ketone marks a time of transition towards restored health—a chemistry clean-up within your heart and blood vessels accompanies those ketones. But the changes don't stop there. Emotional and spiritual changes happen, too. Beginners discover different ways to comfort themselves with and without food. Throughout this transition period, insulin falls the longer you stay in ketosis. The supply of fat rises to a dependable stream flowing into the fat supply-chain. This signals all hormones made from fat to rise. As stated before, these include: peptide YY, ghrelin, cholecystokinin, cortisol, vitamin D, testosterone, estradiol, aldosterone, progesterone, and (.... wait for it) cholesterol. They all transition. During this transition, it's best not to look.

Unfortunately, we oversimplified the education of cholesterol. We practically turned the word cholesterol into an unholy cuss word. In the first week of medical school, my eardrums were bombarded with the rhetoric demonizing cholesterol. The danger of cholesterol and the need to reduce it hijacked every teachable moment related to heart disease for the next decade of my education. Fortunately, I had exceptional tutelage from lipidologist Thomas Dayspring, M.D., early in my career. His mentorship partially corrected my fear of cholesterol.

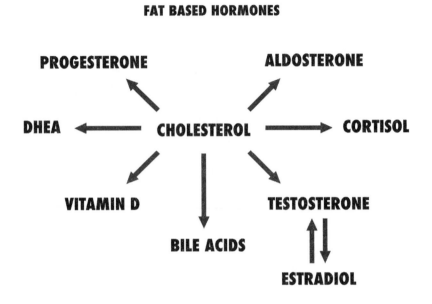

FAT BASED HORMONES

Cholesterol numbers have a logical progression of change, but not to the casual observer. You need the help of a nerd who loves to study fat. Lipidologists are just such people—specialized doctors who study cholesterol and fat-based hormones. Consider consulting an advanced lipidologist if you need to have a thorough examination earlier than a year into your transition.

Let me share what I told my dad when he asked me about cholesterol and keto. He didn't want to know the studies. He couldn't give a hoot about "good" versus "bad" cholesterol. He simply wanted a straightforward answer about his risk of croaking at a young age from a heart event while eating keto.

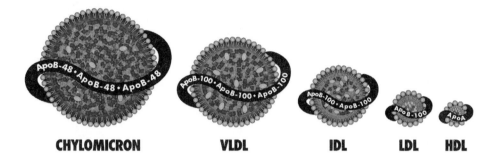

CHYLOMICRON **VLDL** **IDL** **LDL** **HDL**

Cholesterol is Needed for Life.
(... Without it - Life Ceases to Exist)

Cholesterol repairs our bodies and brains. It isn't the curse word associated with early, untimely funerals. This vital hormone mends our skin, chases away brain fog, and furnishes strings of carbons that turn into growth hormone, cortisol, testosterone, progesterone, and estrogen. Cholesterol renders our energy.

What your body already knows, and textbooks fail to acknowledge, is that your body has some rules governing and demanding that you to take advantage of this helpful substance. It isn't the bad guy. It is useful.

The relationship between cholesterol and insulin sets the stage for understanding. For starters, the re-pairing, strengthening, and enhancing part of choles-terol's job occurs only when insulin is not high. Elevat-ed insulin blocks the benefits of cholesterol. If your body overproduces insulin, your cholesterol converts circulating fat into rusty, powerful bullets that shoot you into an early grave. Cholesterol, in the absence of high insulin, is our friendly, fix-it-tool that repairs the human body.

Ketosis, or log-burning, requires delivery of fat to your furnaces. These furnaces, or mitochondria, are in-side your cells. Fat is carried to your cells on delivery vehicles called cholesterol. When I use the word cho-lesterol, think of a delivery truck transporting and of-fering fat to hungry cells. Cholesterol-trucks transport fat from the central fat-packaging plant, the liver, to the rest of the body. The insulin level zealously influ-ences whether or not the cell can receive that package of fat.

Your mitochondria require fuel. Without it, life ceases to exist. Cholesterol delivers fat-fuel for life. Cholesterol-vehicles haul globs of fat to vital parts of your body. The vehicles load up inside the liver and set out along their pre-genetically determined route. The vehicle overflows with fat-fuel as it departs from the liver. Each time the cholesterol-vehicle stops along the delivery route, it offers it's cargo (fat) to the cells. If glucose puffs through the fiery mitochondria in that cell, minimal fat leaves the delivery truck to enter the cell.

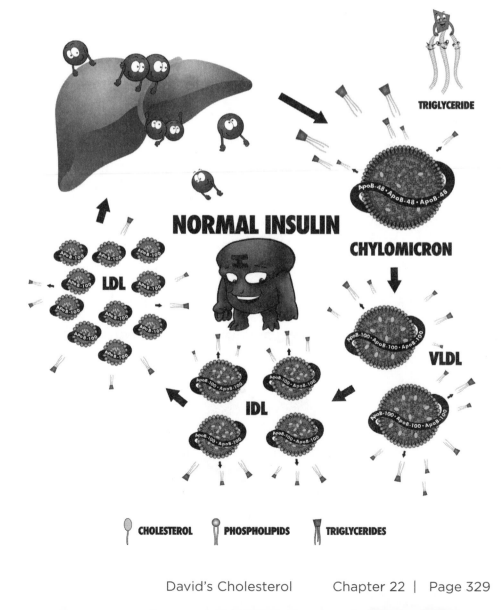

CHOLESTEROL CYCLING WITH NORMAL INSULIN

Liver is the 'Home' for Cholesterol

Intestinal enzymes ooze from the duodenal cells lining the first inches past your stomach to encircle the fat you've ingested. This bolus of goo and lipid get engulfed as it slides from your duodenum to the next section of the intestine, the jejunum. Those morsels of fat filter through the screening protocol of your security team. Once labeled as "safe," they then enter into circulation and head directly to the liver. The liver packages them into triglycerides. Scoops of triglycerides are then loaded into the central part of the cholesterol-vehicles. This triglyceride-loaded cholesterol is called a chylomicron. Chylomicrons are formed in the endoplasmic reticulum in the absorptive cells (enterocytes) of the small intestine. They overflow with the fat you swallowed and offer it fat cells, heart cells, and skeletal muscle tissue. When delivering fat-fuel to the body, triglycerides always win, as the most sought-after fat. They're the tastiest fat in the business.

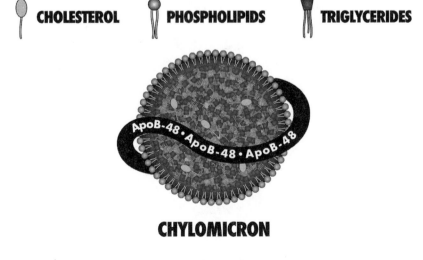

CHOLESTEROL　　**PHOSPHOLIPIDS**　　**TRIGLYCERIDES**

CHYLOMICRON

On the day David snapped Grandma Rose's photo, his triglycerides soared over 300 mg/dl. His blood gushed with these triplet strings of fat almost four times higher than they should be. It had been years since David's triglycerides boasted a healthy range near 60-80. His blood swarmed with these because of his gluttony for carbs and his continuously elevated insulin. Let me repeat so the point is cemented in: Strings of fat bobbed throughout his blood because he consumed too many carbohydrates. David used a magic trick to turn sugars into the body's most prized fat. What's the magical ingredient?

You guessed it: High insulin.

Excess carbs created havoc within David's body. For one he had insulin in excess. This blocked the healthy processes of delivering fat to cells. To compound matters, excess insulin also painted layers of inflammation inside his artery walls and stalled cholesterol-trucks from recycling back through the liver. David's cholesterol-trucks could not empty their prized commodity — triglycerides.

However, keto chemistry acted as the saving grace. For it lowered David's insulin just enough. Enough for what? Enough to allow the flow of fat into his cells. In this slightly improved setting of insulin, David's chylomicrons circulated along their distribution route. The trucks offered triglycerides to cells in dire need of fuel. After the prized commodity left the vehicle, the cholesterol-truck returned 'home' to the liver. The hitch on the outside of the truck changed from ApoB 48 to ApoB 100. Meanwhile, the cargo inside shuffled around and returned to the delivery route as a much smaller vehicle. This smaller cholesterol-truck was called a VLDL.

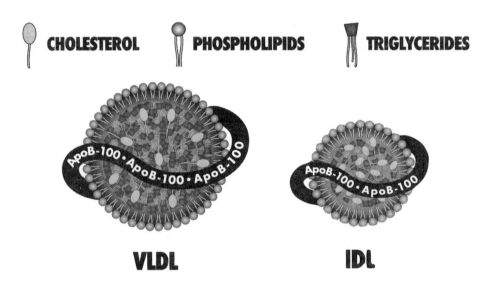

Cholesterol-VLDLs traveled a similar route as the chylomicron trucks. These smaller trucks delivered fuel to more remote destinations. Once again, each stop offered tasty triglycerides to the cells. More scoops of triglycerides were deposited into the hungry cells. The offloaded scoops of fat also shrunk the delivery truck's size even further while simultaneously, increasing the vehicle's density. Yes. It grew denser and smaller. Somewhere in their course of travel, the name of the truck changed from VLDL to IDL.

As the IDL-cholesterol trucks unloaded more triglycerides, they reduced even further — to its smallest and densest carriers. These nearly empty cholesterol-trucks were named Cholesterol-LDL or low-density-lipoprotein. Here enters the bad cholesterol. LDL-cholesterol, commonly called "bad" cholesterol, should head back "home" to the liver. The entrance back into the liver depended significantly on the amount of insulin inside the system.

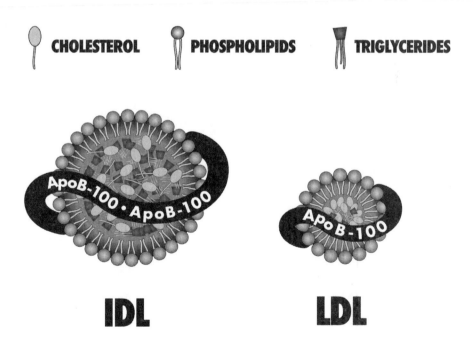

CLASS	DENSITY (g/mL)	DEAMETER (nm)	LIPOPROTEIN	CHOLESTEROL	PHOSPHOLIPIDS	TRIGLYCERIDES
CHYLOMICRON	<0.95	100-1000	ApoB48	8%	7%	84%
VLDL	0.95-1.006	30-80	ApoB100	22%	18%	50%
IDL	1.006-1.019	25-50	ApoB100	29%	22%	31%
LDL	1.019-1.063	18-28	ApoB100	50%	21%	8%
HDL	>1.063	5-15	ApoA	30%	29%	4%

David had lowered his insulin enough to deliver and distribute an enormous amount of fatty-cargo — delicious triglycerides — into his cells. His campfires now had stacks of logs sitting next to his mitochondria waiting to be burned. Unfortunately, in order to recycle his emptied cholesterol-trucks back through the liver he needed to further lower his insulin.

	GOAL	Keto Month 3	Keto Month 15	Keto Month 25
LDL-C	<130	353	221	239
Triglycerides	<150	128	84	91

At the time of his cholesterol blood test, David's bad or LDL cholesterol soared over 350 mg/dl. Many of his LDL cholesterol were waiting to re-enter his liver. Nurse Fright wanted it less than 130. His trucks had delivered all their cargo into the cells and needed to be restocked. The station for refilling his cholesterol trucks resided inside his liver. David's persistently elevated insulin prevented the re-entrance of LDL-cholesterol into his fat-processing plant. With the recycling process blocked, his liver needed more empty trucks to fill and used other means to solve the problem of too few trucks. How? By manufacturing more cholesterol trucks, scooping fluffy triglycerides into them, and sending them out onto the delivery course. This led to higher and higher LDL cholesterol.

If David fell off the keto-wagon, a surge of insulin would return. Years of carb addiction left ample room for his body to rise to the challenge of producing extra insulin. That binge of carbs would further stop the cholesterol trucks from recycling again. If a carb binge landed him at the bottom of a muddy ditch, insulin would dominate his chemistry again.

Chronic high insulin would magically turn those carbs into strings of fats again. These strings of fat would then spin into triglycerides. The abundance of triglycerides would inevitably tap out the storing capacity within David's liver. Without the recycled LDL-trucks returning to the manufacturing plant, the "bad" cholesterol would steadily rise.

In the cholesterol sequence, LDL-cholesterol is the first cholesterol to rise, simply because it was the last one in the sequence. VLDL and IDL-cholesterol follow in short order. The flow of fat would stop returning "home." The longer the bad cholesterol circulated in the presence of elevated insulin, the higher the danger. Too much time spent outside the liver would change the bad cholesterol into a deadly liability. The longer it circulated, the more his delivery trucks "rusted." This became known as the widow-maker. Rusted LDL. Rusted trucks.

RUST: Oxidized LDL Cholesterol

David's trucks rusted from the oxidation of his bad cholesterol, waiting to re-enter his liver. The longer the small, dense LDL cholesterol circulated, the rustier his trucks became.

The root word 'oxidate' sounds like oxygen. To the casual student, that might seem healthy, but don't be fooled. Oxidized LDL really means *unstable, harmful cholesterol.* This particle of cholesterol ought to be feared. Think of the oxidized LDL-cholesterol trucks as bullets.

The higher David's insulin rose, the deadlier his bullets became. The longer his insulin stayed high, the greater the number of bullets circulating in his blood. Adding high blood pressure to his rusted bullets was like sprinkling gunpowder onto them.

BOOM!

CHOLESTEROL CYCLING WITH HIGH INSULIN

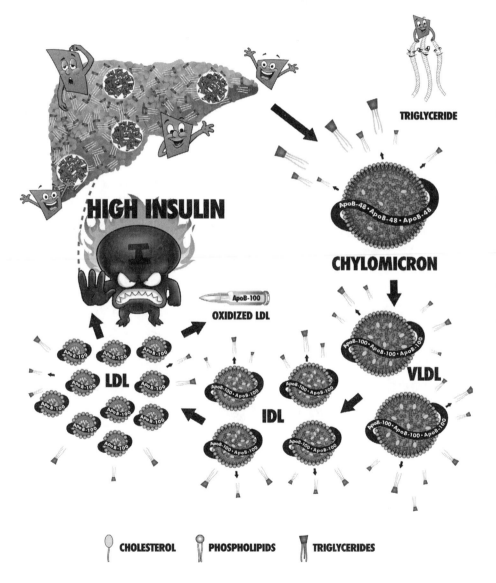

TRIGLYCERIDE

HIGH INSULIN

CHYLOMICRON

OXIDIZED LDL

LDL

VLDL

IDL

CHOLESTEROL   PHOSPHOLIPIDS   TRIGLYCERIDES

Lower the Insulin

David's high insulin starved his body of fat. With high insulin on patrol, resources of his stored fat stayed locked up. But David pushed against conventional wisdom and gobbled up fat which caused his insulin to fall. The flow of fat and the recycling of cholesterol-trucks resumed when keto chemistry swept through his body. His body and mind now had the raw materials to initiate healing, from the inside out. Before keto, his body could not access those strings of fat to help repair things like a torn muscle or a weakened swollen brain cell. Years of denied access left many cells flawed and damaged. Months into David's keto diet, his triglycerides measured 128. Had he looked at his level before starting keto, his triglycerides would have been twice that amount. With the recent weeks of slightly lowered insulin, his cell had processed some strings of fat into ketones and lowered his blood triglycerides under 150 — that's a win! Even though David's total blood cholesterol soared high enough to send Nurse Fright into a panic, it was his history of elevated insulin that should have scared her. Chronically elevated insulin kept his LDL cholesterol circulating in his blood and not recycling the trucks through his liver.

What are David's chances of a heart attack?

FIVE PREDICTORS OF HEART ATTACK

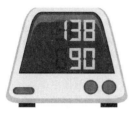

BLOOD PRESSURE
GREATER THAN 130/85

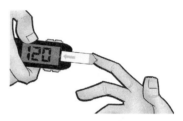

FASTING BLOOD SUGAR
GREATER THAN 100mg/dL
or 5.5/mmol/L

TRYGLYCERIDES
GREATER THAN 150 mg/dL

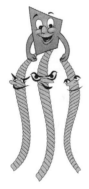

GOOD CHOLESTEROL - HDL
BELOW 40mg/dL FOR MEN
or BELOW 50mg/dL FOR WOMEN

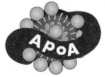

LARGE WAIST LINE
GREATER THAN 40 INCHES FOR MEN
OR GREATER THAN 35 INCHES FOR WOMEN

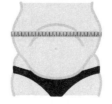

David's cholesterol levels rattled fear through Nurse Fright. A career of watching people like David suffer from heart disease primed her frantic response. Unfortunately, total cholesterol did a lousy job of predicting heart attacks.

Instead of total blood cholesterol, Nurse Fright _should_ have used these five factors to predict David's risk of a heart attack.

1. Blood Pressure
2. Morning Fasting Glucose
3. Triglycerides
4. Good Cholesterol (HDL)
5. Waist Measurement

#1: Blood Pressure > 130/85.

David's blood pressure used to be higher than 130/85. Weeks of ketogenic chemistry reduced his weight by 20 pounds. As the pounds dropped, so did his blood pressure. As a result, the force, or pressure, his heart needed to push blood through the hoses of his body fell into the 110-118s/60-70s. He had lowered his blood pressure in the first weeks of keto-nutrition.

#2: Morning Fasting Blood Sugar > 100 mg/dL

David's morning fasting blood sugar was greater than 100. It took nearly 20 hours without food for his glucose to sink below 100. Further evidence of his elevated blood sugars came through his glycated hemoglobin A1C (HgA1c) lab report. This test reflected David's average blood sugar of about 110 mg/dL. To measure his HgA1c we drew his blood and looked at his red blood cells. Specifically, we looked at the hemoglobin inside his red blood cells. When sugars circulating in his blood were in proximity to his hemoglobin, they spontaneously connected. Like two magnets, the hemoglobin sucked the glucose into it and they stuck together, instantly and permanently. Once the glucose landed on top of the hemoglobin, the glucose rendered that hemoglobin useless. For the rest of that red blood cell's lifetime, that sugar molecule remained stuck to the hemoglobin inside the red blood cell. Hemoglobin was supposed to be carrying oxygen around to the body—but not once glucose gummed it up. The more sugar inside David's blood, the fewer seats for oxygen and the *stickier* his hemoglobin became. HgA1c estimated the average number of blood sugars based on how many sugars were stuck to his hemoglobins. The higher the HgA1C, the higher the blood sugars had been in recent weeks. This higher number also left room for fewer oxygen molecules being carried to David's tissue. David's HgA1c measured 5.4 and correlated to an average blood sugar of 108. Any number with the average blood sugar north of 100 guaranteed a recent history of high insulin.

#3: Triglycerides: > 150.

David's triglycerides were 128 three months into the ketogenic transformation. Before keto, I would bet serious money they drifted north of 300. As his insulin worked back towards normal, his triglycerides would reduce too.

#4: Good Cholesterol HDL: Males < 40 & Females < 50

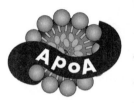

David's "good" cholesterol, also called HDL, depended upon recycling. Once again, insulin dictated how much this activity took place in David's body. Due to elevated insulin, much of David's good cholesterol was destroyed on a suicide mission. In an attempt to lower blood cholesterol while insulin imbibed his system, his kidneys flushed many of his HDL particles from circulation. That's right! In an attempt to get rid of blood cholesterol, his kidneys filtered good cholesterol into his urine. Surprisingly, his lab report came back okay at 60 mg/dl.

HbA1c TEST SCORE

HbA1c	mg/dL PRECEDING 3-MONTH AVERAGE BLOOD GLUCOSE	mmol/L PRECEDING 3-MONTH AVERAGE BLOOD GLUCOSE
4.0	68	3.8
4.5	82	4.5
5.0	97	5.4
5.5	111	6.1
6.0	126	7
6.5	140	7.8
7.0	154	8.6
7.5	169	9.4
8.0	183	10.1
8.5	197	10.9
9.0	212	11.8
9.5	226	12.5
10.0	240	13.3
10.5	255	14.1
11.0	269	14.9
11.5	283	15.7
12.0	298	16.5
12.5	312	18.1
13.0	326	14.5
13.5	340	18.9

REVERSING AGING | FASTER AGING | DANGER

#5: Waistline: Males > 40 in. & Females >35 in.

David's waistline stretched longer than forty inches *before* he lost the 20 pounds. Afterward, it measured 37 inches.

David's score looking for increased insulin =

#1. No #2. Yes #3. No #4. No #5. No

The higher the points on the heart-attack risk-factors list, the greater the possibility of a heart attack. This list better predicted a heart attack than his blood cholesterol numbers.

David scored one of five points on the heart-attack risk factors. This was after being on the ketogenic diet and shedding some of his excessive weight. His risk of a heart attack went up exponentially with each added point. Had he not adopted the ketogenic diet, his numbers certainly would have been four out of five.

#1. Yes #2. Yes #3. Yes #4. No #5. Yes

In three months, he went from a significant threat of heart disease to a mild chance. David had lowered his blood pressure, shrunk his waistline, and burned through a bunch of his triglycerides.

So which was it? Was he a high risk or a low risk for heart disease? Could he really have reversed his risk of heart disease that much in a few short months?

Adding another lab test would improve our understanding of his real risk: hs-CRP.

hs-CRP [Highly Sensitive C-Reactive Protein]

Highly sensitive C-reactive protein, shortened to hs-CRP, correlated to the amount of inflammation lining the inside walls of David's arteries. The hs-CRP indirectly measured how long David's insulin had been high.

Ideally, his hs-CRP should have been under 1.0 mg/L. David's was 2.0. Twice as high as desired. In the spectrum of hs-CRP, this wasn't awful. If his results had showed 10.0, I would have been confident that his heart risk was elevated. Using those five risk factors and adding the hs-CRP, we could see that David's risk for heart disease was elevated—but how much? His slightly elevated hs-CRP offered a hint to the problem, but not a confident answer. Factoring in David's slight inflammation to healthy arteries created a much different risk profile than adding inflammation to arteries calcified with age. If only we could peek inside his heart's arterial walls to see if he has calcified them.

That test exists. It's called Coronary Artery Calcium Score: CAC.

CAC Score

David held an ace in his pocket in this game of predicting heart disease. He had a perfect score on the best test that looked backward, as far as a decade, and computed how hardened his arteries were. If given one test to answer the question, *"Doc, how's my heart been for the last 10 years?"* I would definitely recommend a Coronary Artery Calcium (CAC) score.

Many cardiac tests improved our understanding of David's current heart-attack risk. Certain tests can predict his death by heart attack within the next few hours or days. The best physicians collectively use tests like CAC, hsCRP, triglycerides, and HDL along with measurements of waistlines, blood pressure, and diabetes to predict a patient's risk for heart disease. No single test predicts the future health of a patient. CAC delivers a report card of heart health over the past decade.

David's CAC score was ZERO. The pictures from his scan showed the arteries of his heart contained no calcium deposits. Zero! No hardening of the arteries. Again, Zero! That meant that very few oxidized LDL particles circulated in his blood. Very few bullets rusted inside his veins, waiting to explode. Further translation? David had minimal to no inflammation in his coronary arteries' walls over the past years. A CAC of zero almost guaranteed that a full-blown heart attack during next 10 years was unlikely. That's powerful. Don't get me wrong, David had troubles brewing, and if we didn't address the growing inflammation, it would have wreaked havoc. But sudden death from a heart attack or stroke remained unlikely.

Whatever was happening with his rising blood sugars and thickening inflammation, the damage had started recently and was minimal thus far. If high blood sugars continued to circulate within his body, torching his veins with the fire of insulin, then danger certainly lay ahead. The statin prescription from Dr. Stent wouldn't provide an ounce of protection in this specific case.

Translation: There was time to reverse David's impending health problems.

This equation to predict David's future health was messy and complex. How could I help David grasp the trajectory of his poor health before it was too late? Yet, not overwhelm him with too many numbers and unknown parts of the equation. Ten years ago, his life-

CALCIFYING YOUR ARTERIES

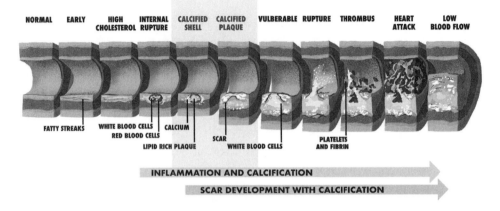

NORMAL EARLY HIGH CHOLESTEROL INTERNAL RUPTURE CALCIFIED SHELL CALCIFIED PLAQUE VULBERABLE RUPTURE THROMBUS HEART ATTACK LOW BLOOD FLOW

FATTY STREAKS WHITE BLOOD CELLS / RED BLOOD CELLS CALCIUM LIPID RICH PLAQUE SCAR WHITE BLOOD CELLS PLATELETS AND FIBRIN

INFLAMMATION AND CALCIFICATION

SCAR DEVELOPMENT WITH CALCIFICATION

TIME   5 YEARS   10 YEARS   15 YEARS   20 YEARS

insurance saw high cholesterol and insured him any-way. He felt fine for all those years. Continuous mea-surement of his insulin would have illuminated the problem for him; but there was no such thing. His blood sugars barely drifted outside the desired range, so he easily scoffed at the numbers as "close enough." His Coronary Artery Calcium score reassured him (and me) that he was safe so far; but how could we measure his risks - going forward?

Even though David's CAC score allowed us to look backward and compute how hardened his arteries were, it failed to predict his ongoing problems. His re-cent spike in inflammatory blood markers warned of the grime and inflammation lining his arteries. This was the real danger. There is another test that helps sort out his recent risks. The recent changes in David's cholesterol could be seen by looking at the skin of his red blood cells. How do you do that?

Answer: Omega 3 index

Omega 3-Index

The population of fats within your bone marrow comes from the foods you eat, your metabolism, your genetics, and a few lifestyle factors. Likewise, the composition of fats within the outer cell membrane of your red blood cells reflects the fats in your bone marrow.

Omega 3 index, a favorite test of mine, analyzes a single drop of your blood to show which fats populate your cells' lining. It peels back the hidden veil to reveal the current state of cholesterol health. Unlike CAC, the Omega 3 Index test focuses on the past 90 days by examining the "skin" or cell lining around each red blood cell. The outer membrane encircling each red blood cell, along with several other cell-types, comes from fat. These fats originate inside the bone marrow. Assembly of those cells begins in the tunnels of your bones. Once built, red blood cells live for approximately 100 days and offer an ideal lifespan to study cellular health relative to the fat resources available during that time. This cellular lifespan also allows us to explore the impact that an intervention, like ketosis, has on red blood cells over the past three months.

Why red blood cells? Their turnover time is ideal. It's long enough to measure a genuine impact made by the patient, yet, not so quick that a whimsical change in diet would change the results.

Each drop of blood contains some young cells just days old, while others dangle at the end of their natural life-cycle. When constructing a red blood cell, fats are selected from the bank of fatty resources within the bone marrow. The composition of fats within your red blood cells reflect the types of fats eaten over the past three months. One by one, fats arrange themselves in proper sequence to make the layer binding the cell together. Fats assemble and weave a blanket of fat proportionate to those housed in the marrow. Saturated fats, unsaturated fats, or trans-fats interlace to make the red blood cell's skin.

Studying red blood cells' fat composition reveals a three-month report card into the health of the fats, or cholesterol, within the body. Unlike CAC, Omega 3 Index measures *current* fat choices as opposed to the last half dozen years. Unlike total or LDL cholesterol, the Omega 3 Index predicts heart disease. Additionally, Omega 3 Index stands apart from many valuable tests as one that doesn't require a doctor's order to obtain it. You can do-it-yourself.

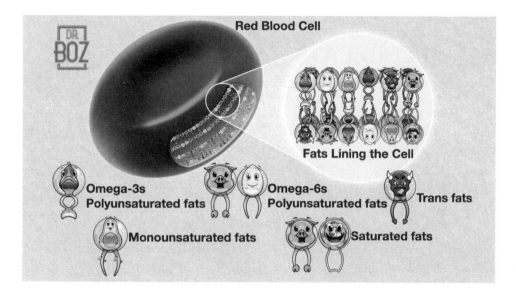

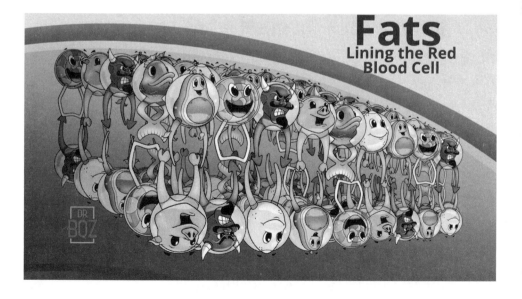

A Brief Lesson on Fat: The Good, Better, & Ugly

SATURATED FATS

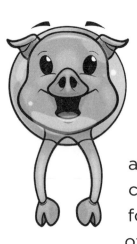

Saturated fats stand alone as the only natural fat that maintains its solid state at room temperature. The amount of heat needed to melt these fats into liquid towers over all others. This makes them desirable for cooking and storing without spoiling. Their chemical stability also wins praise when found inside our bodies. The properties of saturated fats are least likely to produce oxidative stress and form free radicals.

Saturated fats are made inside the liver of mammals. As mammals, our liver makes these fats. When we eat other animals, such as beef or pork, we also digest saturated fats. The strings of saturated fat within our bodies come from swallowing them or making them in our liver. Some of the saturated fats measured in our blood come from eating lots of pork belly, fatty brisket, and chicken wings. However, if you eat NO saturated fats, you still find them circulating in your blood, because the liver synthesizes strings of saturated fat from carbohydrates and protein.

Saturated fats have been demonized and blamed for causing heart disease. The resolution that saturated fats in ketogenic nourishment cause heart disease fills the minds of many health advisors. YES!, But, that's wrong. The focus on saturated fats ought not to be on where the fat originated; instead, the key to understanding their risk comes from what happens *after* saturated fat leaves the liver and bobs around in circulation. Case in point, when you eat that fat-filled steak, saturated fats flow *first* into the liver and then into trucks that circulate around the body. If those trucks swim in a bath of insulin, - plan for a shorter life.

The flames of insulin torch and block saturated fats from offering their resources to the body. Eat carbs, like this lollipop, and you will find saturated fat pumping around your body for an extended period of time — the chances of oxidizing the fat increases with circulation time. High insulin slows saturated fats from recycling through your liver. The longer saturated fats circulate in your blood, the more likely they are to transform into bullets. Once oxidized, these saturated fats stick together and clog the flow of blood. Keep your insulin low and allow bacon fat to convert into fat-based hormones, cholesterol, and ketones.

Only when you turn on the insulin will your saturated fats turn on you - they become the enemy when bathed in insulin. Eat less than 20 carbs per day while swallowing saturated fats, and they are the good guys.

UNSATURATED FATS: Mono (one) Or Poly (many) Unsaturated Fats.

Unsaturated fats fall into two categories: Monounsaturated or Polyunsaturated. Said another way, "monos" have **one** double bond between carbon atoms, "polys" have **many** double bonds. It's a chemistry thing.

Mono-Unsaturated Fatty Acids (MUFA):

MUFAs are frequently marketed as healthy plant-based fats from nuts and seeds. However, red meat, whole milk products, and high-fat fruits such as olives and avocados burst with MUFAs. Algal oil (92%), olive oil (75%), sunflower oil (70%) have hardy amounts of MUFA, but so does beef tallow (50%) and lard (40%.)

We do not require MUFA fats to survive. Like saturated fats, we will not die if we don't eat MUFAs. When we don't eat MUFAs, our liver assembles them out of other resources. However, research shows that consuming MUFAs like olives and avocados contribute to a decreased risk of breast cancer, heart disease, diabetes, brain-problems, and infections.

Today most MUFAs come from oils squeezed from seeds or beans. In my mind, this is where MUFAs lose their healthy image. Brilliant marketers improved the sound of seed oils by calling them *vegetable oils.* Consumers have been duped; How? These oils <u>don't</u> come from vegetables. They come from a highly processed chemistry sequence *that grows inflammation.* If you have bottles of sunflower, canola, or peanut oils in your cupboard, use them to lubricate equipment around the house. *Don't swallow them.* They are hazardous to your health.

Eat non-seed oil MUFAs if you have access to them, but don't fret if they're in short supply in your life.

Poly-Unsaturated Fatty Acids (PUFA):

PUFAs <u>cannot</u> be made by the body. We must eat these fats, *or we die*. The body uses PUFAs to make regulatory hormones.

Omega 3 PUFA:

Every cell in the human body uses Omega 3 PUFAs to keep inflammatory signals doing their job. Each cell depends on Omega 3 PUFAs to both trigger the proteins of inflammation, yet not let them surge out of control. The three primary dietary omega-3 polyunsaturated fatty acids are EPA (eicosapentaenoic acid), DHA (docosahexaenoic acid), and ALA (alpha-linolenic acid). Both EPA and DHA are commonly found in seafood and fish, while ALA is most abundant in high-fat plant foods like flax and chia seeds. Find Omega 3 PUFAs in cold-water fatty fish like mackerel, salmon, cod liver, herring, sardines, and anchovies. The closer you get to the algae on the fish food-chain, the higher the EPA and DHA concentration. These fats best protect against chronic disease. The more of these fats you eat, the more we find blanketing the linings of cells. Higher percentages of these these aforementioned fats in cells' linings, links to longevity and lower heart disease. These fats hold the title of the Omega 3 Index because of their vital link to improved health. They are the BEST fatty acids in the body.

Omega 6 PUFA

Every cell in the human body uses Omega 6 PUFAs to strengthen and activate the immune system. Without Omega 6 PUFAs, we can't fight infection, stimulate autophagy, or repair damaged cells. Examples of Omega 6 PUFAs include animal fats, egg yolks, dairy fats, and seed fats. As with MUFAs, I exclude seed oils from the list of recommended fats in this category. Unlike MUFAs, you can't skip this section of fats altogether without consequences. Omega 6 PUFAs are required for life. Keto menus deliver Omega 6 through lard, tallow, suet, and organ meat.

Most people eating keto nutrition are exposed to lots of Omega 6 PUFAs—usually 20 times as many Omega 6 fats as Omega 3. Both Omega 6 and Omega 3 fats reduce inflammation as long as they aren't coated with insulin. Eating large quantities of Omega 6 fats keeps cells flexible and pliable. Adding more Omega 3 PUFAs further protects the cells from damage and inflammation.

Both Omega 6 and 3 PUFAs are required for life. These fats hold the silver and gold for cholesterol ratings, as long as you don't get them from seed oils. They both rank at the top of the quality scale for healthy cholesterol: Omega 3 wins the gold. Omega 6 holds the silver.

TRANS FATS

If Omega 3 and Omega 6 PUFAs represent the angels of fats, the trans-fats are the devil. These fats rarely occur in nature, and are the cause of horrific problems when laced into the blanket of fats lining a cell. Trans-fats have been concocted by sci-entists via hydrogenated oils. Reigning marketplace leaders drove chemists to invent a synthetic fat with a desirable melting point and an extended shelf-life. Case in point: margarine and Crisco. Our body cannot make these fats; there-fore the amount of trans-fats measured in the lining of the red blood cells directly correlates to how many trans fats were eaten over the past three months. Once the cell lining has been assembled using these fats, the lipids stay there for the lifetime of the cell. Cakes, cookies, pies, and pastries were responsible for the highest amount of trans-fats, followed by yeast-breads, french fries, and tortilla chips. Eat foods with these fats today and find the exact lipids stuck in the lining of your red blood cells 90 days from now.

Trans-fats promote inflammation. High counts of trans-fats predict heart disease, memory problems, inadequate immune systems, and diabetes. The higher these fats, the older your body acts. Trans-fats are stiff and sticky—literally; they fail to flex and bend with the other fats and don't play well with other fats in the tapestry of cell membranes. This rigidity causes damage to other fats within its vicinity and injures the cell in general.

Healthy red blood cells can bend and morph to squeeze through tiny blood vessels without getting stuck to anything else nearby. Not so with red blood cells made with trans-fats. They are highly adhesive. Consequently, their inflexibility adds to their sticky nature, especially when two trans-fats find each other. "So what?" you might ask. But when just a few trans-fats glue to one another, a blocked artery occurs. The more of these devils that line your red blood cells, the closer you teeter on the precipice of a heart attack.

Don't get lost in the globs of fat information. Instead, stay concentrated on reducing your insulin, avoiding seed oils, and choosing foods with PUFA's, - not trans-fats.

You can't manage what you don't measure. Instead of measuring total cholesterol or even "bad" LDL cholesterol, measure these risk factors. Here are the survival metrics:

1. Blood Pressure

2. Morning Fasting Glucose

3. Triglycerides

4. Good Cholesterol (HDL)

5. Waist Measurement

6. hs-CRP

7. Omega 3 Index (Desirable = NO trans fats, and high omega 3s.)

David's LDL reading of 239 and total cholesterol over 300 alarmed Nurse Fright. Her panic came from forty years of medical doctrine that said, *"Elevated LDL cholesterol predicts a heart attack."* That is simply not true. David's heart health strengthened by managing the seven factors listed above. Two years of ketogenic nutrition had shifted the fats circulating in his blood. Before keto, he could not recycle his cholesterol through his liver, because high insulin blocked the re-entrance of cholesterol into his liver. That same high insulin fueled his inflammation. Two years of keto-chemistry:

Lowered his blood pressure under 120/80,

Reduced his fasting glucose under 90,

Dropped his triglycerides under 100,

Shrunk his waistline smaller than 30 inches , and

Lowered hs-CRP under 1.0. mg/dL

Optimizing these risk factors corrected twenty years of brewing heart disease. [See the workbook for parameters of these markers and other recommended blood tests.]

By the grace of God, Grandma Rose's story connected with David and sparked a change. His health was literally at a crisis point, one path diverging onto the highway of danger, the other onto the highway of opportunity. Based on his labs and risks, if he chose the path of abundant insulin, a life filled with aging problems surely awaited him. However, if he chose the path that overflowed with ketones, a life of significantly improved health welcomed him.

The advanced medical testing procedures I've mentioned were just tools that helped me to predict the future of David's health. No single testing method exists that offers the "perfect" health forecast to estimate David's risk of a heart attack. Acquiring and worsening more risk factors can destroy his future—those risk factors matter. By using the collection of tests, and carefully assessing David's current choices, opportunities for a healthier life exists. This future health forecast was messy and required an intimate understanding of David. But that's medicine — messy.

USEFUL TOOLS

Calculator for Omega 3 and Omega 6 contents of food: http://www.fattyacidshub.com/tools-for-fatty-acids/omega-3-omega-6-ratio-calculator/

OMEGAQUANT Order your home kit to test your Omega 3, Omega 6, and TransFats: http://bit.ly/2v2rA9p or https://omegaquant.com/omega-3-index-complete/ref/45/

Chapter 23

KETOCONTINUUM #5 16:8

Heavy cream, warm black coffee, laced with a tinge of salt, filled David with happiness each morning. He looked forward to his coffee with child-like anticipation each morning. His cup of black energy satisfied David, keeping him full all morning. He felt no hunger pangs rumbling throughout his stomach to distract him from his task at hand until early afternoon. When hunger struck, he ate his meal of cheese, meat sticks, a boiled egg, and some roasted nuts. That menu satisfied and energized him until supper—his largest meal of the day.

David's morning fasting sugars predicted poor health. His other risks had slid out of the danger zone. His HgA1c of 5.4% predicted his blood sugar between

93-123 mg/dl, with an average of 108. At first, he denied this reality. Two weeks of pricking his finger each morning educated as well as frustrated him. Diabetes? Not him. Much like blood pressure, he never considered it. This shift in identity swirled in his mind. The awareness of this hidden problem strengthened his motivation. He did not want the diabetes label.

On week three of testing, David ran out of blood strips. A week went by before replacement strips arrived. He noticed temptations creeping into his thoughts as his food choices relaxed. Not checking opened the space to deny that a problem existed. Without testing, his accountability faded, and temptations grew. Strangely, when the meter reported his elevated blood sugar, he felt like the entire world knew.

Optimum health by the end of the year was his goal. But eight months remained until New Year's Day. Could David do this? Could he do all that's required?

Look carefully at this chart. The section along the left separates metabolic skills into beginners, baseline, and stress.

- Beginner's Metabolism: Continuums #1 - #4
- Baseline Metabolism: Continuums #5 - #8
- Metabolic Stress: Continuums #9 - #12

ketoCONTINUUM	
BEGINNER	1. I EAT EVERY 2-4 HOURS
	2. LESS THAN 20 TOTAL CARBS. I EAT EVERY 6-8 HOURS.
	3. I "ACCIDENTALLY" MISSED A MEAL. [KETO-ADAPTED]
	4. EAT 2 MEALS PER DAY.
BASELINE METABOLISM	5. 16:8
	6. ADVANCED 16:8
	7. 23:1 OMAD: ALL IN 1 HOUR.
	8. ADVANCED 23:1/OMAD
STRESSING METABOLISM	9. 36 HOUR FAST
	10. 36 HOUR FAST WITHOUT CELEBRATION MEAL
	11. 48 HOUR FAST
	12. 72 Hour Fast

Steps 1 - 4 = Shift Chemistry

David, along with a majority of beginners, shifted from no ketones to making ketones with ease. Keto-chemistry did the work. David only focused on cutting his total carbs to twenty. He reaped and enjoyed the benefits as his chemistry carried him through keto-CONTINUUMs #1, #2, and #3.

ketoCONTINUUM #1 started when 100% of David's mitochondria fueled from carbs. Pine-needles stoked his fires as he ate every 2-4 hours. Insulin and glucose circulated in high-supply.

ketoCONTINUUM #2 shifted his chemistry. He dropped carbs nearly to zero, and his body intuitively did its thing. As long as he swallowed fat in the absence of carbs, by the end of week one most of his mitochondria burned logs.

Years of squirting too much insulin had affected David's cellular health. The extra insulin led to inflammation, which allowed electrons to leave their circle of energy. Rogue electrons zig-zagged through his cellular atmosphere damaging any tissue in their path. Flawed cells grew in number. Those defected cells lacked enough fat for the repairs needed throughout his body. Instead, these cells divided and copied their flaws.

Errors lived on through generations of cells. The formula for David to fix those flaws required high-fat, low-inflammation, and time.

Comparing his brain from before keto, he shared, "I didn't think I was depressed until I look back at how grey the world was. The sunlight, the colors, the joy had all faded. Ketones added light back into my world."

Logs crackled in more furnaces throughout his body as days turned to weeks. He missed the news-flash when his cells began dumping fat into the supply chain to repair broken parts. He drifted through a surge in growth hormone and a rise in testosterone. Instead of cloning his flawed cells, caused by years of elevated insulin, his ketones offered an advantage: Replicate pristine, healthier cells. All of these transformations took place, in addition to the ancillary benefit of losing weight. David was unaware that he "accidentally" missed a meal. How could this have occurred? His newfound fat-based chemistry not only raised his energy, deepened his sleep, and delivered substantial mental clarity, it also suppressed his hunger. The significance of these changes taking place meant David was now entering into the next keto stage—ketoCONTINUUM #3.

David shared his success of keto-adaption at the weekly support group. Without missing a beat, he looked towards the next step of ketoCONTINUUM #4: Choosing to eat only twice daily. This routine seemed almost natural to him.

With only the rare exception, David found this pattern of eating natural and satisfying. No hunger and rarely a craving, he stayed at ketoCONTINUUM #4 for several weeks. But after David stabilized at two meals a day, he stalled. Almost two months into keto and his scale hovered at the 20-pound loss. No more. No less. Had he not discovered his elevated blood sugars, he might never have advanced to the next ketoCONTIN-UUM.

ketoCONTINUUM

BASELINE METABOLISM	
	5. 16:8
	6. ADVANCED 16:8
	7. 23:1 OMAD: ALL IN 1 HOUR.
	8. ADVANCED 23:1/OMAD

WHY ketoCONTINUUM #5 - #8?

Baseline Metabolisms Reverse Chronic Disease

Metabolism translates from its Greek and Latin origin where it means "to change" or "transform." Units of fat, carbs, and proteins transform into energy for cells to function. Think of metabolism as microscopic exercise for the cell. A further distinction needs to be added. Metabolic health measures the strength of cells and how well they perform their genetically assigned tasks. It measures how: Brain cells think, immune cells defend, heart cells squeeze, and kidney cells clean. Now here's where we get to the crux of the matter.

Baseline metabolism refers to metabolisms that occur on regular days. David often wondered how some people possessed perennial energy throughout the day while others couldn't make it until noon. His mentor came to mind. Did his mentor take a magical supplement, or spike his coffee with triple the caffeine? Little did David know that the credit for boundless energy, robust immune systems, and steady concentration arose from baseline metabolisms. People blessed with healthy, long lives limited their carbs and the hours they consumed food. They limited what they ate, when they ate, and how they ate. What: Rarely did they eat pastries or cake. When: Most consumption happened during daylight hours. How: They chewed their food instead of slurping their food through a straw.

Baseline Metabolisms delivered the secret to superior health: Ketones. Their mitochondria burned without extra grime and consistently used ketones to sweep away inflammation.

David's cells performed much better since he began keto. His "keto-victory" for improved health rang true as he lived life at ketoCONTINUUM #4. But for complete restitution of his health, David needed to "go the distance" and advance further along the ketoCONTINUUM.

Insulin-Resistant to Keto-Adapted

When David's cells operated at peak levels gracefully using ketones, we called them keto-adapted. His unhealthy cells were insulin resistant. Each cell's improvement slid along a continuum from insulin-resistant to keto-adapted. David's initial weight loss coincided with drastic improvement in his insulin resistance. The decreased insulin unlocked the gates to many of his fat cells. This shift in chemistry melted away a layer of his stored fat-energy. Also, this robust chemistry repelled some of the grime of his chronic inflammation.

At ketoCONTINUUM #4, David's metabolic needs settled into the pattern of two meals per day. The chemistry associated with this continuum shifted before then leveling off. The gradient from insulin-resistant cells to keto-adapted ones gradually reduced week by week. Unlike the initial drop, this time, the reduced insulin unlocked only a few fat cells. His weight loss stalled accordingly. David needed to strengthen his metabolism for the next crop of insulin-resistant cells to surrender. They would only open if he slid further along the continuum. How could David pressure those cells to open? By advancing to the next level of ketoCONTINUUM #5, and beyond.

David's cellular exercise plan was outlined in the Baseline Metabolisms ketoCONTINUUM #5-#8.

#5. 16:8 - Eat ALL food, snacks, and supplements in an 8-hour window. No eating, snacking, or chewing for 16 hours. Gum-chewers beware.

#6. Advanced 16:8 - Clean up your morning drink. Remove all calories and sweeteners. Morning drink = no fat, no MCT, no butter, no sweeteners, no calories. 16 hours = salt, water, black coffee, or tea.

#7. 23:1 OMAD - One Meal A Day. ALL calories & sweeteners in one hour. 23 hours = Only salt, water, tea, or black coffee.

#8. Advanced 23:1/OMAD - Move your eating-hour within 11 hours following sunrise to match your circadian rhythm.

ketoCONTINUUM #5 - #8 outlined the general exercise options for David's mitochondria. All four of these metabolisms drew fuel from fat. The longer David spent in one of the baseline ketoCONTINUUMs, the stronger his metabolism grew.

ketoCONTINUUMs #5 - #8 linked to longevity and restored health by pushing rogue electrons back into their proper places. Fixing life at the electron-level took time. Unlike his tornado of a start, David took it slow. Attendance to the weekly support group gave David living testimonial examples of steady progression through their baseline metabolism, versus those who sped through. For some of the successful role models, it took a couple of years to move through the baseline metabolisms. Others reached their healthy biomarkers without advancing all the way to ketoCONTINUUM #8.

The time needed to progress from one ketoCONTINUUM to the next depended upon David's past and present. The past referred to the length of time he'd spent with elevated insulin. According to his hs-CRP (highly-sensitive C Reactive Protein), his average blood sugars, and his Coronary Artery Calcium score,

David was early in his progression. The present referred to David's skills. How successful could David be at saying no? What other coping skills were essential to stay consistently keto? He needed better skills for addressing temptations. His skills required for quality sleep needed tweaking. He needed to learn how to monitor his new behavior and extend himself grace when it didn't go as planned.

Advancing to the next ketoCONTINUUM without mastery of the skill eventually caught up to folks in the fast lane. These desperate students frequently measured their success through the scale. This did not attract David. Instead, he wanted the optimum health seen in the veterans of the group. They had what Grandma Rose had. His mirror neurons watched different examples in the group. Slow and steady won the race. David practiced the skills until he mastered them at each step along the ketoCONTINUUM.

	ketoCONTINUUM	WHO DOES THE WORK?	TEST	GUIDELINES	NEXT STEP
BASELINE METABOLISM	#5. 16:8	YOU - DISCIPLINE NEEDED.	URINE STRIPS	Eat ALL food, snacks, and supplements in an 8-hour window. No eating, snacking, or chewing for 16 hours.	That means no gum during fasting hours. Suck on salt if you need a substitute. Keep your coffee filled with fat.

CHOOSE ketoCONTINUUM #5

The two-meals-a-day plateau wouldn't reverse David's progress nor minimize all he had accomplished. But for continued improvements in his metabolism, David needed to make a choice: progress with ketoCONTINUUM #5 or stall at two meals per day. Unlike the previous ketoCONTINUUM levels, #1-#3, the next phases wouldn't just happen by accident. The wave of keto-chemistry had carried him as far as it could. ketoCONTINUUMs #5 through #8 demanded more than just casual attention to the process. These levels required a conscious choice in order to move forward. Will and intent, mind and body had to move synchronously. Discipline was mandatory, along with time, education, and self-reflection.

ketoCONTINUUM #5, called 16:8, spent sixteen hours of the day without food, snacks, or supplements. Said another way, David ceased all chewing for 16 hours. Eight consecutive hours marked the time he chewed, swallowed, or supplemented his nutrients. The thought of sixteen hours without a crumb rippled anxiety through him. His self-talk chattered, "This isn't me. I can't do it. There's no way." David saw several others in the support group fast for 2-3 days. His mirror neurons must have hijacked part of his choice because he meant to tell the group that he couldn't do it. But his mouth betrayed his thoughts. "I can do this. If you can say no for three days, I can say no for 16 hours. I can do this," he blurted. With the encouragement of his keto support group, David entered ketoCONTINUUM #5.

ketoCONTINUUM #5: 16:8

Eat ALL food, snacks, and supplements in an eight-hour window. No eating, snacking, or chewing for 16 hours.

Use the chart in the workbook to keep track. Track the time you chew or swallow your first morsel of food each day. Set a timer for eight hours. When the timer rings... zip your lips! Gum chewers, this includes gum. Your habit of deferring food by chewing gum needs to be addressed. Use the eight hours each day to chew gum. Then STOP.

ketoCONTINUUM #5 sounds easy. Be prepared to battle old snacking habits, drinking calories, or socializing with food.

I highly recommend a support system from this point forward.

Chapter 24

DR. BOZ RATIO

MEASURE YOUR INSULIN

Two methods of measuring ketones exist: Via urine or via blood. Both paths are backed by science. However the distinction resides in precision. Yes, precision.

Measuring ketones via the urine is quick and inexpensive and reflects the extra ketones that overflowed into the urine. Measuring ketones via blood gives you an accurate, mathematical, real-time report of what's literally taking place inside your body. Measuring via blood shows the amount of fuel—ketones—you have available to burn.

The yellow option avoids a finger-prick and measures the ketones expelled by the body via urine. Due to the oscillating fluctuation of ketones during the early part of the ketoCONTINUUM, urine ketones are recommended over blood measurements. I celebrate with patients using PeeTone strips and remind them, "These are fat calories that just got wasted out of your body — that's a weight loss win!" However, when starting ketoCONTINUUM #5, patients should advance to blood testing to measure their progress.

Measure Your Chemistry

Urine laced with ketones turned David's Pee-TONE strips positive, proving that ketones had circulated in his blood. The darker the pink on the PeeTone strip, the greater the concentration of ketones in his urine. Take note: David's urine ketones DID NOT accurately reflect the amount of ketones in his blood; Urine ketones only confirmed that ketones had been in his blood.

I teach patients how to improve the PeeTONE strip's accuracy when they are the only option. Upon awakening, completely empty your bladder without checking urine ketones. Wait 30 minutes. During that time, your kidneys add a tiny amount of urine into your bladder. Check PeeTONES then. That specific urine ketone measurement best reflects your blood ketones over the previous 30 minutes. Many flaws clutter this approach, but it can work in a pinch.

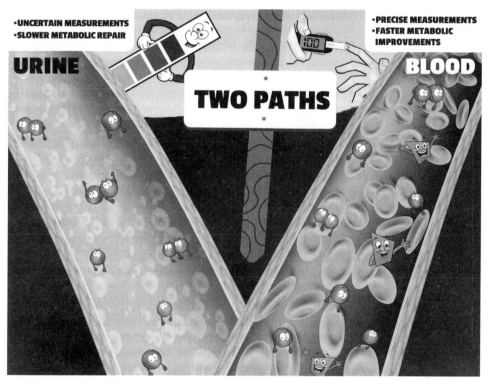

Measuring urine ketones worked well at the on-set of David's ketone production. Initially, his liver made way more ketones than he could use. His kidneys flushed the excess into his urine. But as David advanced to higher levels of the ketoCONTINUUM, too many variables left his urine measurements flawed. Moving to a more robust metabolism required precise measurement of David's chemistry. That data could only be collected via blood-ketone checks.

Ketone Meters

Serum refers to the liquid part of your blood outside of the red blood cells. Blood ketone meters use a drip of blood to measure ketones in the serum. Ketone meters, like glucose meters, empower people to check their data outside of a medical setting. Anyone can purchase this tool, along with the ketone strips. No prescription stands in the way of measuring your blood ketones. Only the cost and a finger prick.

Point-of-care home meters measure one of two types of ketones available in your blood. The device detects the millimoles of the D-isomer structure of Beta-HydroxyButyrate suspended in a deciliter of blood. The units of measurement shorten to mmol/dl. Readings greater than 0.4 mmol/dl indicate nutritional ketosis while reports less than that mean no ketones. The meters provide reproducible results, but the accuracy of point-of-care meters can vary +/- 0.3 mmol/dl compared to the advanced process done in a medical laboratory.

Point-of-care home meter measurements also have several limitations. They do not: Tell us if the Beta-HydroxyButyrate (BHB) came from exogenous ketones or from the liver. Also, this number does not measure the L-isomer structure of BHB, and they do not tell us how long the ketones have circulated in the blood. It does not tell us which ketones are destined for the cells' furnaces or which ones will be filtered into the urine. It merely shows how many ketones of the D-isomer BHB are available in that one drip of blood.

The Skinny on Ketone Blood Meters

The cost of home blood meters and their strips run about $100-$150 to get started. A combination meter measures both blood ketones and glucose and saves the expense of buying two devices. The combination meters detect ketones using one strip and glucose using another.

Most companies sell kits offering the meter for free when you buy their strips. Select a brand with quality test strips. Diabetics understand the importance of this selection. Years of checking their blood sugars offer insight into the importance of quality strips. Low-quality strips fail to withstand extreme temperatures. A 50 test-strip package can cost as little as $30 and as much as $300. Low-quality strips left sitting in an overheated or freezing car will all fail. You prick your finger, place the test strip into the meter, and siphon your blood into the strip. Unsuspectingly, the meter reads back, "ERROR." You test again, assuming one of the common operator errors like the strip wasn't firmly inserted into the meter or too little blood. In the second test, you see "ERROR" again. Frustration sets in by the fourth consecutive error message; you realize the entire, package has gone bad.

Because of their temperature stability, ForaCare (www.Foracare.com) wins my vote. ForaCare's dual meter is called the FORA-6 Connect. This system delivers accurate numbers through their quality test strips despite extreme temperatures. Their beginners Fora 6 Connect Blood Glucose and Ketone Ultimate Testing Kit includes a FORA-6 Connect meter, 50 glucose strips, 50 ketone strips, and 100 lancets costing around $180. This supplies the resources to test blood ketones and glucose for nearly 2 months. At two months, the frequency of testing usually slows down. Ketone test strips cost about $1.00 US, while the glucose test strips cost almost half as much.

Brain Chemistry

As David mastered ketoCONTINUUM #5, he checked his morning fasting glucose. How could such a simple thing like checking blood sugars change the way he chose food?

Before keto and long before he pricked his finger, David selected food based on the signals he received from his tongue. He unwittingly dosed the amount, type, and timing for optimal effect. This practiced private pleasure danced through the neural electrical currents, from his tongue to his brain. By his seventh decade of life, David had spent thousands of hours wiring his dopamine delivery. His dopamine was derived from sugar. Changing his reward circuitry required real-time feedback. Pricking his finger delivered immediate feedback. A more advanced option was to wear a continuous glucose monitor that sent input 24 hours a day, seven days a week. However, David's discipline allowed him to change his trajectory without the 24/7 constant monitoring.

Positive peer pressure from David's keto group coaxed the whispers of his new dopamine source. That new source of dopamine came from the newfound, like-minded relationships he formed in the keto group. He traded carbs for the connected friendships to those trying to improve their health.

Know Your Insulin Level

For 22 years, scientists measured the chemistry of 970 policemen from Helsinki, Finland, to see which factor predicted a severe heart event. In the prime of their lives, men could enter the study as long as they did not have diabetes. Measurements and calculations filled the data-bank over two decades with blood glucose, insulin, cholesterol, triglycerides, blood pressure, indexes of obesity, skin folds, smoking habits, physical activity, and much more.

The metric that best predicted who would have heart disease was (drum roll, please) *insulin*.

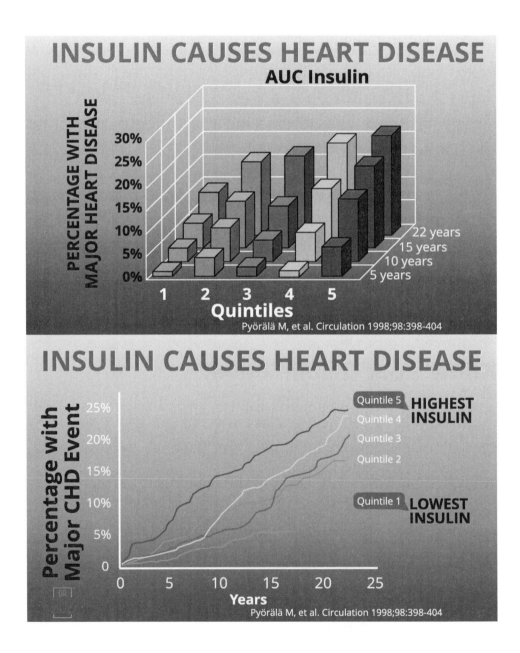

The higher their insulin levels, the greater their chances of heart attack, stroke, or sudden death. The greater the insulin, the higher the problems.

What a punchline! Know your insulin.

Blood Glucose is Not a Predictor of Insulin

Fighting against his history of excess insulin, an enemy he could not see, David focused on reducing his morning glucose. He kept his carb-consumption low, ate high fat, and pricked his finger. Time after time, his morning sugars came back above 100. Decades of excess insulin were the cause. Had David checked his blood sugars during these early years, his blood glucose would have been "controlled." The word control meant that the sugars weren't in the diabetic range.

Meanwhile, David's insulin crept higher and higher as he slowly lost the battle. The early years of the war left his sugars barely outside the healthy glucose range of 55-80 mg/dl. Years of excess insulin burned through his veins as his glucose numbers snuck into the 80-90 range. Gradually his morning fasting blood sugars lofted higher, and sometimes hit triple digits. David remained unaware.

David last weighed in at the doctor's office 15 years ago with 25 extra pounds of stored fat. His doctor reported his fasting blood sugar as "normal" at 95 mg/dl. What wasn't normal was David's insulin. Insulin rang a warning for over 15 years. Extra insulin insulated David's body and helped him pack on the layers. Somewhere in the past couple of years, his morning glucose rose above 100 and stayed there. Finally, his elevated blood sugar 'ratted out' on his insulin.

Elevated insulin acted like lighter fluid and posed a silent, deadly risk to David's survival. His glucose lofted at 115 mg/dL a dozen hours after the last morsel of food. Further lab testing showed his average blood sugar over the previous 100 days crept into the diabetic range. From his liver's size to the volume of insulin produced, David's system stretched to its maximum to protect against his rising glucose.

Had David been a pregnant woman during his 30s or 40s, he might have received screening with a glucose tolerance test. To test for early diabetes, pregnant women swallowed 100 grams of sugar, followed by blood glucose checks at 30, 60, 90, and 120 minutes.

Unfortunately, no one looked at how much insulin it took to control the blood glucose after drinking the sugar-water. Only the blood glucose was checked. Insulin predicted the problem—yet we didn't measure it. We missed many moms, babies, and men like David as we focused on screening with blood glucose instead of looking at their insulin. Their "normal" glucose hid under the blanket of excess insulin.

In the 1970s Dr. Joseph Kraft, a clinical pathologist, blew the lid off of the secret to the fountain of youth. He measured a super-secret weapon that predicted longevity in patients. Dr. Kraft measured insulin. In simplistic brilliance, he added serum insulin checks to the glucose tolerance test. Each time the lab tested for blood glucose, he added a blood insulin check to the list of labs. After several patients, he noticed the insulin rose strikingly at the two-hour check. This prompted him to add measurements at 3 hours, 4 hours, and 5 hours. A shocking reveal showed that behind the normal glucose levels rose a mountain of insulin. Years before the glucose slid out of standard-range, insulin crept higher and higher. The body overproduced insulin to control glucose. Over 75% of the patients tested had excess insulin.

Dr. Kraft autopsied people like David and found 75% of folks with normal blood sugars in the morning had diabetes-like damage in their eyes, kidneys, brain, and heart. Indeed, 10,000 out of 14,000 measured by Dr. Kraft showed soaring insulin levels with normal blood sugars. Like David, extra insulin scorched small blood vessels that peppered their organs. Yet they reported no symptoms. I repeat—the damage Dr. Kraft saw at autopsy occurred in patients with NORMAL blood sugars and no symptoms. As their sugars became abnormal, the damage expanded.

KRAFT GLUCOSE-INSULIN TOLERANCE TESTS

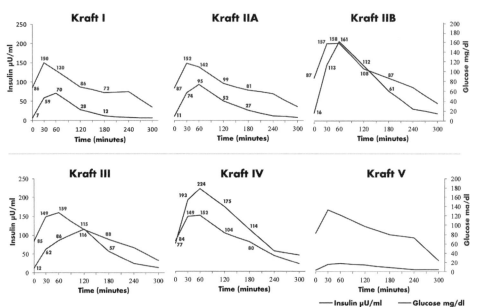

Insulin Grows "Humans"

Grows <u>white</u> fat (not brown fat.)

Grows inflammation.

Grows cancer cells.

Grows brain plaques.

Grows artery plaques.

Insulin signaled David's body to grow, and I mean growth of any kind. This powerful hormone grew David's fat cells, at the same time his skin tags, moles, and extra liver cells grew. If David had any cancer cells hiding in his body, insulin stimulated them to grow too. Insulin also stimulated plaque growth in David's brain, slowed his immune system, and increased inflammation of the kind that led to hardening of his arteries.

Insulin Fluctuation & Cost

Rarely do I order an insulin laboratory blood test for any of my patients. Yes! I just spent all that energy teaching you about the importance of insulin, only to tell you that I never order it. My reasons are as follows:

Cost and Convenience:

Measuring insulin was way out of David's budget. One check of his insulin costs around $70, but he will need at least five insulin assays to know what's happening in his body. The cost of a five-hour insulin assay soared over $2,500. There's more... Insurance won't cover it. In an ideal world David would have tracked his insulin progression using that five hour assay three to four times a year. That's ten-thousand dollars - annually ($2,500 x4). Set aside the burden for him to sit there for over six-hours after fasting for 12-hours, or more, before arrival. The cost and convenience of this test causes me to pause before ordering it.

Accuracy:

Insulin fluctuates moment to moment. Watch it rise from "normal" to three times that when someone has a good scare, a bowel movement, or even the hiccups. When emotions send the numbers dancing all over the page, accuracy of the test comes into question. Experts had a much clearer understanding and a more precise reading of a patient's insulin production when they closely monitored the average insulin output over several hours. Renowned pathologist, Dr. Kraft assessed insulin by checking patients' responses to a specific amount of glucose. He paired a series of blood insulin tests with blood glucose checks. Pairing the glucose with insulin improved the dependability of the score.

In short, checking insulin is complicated, expensive, and a heavy burden on the patient. Rest assured, a better way exists.

Dr. Boz Ratio Measures Insulin

When a hormone like insulin rapidly pulsates, measuring it in the lab fails to reflect its true value. Dr. Kraft studied multiple measurements of insulin to gain understanding of his patients. Another solution to understand this volatile hormone is to measure the substances in the blood that insulin impacts: glucose and ketones.

Glucose:

Continuous arrival of glucose causes the body to produce insulin. Said another way, as glucose rises, so does insulin. However, a normal or controlled blood glucose does not guarantee normal levels of insulin. Continuous stimulation from glucose can push insulin three times higher than expected.

Ketones:

When David's insulin was high, it stopped his ketone production. His liver could not make ketones until his insulin came down some. After years of elevated insulin, ketones first flowed out of David's liver when he reduced the production of insulin.

Glucose didn't directly predict David's insulin. Ketones didn't directly predict his insulin. But measuring his glucose and ketones *together* accurately reflected the function of his insulin. The Dr. Boz Ratio measured blood glucose and blood ketones simultaneously. Combining these two metrics provided a surrogate measurement of insulin.

Glucose Ketone Index - GKI

The Dr. Boz Ratio came from a protocol published in the scientific literature measuring glucose and ketones simultaneously in cancer patients. As my mother battled cancer, we needed to stress and exercise her metabolism via lowering blood sugar and producing more ketones. The stakes were high, leaving no room for guessing. Remarkable outcomes weren't expected without measuring and tracking Grandma Rose's metabolism.

We followed precise calculations to match the protocol published in the scientific literature. We measured her glucose and ketones several times per day. We wanted the therapeutic effect they got in the literature from this protocol. The research teams stressed metabolisms to match one glucose molecule for every ketone. They called it the glucose ketone index or GKI. The successful cases reported a 1:1 ratio.

One ketone for every glucose.

Hold on. Don't freak out. That sounds extreme. Because it is extreme! Every American reading this wants to close the book and throw it away. American metrics were not used in those studies. The scientific studies measured glucose in millimoles per liter, not milligrams per deciliter. Grandma Rose wanted nothing to do with that mess of a mathematical nightmare. She was far too sick for math. In a last-ditch effort to keep her attention, I simplified it.

I plotted out the GKI equivalent using the simplified math, sparing Grandma Rose the mental gymnastics to figure out the rest. I simply told her we needed a Dr. Boz Ratio less than 20. We divided glucose by ketones using the mismatched metrics. The number displayed on her glucose-meter was divided by the number displayed for her blood ketones. "Mom, divide the big number by the little one." That task she could handle. And so was born the Dr. Boz Ratio.

A GKI of one to one equaled a Dr. Boz Ratio of less than 20.   [GKI 1:1 = DBR <20]

The GKI approximated her insulin. In turn, the Dr. Boz Ratio plotted insulin

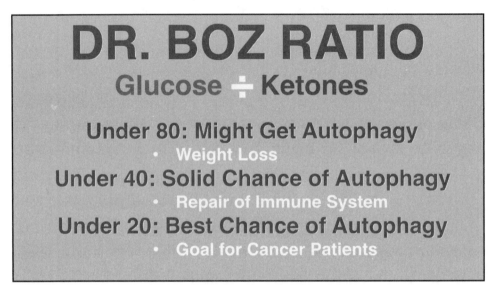

DR. BOZ RATIO
Glucose ÷ Ketones

Under 80: Might Get Autophagy
• Weight Loss
Under 40: Solid Chance of Autophagy
• Repair of Immune System
Under 20: Best Chance of Autophagy
• Goal for Cancer Patients

Weight Loss: Dr Boz Ratio Under 80

On the day this story started, David's blood sugar wavered around 125. To compensate for this excess, his body then produced insulin in abundance to try and push the blood glucose back towards normal. Years of maximum insulin tried to keep up with his gluttony of carbs, but it slowly lost its power and failed to control his sugar. Subsequent tests suggested to me that just a few months prior his insulin had weakened into an inefficient hormone.

Lowering David's carbohydrate intake to less than 20 grams per day, reduced his insulin and he began making ketones. Consequently, residual glycogen released his stored glucose hiding inside his liver and muscle cells. Ketones were now his alternate fuel source.

Diabetics with years, sometimes decades of excess insulin-related issues struggled to improve in less than 90 days of ketogenic nutrition. Their metabolisms suffered from the constant coating of insulin. If David had waited another year to reverse his over-production of insulin, his struggle would have been twice as long, perhaps irreversible. Or prescription medications might have been needed.

During the first two weeks, David's glucose hovered around 120 while his ketone production overshot with robust readings in the 1.5-2.0 mmol/dL range. His Dr. Boz Ratio calculated between 60-80. Those results corresponded with his weight loss. But by week 6, further changes had taken place. Even though David's morning fasting glucose was now 110-115 and his ketones measured 0.7. The dropped ketones with corresponding blood sugars calculated a Dr. Boz Ratio between 140-160. This ratio predicted his stalled weight loss. He could have foreshadowed the stall had he calculated his Dr. Boz Ratio. Simply put, a ratio less than 80 signaled insulin reduction, which meant he was on the path to losing weight. If the ratio was above 80 then it meant a weight loss stall.

David studied his chemistry. In order for him to understand what was happening in his system he had to measure the two substrates that insulin vigorously impacts: glucose and ketones. Learning to be more vigilant in monitoring his Dr. Boz Ratio made David take ownership of his health problem through the direct, accurate feedback at the prick of his fingertip. The Dr. Boz Ratio estimated his insulin. The lower his Dr. Boz Ratio, the lower his insulin. It was that simple. Furthermore, David learned that eating a handful of nuts in the evening ruined his metabolism the next morning and halted most of his ketone production. Keeping his evening hours free from snacks provided better chemistry. Period.

As David's Dr. Boz Ratio decreased, his body naturally healed, and gradually adapted to his newly reset keto-chemistry. But ironic as this may seem, as David's body adjusted, his Dr. Boz Ratio also did the same; it rose. This upward drift in his Dr. Boz Ratio was a signal letting him know that his metabolism was ready for another stress. If he ignored the rise in his numbers, his weight loss stalled. If he reverted to old habits of evening snacking, or too many carbs, his numbers reflected this. When his eight-hour eating-window no longer produced Dr. Boz Ratios under 100, he knew it was time to adjust. He could add a bit of exercise or cut his eating window by 15 minutes. Was the adjustment enough to tweak his metabolism? He would know by watching his morning numbers.

CONTINUOUS GLUCOSE MONITORS

If I could reverse time for David, I would have used a continuous glucose monitor to show him what was happening. Dr. Kraft did not have the advantage of this tool. The complications of measuring and tracking insulin remain an obstacle. Continuous glucose monitors test glucose moment to moment. A high-tech filament snaps into the tissue layer under the skin. The sensor connects to an adhesive that is worn for several days. Communication of the serum glucose registers to a smart phone. What happens when you eat carbs? Meat? Alcohol? What happens when you fast? Real-time data fastens the behavior to the numbers. Your doctor must write a prescription for a continuous glucose monitor.

Chapter 25

KETOCONTINUUM #6

CLEAN UP YOUR MORNING DRINK

For years, low-fat products cornered the market on coffee creamers. Modern chemists concocted imitation creamers from something other than dairy cows. They vacuumed out the fat, milled it into a powder, and promoted it as "healthy." A generation of coffee drinkers stirred this powdered potion into cups across the globe. *Non-dairy, fat-free coffee creamers* slowly hypnotized one mind after another.

Years of low-fat diets had ruined the neuronal wires connecting the sensation of taste inside their brains. Fat should have insulated each brain cell threading messages around the mind. A coating of thick, dense fat blanketing each nerve should channel the electrical communication to its intended destination. Low-fat menus overflowing with carbs, increased insulin production had eroded the insulation. Insulin's fumes had melted divots into their sheaths of insulation as if moths had eaten part of it.

What do patients look like when they have divots in their insulation?

ANSWER: They looked like David. Depressed, brain fog, low energy, and chaotic focus. Migraines ruled their lives. These divots and other brain injuries lingered on for years without the proper setting to heal. When dense, thick fat coated their brain's communications, it worked well. The more moth-eaten their insulation, the deeper their brain trouble, and the longer it lasted. Short-term problems, like headaches and distractedness, led to chronic problems, like Alzheimer's or Parkinsonism symptoms.

ketoCONTINUUM #6:

Clean Up Your Morning Drink

Great coffee began with great beans. David's love for coffee had only strengthened in the past months. He roasted one of the highest quality coffee beans sold in the area. Clean, full flavor lassoed his taste buds each morning with a dark, rich coffee. Before keto, David drank his coffee black. Only after he heard others in the support group instructed to add fat to the morning coffee did he consider it. He tried coconut oil, MCT C8:C10 oil, heavy cream, and butter in his drink. His taste buds said yes to all of them.

Throughout ketoCONTINUUMs #1- #5, David reminded newfound keto converts entering the group of fat's importance. "Fat is important! You need fat for this to work! Put mayonnaise on a hamburger. Add sour cream to pork chops. I put heavy cream in my morning coffee. Before keto, I never did any of that."

Decades of low-fat propaganda hardwired the belief that fat was dangerous. That fear prevented many from gaining advantages from keto-chemistry. Those who cut carbs without adding fat could not withstand the challenges ahead. Without a steady supply of fat entering their bodies, they struggled. Instead of an energetic, robust adaption to ketones, they limped along with a small bump to their chemistry. David's success arose from his plethora of fat-built hormones.

David needed to swallow fat at the onset of his ketogenic nutrition. Thankfully, keto-coffee swooned him with creamy, frothy, liquid fat delighting his taste buds—and brain.

Slurping down fat, while keeping ketones in circulation, restored his lipid supply-chain. Initially, his fatty hormones trickled in low supply as he ate a fat-filled menu of high-calorie, high-fat, low-carb composition. This chemistry lowered his insulin while resurrecting his fat-based hormones. Weeks of consuming heavy cream and slabs of butter restored the hormonal balance of peptide YY, cholecystokinin, leptin, cortisol, and testosterone. These fat-dependent hormones arose from their graves inside David's obesity and danced through his veins again.

During all this chemistry shifting David's calorie intake rose AND he lost weight. How could this be? "This doesn't make sense to me, but it works. I eat fat, don't count calories, feel great, and I am losing weight." But this conversation was about to change. The time had come to remove all calories, fat, and sweeteners from David's morning beverage.

	ketoCONTINUUM	WHO DOES THE WORK?	TEST	GUIDELINES	NEXT STEP
BASELINE METABOLISM	#6. Advanced 16:8	YOU - DISCIPLINE NEEDED.	URINE STRIPS	Clean up your morning drink. Remove all calories and sweeteners. Morning drink = no fat, no MCT, no butter, no sweeteners, no calories. The 16 hours = only salt, water, black coffee, or tea.	Don't remove the fat from your morning drink before this phase. You needed it to get here. Now it's time to let it go.

Remove Calories & Sweeteners from Morning Drink.

Both ketoCONTINUUM #5 and #6 kept all food, snacks, and supplements within eight hours of David's day. This strictly meant that absolutely NO eating, snacking, or chewing for the remaining 16 hours in his day. Those rules stayed the same for both steps.

ketoCONTINUUM #6 brought special attention to David's morning ritual drink—his coffee. For this step in the ketoCONTINUUM, all calories and sweeteners were drained from his morning drink: NO fat, NO MCT, NO butter, NO sweeteners, and NO calories.

Removing the morning fat from a newly revived metabolism bristled many in defense of their coveted fat-filled drinks, especially those who finally absorbed the message that adding fat to their drinks was a good habit to adopt. *"You told me to drink fat. Now you tell me not to?"* This 'opportunity' can spark a war!

Chemistry Before Calories

For the first six decades of life, David believed keeping track of his calories would control his weight. Wrong. He failed to understand the power of excess insulin. High-insulin supported fat flowing into his obese cells and blocked it from returning into his circulation. The only fat David had access to came from the fat he digested. As this fat traveled from his intestines to his storage layer, it impacted his chemistry during those precious but brief moments in time.

David's intestinal juices pumped fatty messages to his body. Swallowed fat announced, "Fat is back in full supply!" Keto-adaption enveloped his mitochondria. Magically, high fat rescued his metabolism and suppressed his hunger. High calorie, high fat rescued David's metabolism. His chemistry shifted —first. Then his rising bile, cholecystokinin, cortisol, and testosterone lifted him out of a long season of a muted, depressed, declining life.

Once this chemistry shifted, David's body capitalized on fat from one of two sources: His existing fat storage, or the fat he swallowed. This minor but distinct difference prepared David for success as he followed instructions to cut calories from his morning coffee.

Restricting David's feeding hours to eight hours per day flexed his keto-enhanced metabolism. His adaption churned ketones from his fat-storage when calories ran in short supply. If David had tried this before keto-adaption, his metabolism would have shifted downward, asking—no— begging his cells to survive with less energy. David had already lived through that miserable experience of dieting without revived fatty hormones. Low-calorie menus left him hungry, grumpy, moody, and slowed his metabolism. Additionally, the lack of calories starved his cells and kept them from doing their jobs. From hair growth to brain repair, his body shut down as many functions as possible. Keto-chemistry and the orchestra of fatty endocrine hormones prevented this mental holocaust and cellular starvation.

No Starving Allowed!
This is NOT a low-calorie starvation diet.

Reduced-calorie diets are a no-no if insulin is still on the rise. Only after insulin begins to decline can you adapt to keto-fuel. If you restrict calories before you awaken the fatty hormones, you will struggle. Keto-adaption must be present before you enter the keto-CONTINUUMs that use time-restricted eating.

How do you know if you have keto-chemistry?

ANSWER: *You <u>accidentally</u> miss a meal.* As fat pours into a system, keto chemistry shoos away hunger. The 'accidental missed-meal' marks a rise in hormones. Several of those hormones message the brain to stop eating. That is keto-adaption. Patients seeking keto-adaption don't always know when their hormones are surging. Listening for hormonal messages requires a quiet, focused brain.

Another sure sign of keto-adaption comes from your Dr. Boz Ratio. If your morning fasting ratios steadily decline, you're keto-adapted. Dr. Boz Ratio approximates insulin. Lowered insulin allows ketones to rise and glucose to sink. Keto-adaption is reflected when patients consistently achieve a Dr Boz Ratio under 100.

David Strengthened Through Discipline

In the mornings, David pricked his finger and calculated his Dr. Boz Ratio. Elevated morning blood sugars continued to rise while his ketones settled between 0.5-1.0. His health had improved substantially from the onset of keto — despite his minor struggles. At keto-CONTINUUM #4 he ate two meals per day. Even though no weight loss took place during that stage, he still felt ready and motivated to step into ketoCON-TINUUM #5. This step squeezed his two meals inside an eight-hour window. ketoCONTINUUM #4 and #5 were not much different in David's case. The calories and meal portions were the same. But the timing of meal consumption was slightly different between the two stages. He also kept his coffee filled with fat each morning. As a result, David saw no weight loss after he advanced.

To lose weight, he needed to use his chemical advantage. He needed to apply stress to his metabolism. Using his keto-adapted chemistry proved more challenging than creating it. Discipline was required.

Unlike ketoCONTINUUM #4, ketoCONTINUUM #5 shut off David's eating for sixteen hours. To flex his keto-chemistry, he needed to stop all calories for a longer time. Advancing to ketoCONTINUUM #6 would force David's body to get calories from his fat storage, not his fat-filled coffee.

ketoCONTINUUM #6 removed heavy cream from his coffee. With quality coffee beans at his disposal, David enlightened the support group with the benefits of cold-brew coffee. Soaking coffee grounds for over 12 hours all but guaranteed the smoothest tasting coffee. Others in the group who had struggled to remove cream from their morning drink shared their tip of adding enriched mineral salt. Salted coffee sounded gross to David. He stuck to his cold-brewed coffee while others added their salt.

The timing of his meals hardly moved from ketoCONTINUUM #5 to #6. His supper finished by 7:30 PM. Afterward, he did not snack. Lunch rarely fit into his day before 1:00 PM. This part of his routine remained stable.

Once David returned to black coffee, he reported hunger pangs the first 2-3 mornings. He had not felt those since the first couple of days of keto. His past habit would have munched pretzels at the first twinge of hunger. Instead, David tucked a small dish of mineralized pink salt next to his computer screen. When his stomach growled, he placed 2-3 salt-crystals on the tip of his tongue.

The mineralized salt flooded his mouth with saliva. Like a magic wand, the desire for food evaporated within a minute of the salt.

Success over that moment rewarded him with improved numbers. Boy, did they improve! Blood ketones rose while his morning fasting blood sugars reduced slightly. David's first week of black coffee produced glucose from 92-105 [5-13 mmol/l], and ketones above 1.0. His best blood ketone hit 1.8 mmol/l.

Checking morning fasting blood markers provided a daily teachable moment. That week his metabolism magnified, and David's stall broke. His number on the scale lowered.

If You're Not Ready Yet

If you can't seem to say good-bye to your buttered, oiled, or creamed coffee, consider this alternate plan. Begin your eight-hour eating window with your fat-filled coffee. The onset of your 8 hours starts with the first sip. As soon as you swallow your first drop, start the timer for 8 hours. If you drink your first cup at 6:30 AM, zip your lips at 2:30 PM.

Fast until the following morning at 6:30 AM. That means no food, gum, or supplements in the late afternoon and evening. No nuts. No broth. No grabbing a meat stick or cheese. Water and salt only in the remaining 16 hours.

I offer this knowing a shared reality. Most struggle with this option. The evening hours hold many social pressures to eat. Eliminating all evening eating rituals challenges the most dedicated students. In my experience, saying goodbye to the fat-filled coffee is much easier.

Chapter 26

KETO**CONTINUUM** #7 23:1

ELEVATED MORNING BLOOD SUGARS

After the initial transition, David found an easy stride with ketoCONTINUUM #6. His black coffee soothed him each morning as he embraced his new identity of checking blood numbers. He took advantage of the spreadsheet shared amongst members of the keto support group. This resource plotted his blood glucose and blood ketones with an automatic calculation of his Dr. Boz Ratio. The spreadsheet contained formatted columns for recording the total daily carb count and the specific times when meals were eaten. This simple yet meticulous act of tracking meal times strengthened David's resolve, instilling him with the power of choice—when and what to eat, or not to eat.

[See workbook]

Three weeks into ketoCONTINUUM #6, the clarity and mental focus he felt and boasted about during the first few weeks of keto, also returned. The numbers on the scale slid downward, bit by bit, making David smile, and emotionally pat himself on the back. But even though his ketones flowed between 0.7 and 1.8 mmol/dl, his morning sugars hardly budged, despite having consumed no calories until early afternoon. David was adamant; he wanted his Dr. Boz Ratio less than 80. For all that he had accomplished, that little voice in his head whispered the fear that his goal might be impossible. The end of the third week of ketoCONTINUUM #6, David started to lose hope that he could ever reach his goal.

"My morning sugars are stuck," David complained at the support group that Friday. "They won't go down." As soon as he proclaimed it, so everyone could hear, he knew what he needed to do. He'd witnessed others in the same predicament. When they encountered a weight loss stall during their keto journey, or could not optimize their Dr. Boz Ratio, they boldly - stepped into the next ketoCONTINUUM. They strengthened their metabolisms by stressing their mitochondria. David's mirror neurons must have taken over his brain because the following sentence came out of his mouth without planning it, "Guess it's time for me to go to ketoCONTINUUM #7."

23:1 OMAD

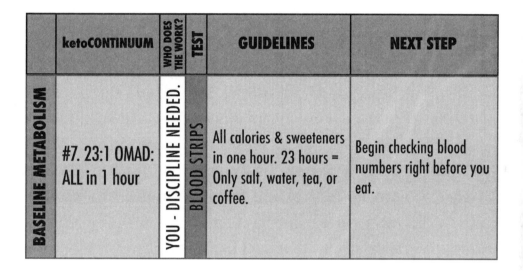

	ketoCONTINUUM	WHO DOES THE WORK?	TEST	GUIDELINES	NEXT STEP
BASELINE METABOLISM	#7. 23:1 OMAD: ALL in 1 hour	YOU - DISCIPLINE NEEDED.	BLOOD STRIPS	All calories & sweeteners in one hour. 23 hours = Only salt, water, tea, or coffee.	Begin checking blood numbers right before you eat.

OMAD stands for One Meal A Day. I like **ACIOH** instead. ACIOH means All Calories In One Hour. It's not as pleasant to say, but that acronym delivers a more exact message. All calories slide down your food-pipe in 60 minutes or less. The other 23 hours of the day remain void of calories and sweeteners.

None.

Zip. Zero.

Many students claimed to be OMAD for months, complaining that keto wasn't working, "I've been OMAD for six months, and the scale will not move." Their problems started with OMAD not being ACIOH. 23:1.

In their rulebook, OMAD meant eating one daily keto-meal. Keto-style eating suppressed their appetite and whittled their eating down to one satisfying meal per day. But only upon closer inspection of their eating habits could we see the trouble. Their day started with a dollop of fat in their morning coffee. By mid-afternoon, they craved "a lil' somethin' somethin'." They wouldn't call it hunger. They didn't need to "eat." These keto students thought they just needed a bite or two. "With one bite, I am better, Doc. It doesn't take much to make it go away; but I needed that something." They felt better after sipping on salty bone broth, nibbling a handful of nuts, or even chewing gum. Within minutes of one of these antidotes, their sensation passed.

Cravings vs Hunger

That afternoon sensation was a craving. How do I know?

Three reasons:

1) Length of time the sensation lasted

2) Timing of when it occurred

3) The antidote to make it go away

Hunger differs from craving in many ways, but these three points offer the greatest separation. A downward drift in blood sugar unleashes a surge of hunger-hormones. A genuine feeling of hunger uses hormones to summon the body to eat. Hunger hormones cause your tummy to growl. You may start to tremble, feel light-headed, and even break out in a sweat if you don't eat. YOU MUST EAT. Hunger-hormones oppose the fat-based hormones used by the trolls in the previous chapter. Refueling with carbohydrates elevates the glucose levels and temporarily shuts off those hunger-hormones. Rapid consumption of "pine-needle-fuel" satisfies hunger for a short time with bursts of energy. As that energy burns, glucose plummets as hunger hormones spike again. That drop in power signals it's time to eat again. Swallow some calories, and within ten minutes, the feeling of danger subsides. That pattern is genuine hunger, not a craving. The fluctuation of glucose leads the cycle, and the hormones' rise and fall sustain the process. The best block of hunger hormones is a stable, steady glucose level. Use ketones as the fuel, and the glucose holds quite steady keeping hunger away from the equation.

In contrast to hunger, cravings are much quicker. They onset quickly and resolve quickly, lasting less than a few minutes. <u>Cravings don't involve blood sugar</u> nor any endocrine hormones pulsing through your veins. <u>They are born from thoughts, patterns of behavior, and emotions.</u> Cravings often happen at similar times of the day. Frequently, they link to a pattern of eating from your past. If you've comforted yourself with food routinely every night before bed, cravings will haunt your thoughts when you stop eating at night. Unfortunately, if you can't control your mind and chase away those thoughts of the food, the cycle repeats again and again. A dramatic pity-party can churn cravings through your mind for 20-30 minutes. Don't mistake this perpetual thought-loop for genuine hunger.

Learn to distinguish cravings from hunger. When sorting the differences, focus on how to abort the sensations. Cravings vanish when the mind is distracted. Meditation, singing, a splash of water to your face, or a hearty dose of salt to your tongue can melt cravings. All these tactics warp your mind with strong signals in other areas of your brain. In fact any meaningful stimuli will mute the craving desire by drawing your attention to something else other than this momentary emotional spell.

Hunger leans more towards physiological than the emotional. It takes approximately 10 - 15 minutes for messages of hunger to arrive and pass. Yes. These pangs are much slower than cravings. If you apply the tactics used to abort a craving when a real hunger wave hits, you will see some improvement. They don't ameliorate the feelings, they simply decrease it.

To master ketoCONTINUUM #7 or any time-restricted eating, you must sort your cravings from a hormonal desire for food. Success pivots on figuring this out.

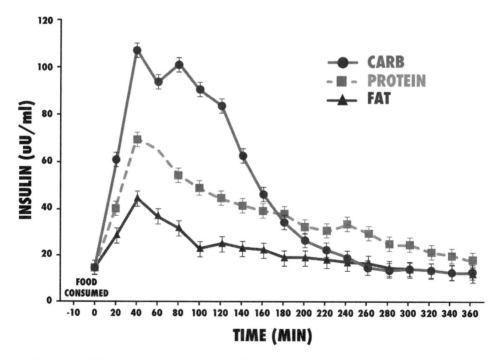

The Journal of Clinical Endocrinology & Metabolism | Volume 93, Issue 5, 1 May 2008, Pages 1971–1979
https://doi.org/10.1210/jc.2007-2289

Serum Insulin Levels

Have a look at this seminal study measuring insulin. It shows the amount of insulin circulating in healthy subjects after they ate different types of food. Patients of a healthy weight (that means not overweight) and no history of insulin resistance fasted overnight. Upon awakening, researchers then tested their blood levels for insulin, glucose, ketones, and ghrelin. The participants received one meal each morning. Blood tests were repeated every twenty minutes for six hours as they fasted throughout the day. The first day participants were fed a pure carbohydrate meal. The following morning the menu was pulverized protein. No carbs. No fat. On the third day, they ate only fat. The graphed line with the circles shows their insulin after eating the carbs. Squares show their insulin response to the protein-meal, and triangles follow the fat-meal.

Carbs stimulated the highest insulin blood levels. Eating only protein caused a moderate amount of insulin production. But as you can see, feeding on fat alone released the lowest amount of insulin. Many keto-lovers mistakingly think that eating fat produces no insulin. Eating *nothing* produces no insulin. In relative comparison, much less insulin flowed from the pancreas after eating fat, but insulin still oozed out from their endocrine organ. Let me remind you, these were healthy patients. They were not overweight with chronic health problems.

Insulin resistant patients demonstrated excessive insulin secretion. Years of high demand turned their spigot into a fire hose. Their body grew accustomed to the shower of insulin each time they ate. When they swallowed protein or fat, they made plenty of insulin. When insulin-resistant patients ate carbs, they pushed maximum insulin out of their pancreas, up to ten times higher than lean patients.

In his twenties, David's young endocrine system added a teaspoon of insulin into his system after eating an apple. Fifty pounds and three decades later, he used two-thirds of a cup of insulin for the same food. Similarly, eating two tablespoons of pure butter once evoked a few drops of insulin. With his age grew his insulin resistance. Now, that butter would stimulate spoonfuls of insulin.

David needed to unlock another layer of fat in order to see further weight loss. For this to take place insulin had to decline — even further.

How could he lower his Dr. Boz Ratio?

ANSWER: Stress his metabolism to the next ketoCONTINUUM. Lowering David's Dr. Boz Ratio re-

quired a reduction in his glucose or a surge to his ketones. Either option worked.

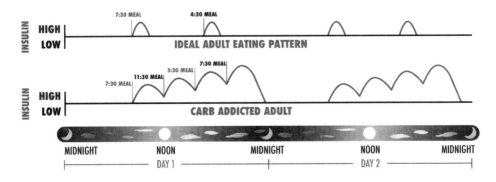

Before adapting to ketosis, David's mitochondria
burned only glucose. Ketones didn't enter his campfires. Only pine-needles crackled away. David spent an
enormous amount of time shoveling kindling into his
mitochondria. Once several logs began to burn inside
his mitochondria, his blood glucose numbers stabilized. Instead of the rise and fall every few hours, the
combination of ketones and glucose offered a stable,
albeit elevated, blood sugar. David's hunger hormones
stopped surging because his glucose stopped fluctuat-
ing. Without that constant signal of hunger, time-re-
stricted-eating happened naturally. David's obstacles
to this came from his old habits, not from hunger
pangs. Watching his blood glucose assured him that
he had plenty of fuel swimming around his blood to
skip meals. Frustration with his abundant morning glucose drove him to closely study his data. His numbers

from the first two pages of his Dr. Boz Chart showed him a pattern. His blood sugars were stable, around 95-110. He saw with clear and specific evidence that he needed to lengthen the time between feedings. When he ate late at night, they were the highest. If he skipped supper, they were the best. The chart boosted David's understanding that he needed to do this—twenty-three hours without food.

David left that week's keto-support meeting, wondering how to approach this. His mirror neurons triggered a memory of someone else's advent of a new restriction, "When you restrict food for the first time, success happens in the setup. Look for the timing associated with fewest temptations." David looked at his calendar. After considering his job, family, and social settings, he planned to start ketoCONTINUUM #7 the following weekend. Over the next six days, he stretched his time-restricted eating from ketoCON-TINUUM #6 towards 23 hours. He was pretty good at holding off food for 16 hours. Lengthening that time intimidated him. On his first stretching attempt, he chuckled when he glanced at his watch within minutes of the 16th hour. He could feel his desire for food rise and wanted to eat. He pushed himself to 17 hours, leaving 7 hours for eating. By Tuesday, he was closer to 18 restricted hours with six hours for eating. By Friday, he was ready.

Friday marked his first day of 23:1. David and his wife had evening plans on Friday and Saturday. He co-ordinated his one hour of eating with those social engagements. David filled his day with busyness. His list of distractions kept him away from the snacks with very little time in the office. He hustled through the Cathedral's door for 4:30 mass. In the past, the dim, calm sanctuary had coaxed him to sleep. David leaned in to capture the mindfulness of this ritual. He focused on the words as they left Father's mouth. Shooing away distracting thoughts, he prayed for strength and channeled any suffering through his faith. On the way out, Father said, "You're sure looking healthy, David. So good to see you." David smiled as he wondered, "Did mass make fasting easier? Or was fasting making mass easier?"

He joined Kat and the others for supper. The traditional Midwestern menu hid some high-fat, low carb items. He ordered the artichoke-spinach dip for an appetizer and ate it with a spoon. No chips or bread. Their brisket tasted delightful, and he traded the russet garden potatoes for grilled asparagus with hollandaise sauce. His choices surged the hormones of satiety. As others ate desert, he focused on his body's endocrine communication. He was full. Nauseatingly full. He followed a similar plan on Saturday night and made it through Day 2.

On Sunday, David's family shared an afternoon meal at 1:00 PM. He shifted his one meal to match his family's plans. Like the meals on Friday and Saturday, he ate until he felt that surge of satiety. Months of keto eating had made that sensation familiar to David. He knew what to look for and detected the rising signal to stop eating.

Sunday evening, David felt tempted to eat. Not from hunger. From habit. David placed a kernel of salt on the tip of his tongue as he grabbed his Rosary. He resisted the urge as he focused on the first few prayers linked to the beads. Gone. The desire to eat vanished by the third one.

Day Time:	Time since last bite	Blood Glucose	Blood Ketones	Dr. Boz Ratio
Sat 6:30 AM	8 hours	103	0.7	141
Sun 6:30 AM	9 hours	109	0.8	136
Mon 6:30 AM	18 hours	101	1.3	77

His morning Dr. Boz Ratio on Saturday and Sunday rose above 100, but Monday's number hit a home run: a Dr. Boz Ratio of 77. David was hopeful that his elevated morning sugars were about to meet their match.

That next week, David's morning fasting sugar read 107, 115, 99, 104. ANGRY. Disappointed. Frustrated. David was downright MAD. He'd followed the rules and refrained from every stinkin' bite of food for 23 hours. He did not cheat. Salt. Black coffee. Tea. Water. That was it. Those numbers stung and felt like a betrayal of his own body. How could they still be high? Maybe something glitched inside his blood meter. He changed the batteries in his meter and rechecked. Same. Still high. Despite effort, despite his faithfulness to manipulate his blood sugars under 100, it fell short. Restricting his eating to one hour a day was a real sacrifice for him. He wanted perfect numbers in return for his offering.

He returned to Keto Group the following Friday. "Doc, I haven't eaten anything in hours. How can my blood sugars be that high?" he asked in a wilted voice. "I'm doing everything you asked."

The answer was cortisol, glycogen, and gluconeogenesis. David's metabolism chalked up years of suffering to tolerate his level of insulin. These other three terms played significant roles in orchestrating his current dilemma.

HbA1c TEST SCORE

HbA1c	mg/dL PRECEDING 3-MONTH AVERAGE BLOOD GLUCOSE	mmol/L PRECEDING 3-MONTH AVERAGE BLOOD GLUCOSE
4.0	68	3.8
4.5	82	4.5
5.0	97	5.4
5.5	111	6.1
6.0	126	7
6.5	140	7.8
7.0	154	8.6
7.5	169	9.4
8.0	183	10.1
8.5	197	10.9
9.0	212	11.8
9.5	226	12.5
10.0	240	13.3
10.5	255	14.1
11.0	269	14.9
11.5	283	15.7
12.0	298	16.5
12.5	312	18.1
13.0	326	14.5
13.5	340	18.9

REVERSING AGING

FASTER AGING

DANGER

Insulin Resistance

Unless you counted David's decreased metabolism, obesity, sleep apnea, high blood pressure, arthritis, depression, and scattered mental focus, he had no symptoms of insulin resistance. He didn't know he was insulin resistant. But I knew. Other indicators of his resistance were: The length of time, (decades) that he'd struggled with his weight; his body's shape, and the rapid weight loss during the first phase of the ketogenic diet. What clearly fortified my certainty was David's elevated hemoglobin A1c of 5.4.

Readers ... Don't make the same mistake as David. He assumed insulin resistance was for someone else. He had never checked his sugars. He rejected labels linking him to problems with insulin, diabetes, or pre-diabetes. His resistance started when his blood sugars averaged 100. Truth be told, David's love-affair with carbs began forty years ago. His body required a few more drops of insulin every time he ate them. This forced David's pancreas to work overtime, adding insulin into his blood to keep his glucose in the semi-normal numbers. In his 20s, he needed 30 drops of insulin to match 30 carbs. In his early 30's David needed 45 drops of insulin to do the same job. His pancreas topped out in his mid-50s. For years, maximum insulin burned through his veins. His lack of awareness mixed with denial resulted in many sticky red blood cells — stuck full of sugar. A healthy blood sugar averaged around 80 mg/dL [4.5 mmol/L.] That matched a HgA1c of 4.5. David had been north of that for years. Reversing that was going to take steady keto-chemistry.

Seeing others in the keto group struggle with the exact same concerns, David accepted the reality of his problem one harsh fact at a time. Testing his blood sugar in front of the group riveted his attention. That scene sent shockwaves through his self-talk, "She said I was diabetic. I can't believe that. Not me." His recently stalled weight, combined with the stubborn sugars, fit the pattern of insulin resistance. Now, that he'd removed the fat from his morning coffee and stopped eating for 23 hours a day, how could those morning sugars stay elevated? It would have been easy to lose hope.

In recent weeks David had received so much praise for the weight he'd lost. Neighbors, clients, and family had approached him, asking, "How are you losing so much weight? You look so good and seem so happy. What's your secret?" These compliments encouraged him. He found that educating his friends and family to count carbs and eat fat strengthened his commitment. He was determined to figure out this hurdle to lower his morning blood sugars.

David's afternoon Dr. Boz Ratios were much better than his morning ones. This made no sense to him. His Tuesday morning sugar rose above 100, eighteen hours after his last bite of food. How could he go nearly a whole day without a lick of food and still have that much sugar in his blood?

ANSWER: Glycogen.

DAY Time:	Time since last bite	Blood Glucose	Blood Ketones	Dr. Boz Ratio
Mon 2:30 PM	23 hours	98	1.2	81
Mon 8:30 PM	2 hours	118	0.5	236
Tues 6:30 AM	12 hours	105	1.1	95
Tues 3:30 PM	21 hours	88	1.4	62

Glycogen

If David drained all of his blood into a container and sorted out the glucose molecules, his blood held about one teaspoon of dissolved sugar. Whenever he ate more than about a dozen carbs, glycogen caught his overflow. Whenever he ate more carbs than his blood could hold, his body lassoed the extra glucose into a string and wound it into glycogen. He stored bubbles of glycogen in his liver and muscles — close to the campfires that burned glucose. As soon as the circulating glucose dropped, he unwound those strings of glucose and used them as fuel.

If David were a stone-age man he would have used that extra energy within a few hours after storing it. The quick access to glucose ensured that Caveman-David would have the fuel to survive. After a hardy feeding of carbs, tightly packed glucose morphed into glycogen bubbles. These bubbles nestled into cells when his glucose rose. Insulin commanded the circulating blood glucose to stay within range. As it approached the upper limit of healthy, insulin swiftly stuffed glucose into storage. Both Caveman-David and Modern-Day-David popped glycogen bubbles to release the storage.

Glycogen bubbles snuggled right next to the mitochondria in David's muscle and liver cells. As soon as his insulin dipped, 'POP' went a few bubbles. As the strings of glucose unwound, flames of pine-needles burned through his mitochondria.

David stored one-fourth of his total glycogen inside his liver cells, while his muscle cells hoarded the rest. Minimal glycogen bubbles awaited popping inside Caveman-David, simply because his Neanderthal menu offered seasonal carbs in limited quantities. But modern-Day-David added more carbs in a single day than his stone-age ancestor consumed in an entire month. Extra carbs delivered extra insulin. Decades of this hormonal abuse overloaded his body with glycogen. This signaled his liver to grow more cells. Yes - remember, insulin GROWS things: Skin tags, fat cells, cancer cells, and liver cells. Over time, David's modern-day liver doubled in size when compared to his ancient ancestor. His steady supply of insulin demanded more storage space. David wasn't born with extra liver cells. He grew them.

David's ketogenic nutrition lowered his insulin. Each notch down on the insulin gauge opened a new crop of bubbles. David's over-populated glycogen supply was the sole reason his blood glucose remained high, despite fasting for 24-hours.

How do you pop glycogen bubbles?

One of two ways:

1) Drop the level of insulin.
2) Add cortisol.

Cortisol

Things in life seem unconnected and unrelated. Oftentimes they are. A closer inspection reveals the order of nature's rules. Take for example the cycles of:

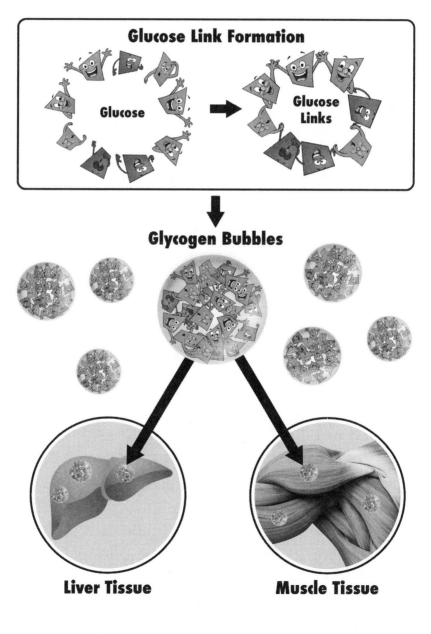

sleeping and awakening; night and day; lunar and so-lar—and our hormones, namely cortisol.

Cortisol was not the name of his ancient Saber-Toothed dog. Cortisol was the hormone that instructed caveman David to wake up each morning at sunrise. About an hour before awakening, this hormone sparked a message from his brain to his liver. The statement translated, "Wake up."

Millions of generations ago, David's brain evolved to synchronize with sunrise and sunset. Sunlight has led humanity for millions of years. Not even modern dark curtains could block David's mind from communicating with the sun. If he overslept or worked the night shift, his day-night rhythm faithfully delivered cortisol right before sunrise. This happened without fail.

As the sun crested the edge of David's world, his cortisol transcended a message upon his liver. It sent vibrations through David's glycogen bubbles. The alarm wiggled his strings of stored glucose to release from the glycogen bubbles. "Snap, crackle, pop!" Cortisol sparked a fire of pine needles every morning.

As a teenager, David's brain sent the same message of cortisol to his liver. At that age, a fraction of glycogen bubbles awaited his hormonal signal. With the help of a dozen years of processed carbs, a modern-day teenager's liver looked like the mature liver of Caveman-David's. Cortisol chimed through the liver popping bubbles. Strings of glucose flowed into his circulation, lifting his glucose from 60 mg/dL [3.3 mmol/l] to about 85 mg/dL [4.7 mmol/l]. This chemical ritual happened every day at dawn. Through the decades, David amassed significant quantities of glycogen bubbles. The abundance kept the level of glucose in his bloodstream above 90 mg/dL, where as a healthy range averaged at least less than 90.

Decrease Insulin to Break the Cycle

Which would decrease first, David's blood sugar or his insulin? They both needed to come down. Yet, the insulin imprisoned his stored sugar, and the sugar drove up his insulin. How could he break this catch 22 predicament? Willpower hadn't worked. Despite all of his wanting and willing, his morning blood glucose hovered above 100 with a rare exception. How could he decrease his glucose to unlock the gates of glycogen?

ANSWER: Begin each day with a few ketones.

Throughout David's growth years, his liver held a bubble-bath of glycogen. His liver cells were now stuffed beyond their limits with stored sugar. Each week spent in ketogenic chemistry, lowered David's insulin closer to its normal, baseline level. The first time he stressed his metabolism with the 23 hours of fasting, glucose burst out of storage and simultaneously entered his circulation. Once emptied, his body replaced those glycogen bubbles after his daily hour of eating. Each day spent in 23:1 emptied and replenished glycogen with slightly fewer glycogen bubbles than the previous day. The 23 hours without food emptied more glycogen bubbles than he made from the one hour of eating. The daily cycle of emptying and then replenishing glycogen resulted in fewer glycogen bubbles each day spent in 23:1. As a consequence David's liver grew healthier each day. POP!

David needed lower levels of insulin to unlock the gates of glycogen. Only after his insulin dipped could glycogen be released from his liver and muscle cells. The first time his insulin dropped, oodles of glycogen storage were unlocked. After years of constant insulin, declining levels exposed another layer of old glycogen. As long as David's insulin lowered a little bit every day, glucose gushed from the bubbles. Glucose finally began moving out of storage.

David had shoved glycogen into every corner of his storage cells. Stuffed to the max, glucose burst out of storage the first time he fasted 24 hours. A bountiful amount of glucose entered his circulation all at once. These morning waves of glucose deceived David as to what was happening inside is body. He wondered if the keto diet was working. Despite following the keto way of eating, his morning sugars rose over 100 nearly every time he checked them.

David's morning fasting blood glucose did not measure David's cortisol. Instead, it measured the amount of glycogen released from storage. His cortisol changed minimally from one day to the next. Meanwhile, his ketones crept up by the slightest amount.

Increasing ketones showed evidence that his metabolism was not dwindling, but strengthening, Using ketoCONTINUUM #7, David began each morning with a tiny trickle of ketones on his side. Although he frowned at how few were in his blood when he measured, he was winning. That tiny yet nuanced trickle made the difference between time-restricted eating on a low-carb diet versus a low-fat, high carb menu.

David's body improved using his steady, albeit small, supply of ketones. The pace was measurable, not dramatic. David's triumph over his morning fasting sugars grew with the rising ketones, his whisper of fatty-hormones, and plotting his data carefully.

First 3 Weeks at ketoCONTINUUM #7

Study David's first three weeks at ketoCONTIN-UUM #7. The ketone numbers increase slightly over time. Pay attention to the relationship between the length of time since David's last meal and its impact on his Dr. Boz Ratio. *The attrition of his ratios reflected his declining insulin.* Had David digested an exorbitant amount of carbs within his sixty-minute eating-window, his ketones would have vanished. He improved his health *one ketone at a time* by staying the course. His consistent ketone production would win.

DAY Time:	Time since last bite	Blood Glucose	Blood Ketones	Dr. Boz Ratio
Sat 6:30 AM	8 hours	103	0.7	* 141
Sun 6:30 AM	9 hours	109	0.8	* 136
Mon 6:30 AM	18 hours	101	1.3	* 77
Thur 6:30 AM	12 hours	107	0.5	* 214
Fri 6:15 AM	12 hours	110	0.7	* 157

DAY Time:	Time since last bite	Blood Glucose	Blood Ketones	Dr. Boz Ratio
Sat 8:00 AM	12 hours	118	0.6	* 196
Sun 2:00 PM	22 hours	100	1.0	100
Mon 2:30 PM	23 hours	98	1.2	81
Mon 8:30 PM	2 hours	118	0.5	236
Tues 6:30 AM	12 hours	105	1.1	* 95
Tues 3:30 PM	21 hours	88	1.4	62
Wed 6:30 AM	11 hours	108	1.4	* 77
Thurs 6:30 AM	11 hours	111	1.2	* 92
Fri 6:15 AM	11 hours	110	1.1	* 100
Sun 3:00 PM	22 hours	99	1.4	70
Mon 6:30 AM	14 hours	102	0.9	* 113

DAY Time:	Time since last bite	Blood Glucose	Blood Ketones	Dr. Boz Ratio
Tue 6:20 AM	12 hours	99	0.9	* 110
Wed 6:25 AM	11 hours	105	1.1	* 95
Thurs 6:40 AM	11 hours	98	1.3	* 75
Fri 6:15 AM	12 hours	101	1.2	* 84
Sat 7:45 AM	12 hours	103	1.1	* 93

* A Dr Boz Ratio measured during the morning cortisol surge.

Use the workbook to plot your data. During struggles, times of fading hope, or a stall, use the worksheets. Keeping track of your data helps increase the mindfulness of your journey. Studying a chart like this can reveal the subtle improvements in the war between ketones and inflammation.

Stay the course. You can do this.

Chapter 27

KETO**CONTINUUM #8**

ADVANCED 23:1

David's tidal wave of bursting glycogen bubbles happened the first, second, third, and fourth times he restricted eating. His fasting blood glucose of 105, 98, 101, and 103 could have discouraged him. He expected instant improvements after denying food for 23 hours. His improvements stayed hidden if he only looked at his blood glucose. Adding blood ketones to the equation showed the progress in reversing his insulin resistance. David's Dr. Boz Ratio often dropped into the double digits. Each day at 23:1 added slightly more ketones to his metabolism. His last four morning ketones measured 1.1, 1.3, 1.2, and 1.1 mmol/L.

If David had presented to a modern medical clinic with insulin resistance, prescription insulin most likely would have treated his elevated glucose. But more insulin would have fattened him up and dialed down his metabolism. Instead, he applied keto chemistry. Week after week, his insulin signal reset as it drifted downward.

23:1, flanked by ketogenic chemistry, strengthened the power of David's insulin. He now required a fraction of insulin to keep his sugars under 110 mg/dL. His insulin delivered twice the power it did when he started. The attrition of his insulin, measured through his Dr. Boz Ratio, was gentle and slow.

David measured his Dr. Boz Ratio first thing in the morning. Pricking his finger and plotting his numbers was his least favorite part of the keto journey. He didn't like the cost of the strips, or the blood, or the charting. But he did it anyway.

One afternoon, David pricked his finger and found his best Dr. Boz Ratio. "How could this be?" he thought. Curiosity pushed him to check a few more mid-afternoon numbers. They were superb, way better than his morning numbers. The morning ratios spiked when compared to the afternoon. His morning-fasting blood sugars were to blame.

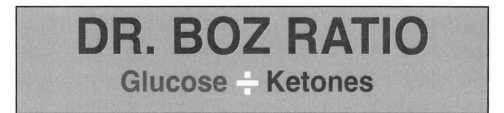

DR. BOZ RATIO
Glucose ÷ Ketones

That extra squeeze of morning cortisol popped liver glycogen like wringing a sheet of bubble wrap. Glucose flooded his system as it exited the storage.

How long would his spiked morning glucose continue?

Crystalized Glycogen

Have you ever lost a bag of brown sugar to the dark bottom corner of your pantry; then upon discovery you realized it had crystallized into a brick? Stored glycogen acted like this.

If David had filled his glycogen bubbles yesterday, only to empty them hours later, he would have found flexible, squishy, plump glycogen-bubbles. His older glycogen bubbles, trapped behind a thick coat-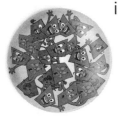ing of insulin, crystallized. These crystallized glycogen-bubbles not only hardened David's liver, they spun free-radicals into orbit, and aged his body.

David smoldered on the edge of diabetes before he summoned ketones to the rescue. His liver held so much stored sugar that fasting for a dozen days surely would not empty it. Two weeks of salt and water might get rid of 90% of his bubbles. The final 10% morphed from bubbles to marbles. Inside the liver lurked the oldest, hardest, most destructive fuel.

The drop in David's insulin over the first five steps of the ketoCONTINUUM popped the first ten percent of his glycogen bubbles. During that same time, he opened the first layer of stored fat-energy. Ketones unzipped from chains of freed fat. This recent phase of elevated morning blood sugars irritated him. David coped by reminding himself that those elevated sugars represented recently destroyed glycogen. As long as blood ketones were present, he would prevail.

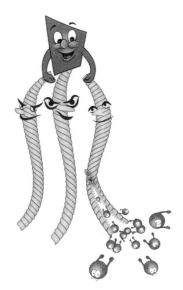

Morning Cortisol Delivers a Meal of Glucose
... without eating.

The following week, David received bad news. His sister, Aunt Know-It-All, called to tell him that their older sister had received the diagnosis of Alzheimer's. She lived on the East-Coast, and it had been a couple of years since he saw her. Their frequent and lively phone chats had dwindled. He recalled how unsettled their recent conversations made him feel. She repeatedly asked the same questions, and could not connect to the visit the way she used to. Her immediate family was struggling with what to do with her. She wasn't safe to be alone. A deep sadness weighed on David. Her situation was not uncommon. Several of David's associates had been down that path in recent years. "Once the brain goes," he said to his wife in a gloomy voice. "Their lives get rough."

Driving home from the studio that evening David wondered how the ketogenic diet might help her. He knew she wouldn't be able to endure the keto-journey by herself, and wondered if her kids could do it with her. "Was it even worth it?" he thought. "Was her brain too damaged to try?" Thoughts of his sister made David restless. He comforted himself with macadamia nuts. He was unaware that he ate more than he had planned to and muttered to himself, "At least I didn't eat the entire bag."

The next morning his blood sugar was 122—his highest since starting ketoCONTINUUM #7. That feedback was a clear message: NO LATE NIGHT SNACKS. Morning fasting glucose became David's reality check. As much as he didn't like testing, his results reflected the sum of two things: Morning blood sugar before cortisol PLUS the blood sugar released because of cortisol. Eating those keto-friendly nuts late in the day boosted his pre-cortisol sugars the next morning. Poor sleep kept his cortisol high throughout the night. Adding his scheduled jolt of cortisol to already elevated morning blood-sugars meant double trouble. There was no avoiding the fact that the earth spun around on its axis daily. The rising sun whacked David's brain to produce the same dose of cortisol every morning. But unlike the sunrise, his evening snack was avoidable. They were the devil, just as restless sleep was. Both ruined his keto-chemistry.

David needed to empty lots of glycogen and an equal number of his fat cells. By monitoring his numbers, he quickly learned what worked for him and aimed for a Dr. Boz Ratio of less than 80. Like many, he did not feel hungry when he awoke. Once he saw how much glucose circulated, he understood why he felt no hunger. His cortisol level each morning was responsible for this sense of satiety. Cortisol released as much glucose from his liver as eating a full meal. The exodus of glycogen flooded pine-needle-fuel throughout his body every sunrise. Without one stinkin' bite, his cells feasted. Cortisol supplied David with sugar-energy for nearly five hours, which he burnt through without much hunger. His busy morning schedule distracted his mind away from thoughts of food and kept the cravings low.

David crusaded on his mission to pulverize his glycogen bubbles. His slight improvements along the ketoCONTINUUM lowered insulin and his Dr. Boz Ratio. Each dip emptied a few more. Keto-chemistry also unlocked more fat cells. A steady stream of ketones came each day of 23:1, and fat-based hormones washed away most of his hunger. Immediate feedback from his finger-pricks helped David conquer this new skill. For 23 hours, he ceased all intake of calories and sweeteners; that meant - no snacking, only black coffee or water. David was surprised at the power a crystal of salt had in suppressing his desire for food. His ketogenic chemistry mimicked fasting while strengthening his metabolism. Each 23-hour fast acted like a workout for his mitochondria. When his blood sugar rose during fasting times, he knew it meant he'd hit a lower notch of insulin and had unlocked more glycogen.

David wanted to reverse his diabetes completely; he wanted it gone - immediately. Fasting for a whole week to chisel away the old, crusted glycogen crossed his mind. I dissuaded that idea, explaining, "Your chronic problem took time to form. A one-time-marathon fast won't magically fix it. Chip away at your messy liver with ketoCONTINUUM #7. For faster results, advance to ketoCONTINUUM #8 or stress your liver with ketoCONTINUUM #9."

Advanced 23:1

Move your meal closer to the highest sunlight

	ketoCONTINUUM	WHO DOES THE WORK?	TEST	GUIDELINES	NEXT STEP
BASELINE METABOLISM	#8. Advanced 23:1/OMAD	PSYCHOLOGY - USE TRIBE.	BLOOD STRIPS	Move eating-hour within 11 hours following sunrise to match your circadian rhythm.	Record the Dr Boz Ratio first thing in the morning. Repeat before eating.

David acquiesced against his idea of a week-long fast. He stayed at 23-hours of fasting per day. Except for Sundays, David ate his meal in the evenings around 7 PM with Kat and John. He had tried talking them into eating an hour earlier. This shift in their schedule had the unintended effect of sparking a conflict between all of them. David had advanced solo along the keto-CONTINUUM. His wife was at her goal weight and felt good at ketoCONTINUUM #5. She saw no reason to advance further. John also used the guardrails of keto-CONTINUUM #5. Containing his food consumption within those 8 hours was proving to be a challenge. Both John and Kat supported David to reverse his diabetes but bristled when he interfered with suppertime.

They did give it an all American try by eating at 6 PM instead of 7 PM, giving more free time between supper and bedtime. John and David both caught each other snacking more during that time. Their snack choices were bacon bits, cheese, or macadamia nuts, because the cupboards were pretty bare. David worked through that struggle. The key to his success orbited around keeping snacks out of his house. As he moved that mealtime further away from bedtime, he noticed another pleasant change occurred. He had quite a bit of energy after eating. Six months prior, his brain fueled solely from carbs. Eating late at night had helped him sleep, "I ate ice cream about an hour before bed and slept like a baby. If I skipped it, I could feel the hunger pains keep me awake. I was sure my body needed the sugar to fall asleep. It was like my sleeping pill — a bowl of ice cream."

Why did that sugar rush make him sleepy?

ANSWER: Swelling of his brain.

An insurgence of carbs added another dose of insulin to his already insulin-soaked system. He timed that bowl of ice cream just right. That burst of sugar topped off his brain with as much glucose as it could take. Along with the glucose flowed the water molecules. The orchestration of rising glucose, chased by insulin, furthered the inflammation that chronically slowed David's mind. On a cellular level, that added wave acted just like being hit over the head. Snooze, he fell right asleep.

A closer look at his sleeping habits revealed his low quality of sleep. To an observer, it looked like sleep. To David, it felt like sleep. His eyes were closed, and he did not struggle to shut off his brain. Yet, that type of sleep mimicked a concussion. Electrodes tracing his brain waves looked like the sleep seen after drinking alcohol or a recent blow to the head. His swollen brain cells governed his depth and quality of sleep. Swelling prevented him from filing new memories or organizing his thoughts. His "fake" sleep prevented his brain from performing the daily repairs needed to keep depression away and ward off Alzheimer's.

David praised the keto diet for his improved vigor. His energy cycles had changed again after he started 23:1. Instead of the previous carb-slump, he found a rise in his energy after eating. One obstacle to his six o'clock suppertime was his bountiful energy at bedtime. The quality of his sleep deserved just as much praise thanks to keto chemistry. Deep sleep gradually repaired his neurons each night. He no longer used the destructive swelling triggered by sugar to suck the hypnotic fog into his brain. He slept every night without that mini-concussion.

On Sundays, David's extended family gathered for a meal in the mid-afternoon. This weekly shift in his meal provided an easy comparison and taught him quite a bit. For starters, his post-meal energy hit during daylight hours. Eating before 3 PM stoked his furnaces—no afternoon slump. Reliable energy lasted until sunset. He fell asleep quickly at bedtime on Sundays.

Next, his Monday morning numbers looked fantastic compared to the rest of the week. The first time David's morning blood sugar registered in the 80s came on a Monday, sixteen hours since his last bite.

After several attempts at inching his evening meal earlier, he gave up on that approach. He broached the topic with Kat and John about eating his one meal per day before 3 PM for a whole week. He quickly assured them that he would be doing this on his own. They did not need to join him. Reluctantly, they agreed to eat their evening meal without him for the next week.

This change to his schedule caused ripples in other areas. Eating before 3 PM meant he would eat around 2 o'clock. This proved harder than it sounded. He tried eating at the local restaurant, but not all restaurants served folks in the middle of the afternoon.

A couple of days, he ate leftovers that he reheated at the office. Unlike his previous packed lunch of cheese and pepperoni, his 23:1 meal disrupted the workflow.

To avoid the temptation of John and Kat's evening meal, he stayed at the office until after supper.

His productivity stepped up nicely for those days, and his extended concentration all but eliminated his "someday" stack of paperwork. Twenty-three hours per day without food fixed something. Moving his hour of eating into his afternoon added more power. He picked up momentum like a massive train, gently tracking down a 100-mile-hill. Slowly, his metabolism strengthened. Today's success stacked on to yesterday's. He burned ketones like an 1850 steam locomotive burned logs. The force felt unstoppable.

David's 7-day experiment showed him the impact of eating in the afternoon. Eating mid-day flaunted the best numbers his metabolism had ever measured. His Dr. Boz Ratio dropped below 50 the final four days of his experiment with morning fasting blood sugars all under 100. He was delighted with the mathematical side of this experiment. The social side was not fun.

He ate alone. He worked late alone. He scheduled a couple of business meetings over his mid-afternoon meal. The pattern of eating was not ideal for clients, his business, or his wife. The stress of not sharing his wife and son's eating-time created tension at home that was not worth it. Socially, this wasn't sustainable. He liked being married. He enjoyed spending time with his wife. He loved the food his son prepared.

Eating between 2-3 worked for David's metabolism, but sent an earthquake through other parts of his life.

Sharing this struggle with his wife, they compromised with mealtime in the middle: 5 PM. For four weeks, they agreed to have supper at 5 PM. Trouble hid around the corner.

Supplement Your Mistakes

That steam-engine momentum carried David through a terrain of temptations, but then he stumbled. He succeeded for a bit, and then carbs doused his blaze. Not birthday-cake carbs. Not mashed-potatoes-and-pancakes kind of carbs. Snacking carbs. They sort of snuck back onto his menu. The 5 o'clock meal only worked if Kat and David dined out. The first week they left their office in time to be eating by 5 PM. The restaurant options were pretty good, but little compromises started to happened.

David knew that his meal choices mattered; timing mattered even more.

At the end of week two, they weren't getting out of the office on time. Several events planned for the evening hours tugged them out of their routine even further. Somehow the 5 o'clock meal was eaten at 7 PM.

His morning numbers tanked. Ignoring his reality by not pricking his finger didn't work either.

At a couple of gigs, he threw caution to the wind and just ate "normal." The next morning he could feel it. Like a hangover, his brain regressed to the foggy state of mind. His ghastly mental performance haunted him for days after he fell off the carb-wagon. Compared to Day 1 of his story, he felt amazing. Yet, relative to his recent improvements, his brain's downward shift felt like the eternal burden of king Sisyphus, whose punishment was to roll a boulder uphill - forever.

A pattern of derailments had infiltrated David's success. It all started with a few bites of food outside his one-hour eating window. Consuming an evening meal, instead of his standard afternoon meal followed. This one-two punch concluded with an evening binge. The morning after a community fundraiser, he felt a literal hangover. One taste of a carbohydrate-delight led to a full-blown crash. After two servings of carrot cake, he finally stapled his lips shut at 11 PM. The next morning his blood sugar was 113, and his ketones limped in at 0.3. His #DBR had been in the 40s for the past five days, but that morning his ratio soared over 300. It killed his productivity, like dumping a barrel of water onto his fiery logs. Crash! There went all his momentum. So powerful. So confident. So strong. Now all gone. Vaporized.

He longed for that momentum again. The ambition to recreate his keto-metabolism daunted him. Ugh. Regret added to his suffering. He pouted and moped about grumbling to himself, "Why did you do that? One bite is never just one bite."

It took three days of perfect choices to lift him back to his power-zone again. Temptations rarely bothered him when he was in his rhythm, but the enemies popped up everywhere after he'd crashed. Cravings spun through his mind, and his Dr. Boz Ratios bounced up over 150 for a couple of days. His confidence wilted. Yuck.

As awful as that carb-hangover felt, he pledged, "Never again." But it happened again—another stumble.

This time, David supplemented his stumble. He awoke the morning after late-night eating with friends. The telltale sign of a sluggish mind prompted him to stir ketones-in-a-can into a glass of water. The first swallow puckered his cheeks. Too strong. He threw in a few ice cubes and added some heavy cream. A twist in the blender left his taste buds much happier. He'd been warned not to guzzle it, but wanted to feel better. He drank the rest within minutes and headed to work. Minutes later, it hit. Like a tidal wave plunging through his gut, a sudden urge to empty the liquid from his backside became priority number one. He swung the car into the gas-stop and squeezed his butt cheeks as he scurried to the toilet. Whew. That was close.

Relieved, he strolled back to the car when another unexpected, yet unmistakable sensation hit his brain. This one he knew and liked. Drinking ketones-in-a-can poured lighter-fuel onto his drenched logs. It re-ignited his fire. The warmth of burning logs awoke his brain. Wow. The colors brightened. His awareness improved. The steam-engine had turned back on as the smile stayed plastered to his face for hours.

David had never used drugs, but this must be the sensation they chased. Euphoria flowed through his day. Life felt jubilant. Maybe he appreciated the joy after years spent in a grey fog. Maybe his depression had been more profound than he admitted. Perhaps this was how happy people always felt. He didn't care. He wanted it to stay.

David found better ways to handle the evening temptations. He learned to eat a high-fat meal before entering any event at night. When fat-based hormones pulsed on his side, he resisted that first bite. He also kept supplements stashed in the secret compartment of his travel bag: Ketones-In-A-Can, Ketones-In-A-Capsule, or MCT C8:C10 soft-gels.

Powdered Ketones: At first, he added powdered ketones BEFORE his evening event. He slowly sipped on them to avoid diarrhea. The exogenous ketones lasted 2-3 hours. Getting the timing right took some planning. He sipped on his iced mixture while he set up and then tried to keep the drink near him for most of the night. Sometimes, it just didn't work to keep sipping on ketones while he worked. The extra ketones suppressed his hunger, and he denied the temptations. Even when carrot cake flirted with his nostrils in an attempt to seduce his tastebuds, he stopped at a few bites instead of a few pieces.

Ketones-in-a-capsule worked somewhat similarly. These capsules filled with powdered exogenous ketones had no flavor and no sweeteners. He stashed half-a-dozen capsules in his bag. If he didn't have the privilege of mixing his drink, he could swallow 4-5 capsules to get out of a pinch.

MCT C8:C10: David learned that the MCT C8:C10 increased ketones for 5 to 6 hours. If he swallowed several soft-gels on his way to an event, he handled the temptations better. The timing was much more forgiving too. If powdered ketones burned like lighter fluid, then MCT C8:C10 oil burned like kerosene. Instead of the flash-flamed energy of BHB, MCT C8:C10 oil doubled the ketone production flowing from his liver for hours. If he used both MCT soft-gels and Ketones-In-A-Capsule, he was protected. No cravings. No tiredness.

Most of the time, David used no supplements. His liver made far more ketones than any supplement could deliver. However, he learned that having resources on hand lifted him back on track after a stumble.

Chapter 28

KETOCONTINUUM #9

36-HOUR FAST

At ketoCONTINUUM #8 [Advanced 23:1], David's Dr. Boz ratios sank under 100 as his morning ketones rose. He found uniquely creative ways to reject temptations. For example, when offered carbs, he responded, "I'm allergic to carbs. My doctor says I can't have that." or, "Some people are gluten-free. I'm carb-free." He used the word "N-O" - <u>as a complete sentence</u>, attended the local keto support group, and kept his coffee black. Supplements also pulled him out of the ditch when he stumbled.

David pushed himself into ketoCONTINUUM #8 to reverse his diabetes and achieve ideal body weight. The Dr. Boz Ratio measured his metabolism and tracked his progress. His persistence rewarded him with another ten-pound weight loss. The change in his outward appearance

was so striking that even casual acquaintances complimented him. The positive attention toward his health encouraged him and reinforced his behavior.

After two weeks at ketoCONTINUUM #8, David's ratios dropped under 80 as his army of mitochondria
strengthened. However, he soon learned that ketoCONTIN-
UUM #8 proved to be a difficult challenge. The social limitations of keeping 23 hours devoid of food peppered his
resolve. His desire for optimal health conflicted with his
marriage, business, identity, and extended family. David's
evening meal drifted from 5 to 6 PM, and before long, the
whole crew ate at 7 o'clock again. David regressed back to
the eating window found between ketoCONTINUUM #6
and #8. David's recent attempt to restrict food to one hour
a day had emptied his social capital with Kat. They agreed
that a six-hour eating window was a better compromise—
all things considered. When David opened his eating window from one hour to six hours, his glucose inched upwards while his ketones settled between 0.7-1.4. Most of his
Dr. Boz Ratios that were in the 80s soon returned to the
default triple digits.

His invigorated metabolism did not disappear after
he stepped down from ketoCONTINUUM #8 to #6, but his
body's repairing system slowed its pace. The ketoCONTIN-
UUM offered four options for David's daily, or baseline eating pattern. Baseline ketoCONTINUUM's #5, #6, #7 and #8
promoted longevity, improved health, and lowered insulin
levels. However, these levels differed in the speed in which
they reversed his insulin resistance. While ketoCONTINUUM
#5 had the slowest rate of correction, ketoCONTINUUM #8
held the medal for having the quickest.

Although ketoCONTINUUM #6 fit much better for his lifestyle, he wondered how long it would take to completely reverse his diabetes. To correct his average blood sugars, further pressure needed to be applied to his mitochondria. He had learned that an A1C of 4.6% calculated an average blood sugar of 85 mg/dL [4.7 mmol/L]. But his last measurement averaged a blood sugar near 108 mg/dL [6.0 mmol/L].

David had another option to advance his health. This one would stress his metabolism like a sprinter instead of a long-distance runner.

	GOAL	Keto Month 3	Keto Month 15	Keto Month 25
A1C	**<4.6**	5.4	5.5	5.3
Average Blood Sugar [mg/dL]	**<85**	108	111	105
Average Blood Sugar [mmol/L]	**<4.7**	6.0	6.2	5.9

	ketoCONTINUUM	WHO DOES THE WORK?	TEST	GUIDELINES	NEXT STEP
STRESSING METABOLISM	#9. 36 Hour Fast	**PSYCHOLOGY - USE TRIBE.**	**BLOOD STRIPS**	Fast for 36 hours. No calories. No sweeteners. Start in evening as to use 2 cycles of sleep during the 36 hours.	Begin fast after evening meal. DANGER: If on blood pressure meds or blood sugar lowering meds. ASK YOUR DOCTOR.

ketoCONTINUUM #9: 36 Hour Fast

Why would anyone go for 36 hours without eating? Most importantly, why would David take the next step up to ketoCONTINUUM #9 after the tensions from ketoCON-TINUUM #8 had emptied his social capital?

ANSWER: Because his numbers said so.

David never imagined pricking his finger a few months prior. Nor had he imagined going 36 hours without eating. Much like the moment a lancet darted through his skin to check his blood sugar, the idea of fasting was not his. He did not want to fast any more than he wanted to check blood sugars. But that's exactly what he did when he chose ketoCONTINUUM #9.

After hearing the benefits of the 36-hour fast, David agreed that the "sprint" analogy of a fast better suited his current situation.

I broached this subject by explaining to David that thirty-six hours is only one day.

Yes. Not one and a half days - it's ONE DAY.

The method was this: Place 36-hours without food over two nights of sleep. This meant eight hours the first night, plus eight hours the second night. Strategically utilizing 16 hours of the fasting-time during his sleeping hours left one day of fasting. David needed to flex his fasting skills from sunrise to sunset. That's it.

David recalled a story from the keto support group. A widow began the ketogenic way of eating several months after her husband had died. The anniversary of his death approached. She shared her plans to fast and pray through this difficult time. As the lady endured the pain of remembering her husband's death, she fasted for 72 hours. Each time a wave of sadness chained her spirit, she prayed. She reported a near-absence of hunger during those 72 hours. The woman chuckled that before her husband's death, she never missed a meal. He only known her as a carb-loving woman. Successfully denying food for 72 hours would have killed her before keto. Ironically, she drew strength in fasting as she endured the painful memories from a year ago. In short, a highly motivated reason for fasting helps to endure this temporary tribulation. This goes back to the earlier process we did in 'Discovering your WHY.'

For thousands of generations, prayer and fasting have been linked together. Fasting and prayer share many similarities. They both orbit around rituals designed to help people push through difficult seasons of life. Often first-time fasters go the distance alone, similar to the first time someone prays. As they mature in their fasting skills and confidence, they invite others to join. Like prayer, our strength multiplies when fasting with others.

David had a lifetime of prayer. Fasting intimidated him, yet the challenge stirred a little excitement. As he considered his first fast, David wondered how he could mentally frame his fast towards a greater purpose. His oldest sister came to mind. A diagnosis of cancer had compounded her memory problems. He pledged to himself that when a pang of hunger hit, he would start with salt, and pray for his sister as the salt crystals dissolved inside his mouth.

David selected a day to fast that overflowed with busyness. He built a checklist that would distract his mind away from food. His evening meal with his family was as usual. He officially began his fast after taking his last bite at 6:15 PM. He then retired to bed that night without sharing with his family that he was fasting.

Months of navigating his new eating choices taught him the value of "Head down. Mouth Shut." This slogan did not refer to his eating pattern. This mantra guided him on the best way to test out a new eating idea. Involving others in a new food ritual created drama. Stirring their opinions felt overwhelming — too heavy. Besides, David wasn't sure he could fast for 36 hours. He chose to go it alone the first time around and see what happened.

David awoke the next morning and prepared his black coffee as usual. Breakfast had long faded from his morning routine. He put a couple of tablespoons of salt crystals into a small tin and slid it into his pocket. While reading the morning news, he shared a few highlights regarding his busy schedule for the day. He then told his wife and son that he'd scheduled a 90-minute magnesium Float Spa that night at 6 PM. He would be on his own for supper.

The first wave of hunger hit around the time he usually ate, 2:00 PM. David checked his pocket for his tin filled with salt and announced he would be back in 15 minutes. He burst out the side door, and a crisp South Dakota wind filled his first breath. He cornered the building as he popped several salt crystals into his mouth. The tip of his tongue rolled the salt against the back of his teeth. Saliva poured in as he prayed for intercession for his sister, "Hail Mary, Full of Grace, The Lord be with Thee." His prayer continued as he walked. Twice more, he added the salt. In under 10 minutes, he returned to the studio, feeling enlightened. He wasn't sure who or what deserved the credit, but he felt great. His blood ketones offered proof when the number read 1.7. That's an excellent number for him. Another wave of hunger washed through David's body at 4:30 PM. Again, he excused himself and repeated his salty-Hail Mary-walking ritual. Success! The hunger evaporated.

As he finished out the final edits of the day, he looked forward to the float spa. "Vacation in an hour," rang through his mind. That wasn't quite how he felt the first time he soaked in magnesium. The experience left him outside his comfort zone. For starters, most people floated naked. David took his swim trunks. Several in the keto group raved at the experience. On his first float, he thought the oval-shaped pod holding the saltwater looked like a space-age machine. The pod had stretched to twice the size of his bathtub as blue light shimmered through the eight inches of water. A domed lid hinged over the aquatic coffin. David followed instructions and rinsed off in the shower before placing wax earplugs tightly into his ears. He sat down into the pod and wondered when the floating started. He closed the lid, trapping in the blue light and shutting out the darkness from the rest of the room. He played with the controls for music and light. His anxiety rose as he trusted the prerecorded announcement, "Lay down, and you will float."

Indeed, he floated. The first float left him wide-eyed for the first half. Eventually, he embraced the darkness and silence by dialing off the lights and sound. This time he anticipated the sensory-deprived reset. No sound. No light. Just floating on top of the water; alone with his thoughts. A 90-minute vacation.

David reflected to the Friday afternoon before starting this keto way of eating. His thoughts bounced along the timeline since then. The weight loss. Better sleep. Clearer focus. Happier. He was definitely more optimistic. Images of magnesium seeping into his body calmed him. He returned to the prayers for his sister as he floated away inside the darkness. Somewhere along with those thoughts, he drifted to sleep.

David entered the house after 8 PM that night. Magnesium therapy worked like a hypnotic charm. As advertised, he felt relaxed. His mind smoothly shifted to thoughts of going right to bed. He had completed 26 hours of his 36-hour fast. Ten hours to go.

David chatted with his wife about his floatation experience as the smell from supper hit his nose. His proximity to the refrigerator pulled his thoughts towards the food. His nose and mind betrayed his intentions not to enter the kitchen. He could feel his vulnerability rising. "Go to bed. GO STRAIGHT TO BED." He started to hear the words other group members said. "Do not enter the kitchen. Stay away. Go to bed."

With every purpose-filled drop of willpower, he walked away from the kitchen towards his bedroom. As he slid between the sheets, David felt empowered. He won.

A Night For Ketones

Sleep came quickly that night. David sunk into such a deep sleep that he failed to hear his wife come to bed. Was it the magnesium that soothed his nerves and relaxed his muscles? Maybe the extra Hail Mary's had settled his soul. Or was it those mighty ketones that swept away his aches and pains of inflammation?

3:30 AM, a switch snapped. Without warning, his eyelids abruptly opened to their fullest extent. David was awake. Not groggy. Not restless. AWAKE. Not even four shots of espresso had delivered this intense alertness so quickly. One minute ago, he slept soundly. Now, the opposite.

David recalled the testimony from a guy at group that fasted for a week counting down to Easter. He practiced low-carb eating most of the year and pressed his metabolism for the week preceding Easter. On the third or fourth day of his fast, he could not sleep. This wasn't merely a struggle of an insomniac. His brain functioned with a 100% charge, and there was no shutting it off. The cause: his ketones had launched into the 3.0 range.

David rushed to check his ketones. He was right! His blood glucose was 77 [4.2] and his ketones hit his all-time record at 2.6. A Dr. Boz Ratio of 29. His metabolism had just leveled up!

His glucose dropped, and ketones soared. He had oodles of energy, especially for the predawn hour. Returning to bed was a laughable idea. David wanted to use this tidal wave of ketones to celebrate. Then he remembered, no one knew he'd fasted.

He sat wondering when the last time he awakened before dawn with an outburst of energy. Maybe never. Middle of the night awakenings for pain or even for hunger regularly occurred before ketones bathed over his nerves. Those awakenings had led to a carb-snack in the darkness to quiet his brain back to sleep. Not this time. The opposite effect traveled through his body now. He had no pain, no hunger, and lots of energy.

The clock read 4AM. David considered taking a walk. It had been years since he strolled the neighborhood before sunrise. A walk could use up some of those ketones. They were fuel, and he had lots of it right now. Exercising during a fast had been talked about at the group. Apparently, it wasn't that awful.

David grabbed a hat, gloves, and a flashlight. He walked for almost an hour. As the sun crested the morning, the final minutes of his 36 hours approached. David felt a natural high. He was going to make it. The energy, the walk, and the ketones created the perfect combination.

Wash, Rinse, Repeat

David made it! He stopped all calories and sweeteners for 36 hours. He surged his metabolism, emptied another layer of old glycogen bubbles, and unlocked a new fat cell section. David waited for Kat to awaken and made eggs for breakfast. As he shared his fasting experience with his wife, he admitted that he wasn't hungry. Not even a little. He ate fried eggs with some bacon and enjoyed the first morning meal he'd had in weeks. If David wasn't hungry, then why eat? "Because it was time to eat," he said with a laugh. The whole experience blew David's thinking wide open.

His Dr. Boz Ratio stayed under 90 the four days following his fast. All of his morning fasting glucose numbers were under 100, and his ketones ranged from 1.1-1.6. In addition to those numbers, he felt more confident in his ability to say NO.

The rest of the week, David resumed his baseline metabolism of ketoCONTINUUM #6. He easily kept his eating window under eight hours. Most days, he tucked food into a six-hour window. Somedays, without even trying, he closed the window even further — to four hours. Eager to fast again and proselytize the benefits, he invited his family to try it. No takers. They were supportive but not prepared to join him.

David shared his experience at the keto support group. His success entranced others in the support group, as well as inspired those teetering on the decision whether to fast, or not. Seeing their attraction, David warned, "This would not have turned out so favorable had I fasted two months ago. My metabolism is much stronger than it used to be. I now understand the importance of practicing a baseline metabolism for weeks before fasting."

He was right. Fasting super-charged David's metabolism. Had he revved his system too soon, he would have failed. He succeeded because he did not launch a fast from his crippled body found on Day 1.

"Don't fast until you've been at your baseline metabolism for four weeks," he warned. "Don't fast if you take blood-pressure-lowering medications. Don't fast if you take blood-sugar-lowering medications."

David's eating pattern alternated between fasting and restricted-eating. He said "No" for a pocket of time. Then he resumed the time-restricted eating that matched his life. This blend fit socially and metabolically for him.

The next fast was easier for David. The early hour awakening sparked him out of bed again at the 32-hour mark. This time he agreed to resume eating when he felt hungry. He made it 42 hours before a wave of hunger hit. Surprisingly, adding those few extra hours of fasting fit better in his schedule than the 36-hour fast did. Morning meals had become a rarity in his world. As he stretched toward noon before eating, he matched up with his wife, lunch meetings, and desire to eat.

After each fast, David won. Each restriction depleted his glycogen and opened up more fat cells. This back and forth combination between his baseline metabolism and fasting made great strides towards reversing David's diabetes.

He wasn't there yet, but victory lay ahead.

WARNING: Fasting is NOT for everyone

Do not fast for 36 hours without supervision if you take medication for blood pressure or diabetes. Do not fast for 36 hours until you are keto adapted.

Folks with flowing ketones race to reverse chronic health problems. Galloping into a 36-hour fast too soon can buck you off the path to recovery. They crash in the middle of the night. Not a metaphorical crash, a literal crash. Their head crashes against the floor.

They flexed their metabolism and ketones rose while glucose lowered. In addition, their circulating blood volume dropped. They'd wrung out every droplet of inflammation from their body. Like David, they reached a new low for blood glucose during the final hours of that fast. Their dip in glucose left fewer molecules of water in their blood. Less water in the blood vessels resulted in lower blood pressure.

Healthy people compensate when their circulating fluid decreases. The muscles tracing their blood vessels squeeze down and reduce the size of those hoses. Many modern blood pressure medications manipulate those tiny muscles around the arteries of the body. If you take blood pressure medication and fast, be warned. Ask your doctor to hold the blood pressure medications during the fast.

Yes. Tell your doctor you are planning a 36-hours fast. When you pick your doctor up off the floor, ask what she recommends to do with the blood pressure medication. If you're worried about having this conversation with your provider, explain that it's for spiritual reasons. Then be sure to pray at least once during your fast.

Own the responsibility to look at your blood pressure. Blood pressure medications lower the pressure. Fasting lowers the pressure too. Combining them can lead to a head injury. Fasting improves your health. A head injury is the opposite of improved health.

The same warning goes for medications that lower blood sugar. I do not give my diabetics permission to fast for 36 hours until we remove nearly all of their diabetic medications.

Chapter 29

DAVID'S AUTOPHAGY

Following the ketoCONTINUUM, David reached his new normal. Eating fat, pricking fingers, and fasting happened without siphoning all of his attention. With a little planning, he successfully fasted about once a week. David scheduled his fasts based on social pressures. His success pivoted on how much the choice not to eat affected the people he loved. His 36-hour fast sometimes lasted 45 hours. Each span of time without food enhanced his metabolism, his confidence to say NO, and mostly his faith. When not fasting, David limited his eating to a four or five-hour window of time.

David's extra body-fat melted away week after week. So did his skin tags, wrinkles, and sunspots. His wife wondered if he started using colored shampoo.

His dingy, grey hair shined with more color. Was that possible?

Autophagy means 'to eat thyself.'

In 2016, Yoshinori Ohsumi won the Nobel Prize for explaining this phenomenon called autophagy. Ohsumi explained how our body degrades and recycles damaged or old cellular components. It removes misfit proteins cluttering inside the cells of an aging body. Autophagy is a normal process where your body 'eats thyself.'

As fat evaporated from his body, the lines defining his muscles returned. David knew losing weight correlated with improving his health. It went without mentioning that he preferred losing *fat* from his body, not muscle. David learned that autophagy meant removing proteins from the body. He assumed that meant losing muscle. If autophagy destroyed the muscle, David wanted nothing to do with it. He had made the common mistake of interchanging the word protein with muscle.

David's *amino acids* stitched together to make proteins. His *proteins* then strung together to make fibers. Those *fibers* then ganged up to make his muscles, tendons, and ligaments. Specialized protein-fibers arranged themselves in honeycomb formation to shape the cartilage of his nose. Proteins whisked into threads crisscrossing within his cells to provide their shape. Other unique proteins linked together to form the near-invisible slime lining the inside tunnel of his blood vessels. Some gelled together to create the protective grease inside David's guts. The transparent cling-wrap that once held David's fat in the jolly-center of his tummy came from sheets of protein. The dimples puckering David's skin into cellulite, that's protein too.

After his proteins expired, they lingered throughout his body until autophagy recycled them. Autophagy snipped his strands of defective, inferior proteins into amino acids and *reused* the components. Without autophagy, David's cells looked older, wrinkled, and ragged. Autophagy smoothed and straightened crooked cell membranes and restored chromosome telomere length. Unlike the drugstore's anti-aging potions, each trigger of autophagy improved his cells' deepest layers. David's recycling process "ate himself" to reshuffle proteins into youthful, flexible, healthy-looking replacement cells. In essence, he swept away his age.

Remember, ketosis is not a diet. It's chemistry. As long as David kept his chemistry keto, he won.

David's fear of lost muscle mass was right. Muscle breakdown was against the rules. Especially for folks who have orbited the sun more than fifty times, "Ye who loses muscle, dies faster."

With keto-chemistry, David's weight loss ignited autophagy and reversed his age. Previously, when David and his son ate packaged food for a year, the recycling process of autophagy did not happen. Calorie-restriction in the absence of ketones sacrificed his muscles for those resources. Low-calories without keto-chemistry shrunk his muscles, slowed his brain, weakened his immune system, and dialed down his metabolism.

What was the difference? One used keto-chemistry, the other did not.

When David lost weight with packaged food, he used calories as his guide instead of chemistry. The packaged food delivered the perfectly calculated number of calories to lose weight. If that formula held the key to weight loss, David would have succeeded. Unfortunately, the program cut calories before fixing his endocrine system. Limited calories left his cells fighting for resources. A meager amount of calories without a storage bank of fatty hormones triggered his back up survival defense system, "Turn off the heat. Turn down the immune system. Brain cells, drop your function to 80%. Muscle cells, cut two-thirds of your motors. Shut them off, now!" These messages rang throughout David's body every starving day.

Even after throwing those packages into the garbage, his mitochondria whimpered along the edge of survival. David's starvation-chemistry scorched his health from inside his cells. He lost muscle cells during that fiasco and carried the burden of damaged metabolism for years. Without keto-chemistry, he replicated generations of broken cells. He copied the dents and worsened the cracks with each cell division. He limped away from his starvation diet with decreased power to his heart and a foggy brain. He could have prevented this had he restored his fat-based hormones first.

Autophagy Rescued Thick and Thin

David used the baseline ketoCONTINUUM to set the stage for a powerful reversal against his years of malnutrition. The size of his body failed to reflect his nourishment. David's obese size easily misled the assumption that he was over-nourished, not under-nourished.

Chronic inflammation swamped his cells. They lacked vital minerals and micronutrients needed for repair. The tight-junctions in his gut leeched unchecked nourishment into the drain. David blamed his age for his growing arthritis, poor sleep, and lagging energy. His damaged cells further betrayed him by allowing infections to enter without a fight. When his immune cells mounted a response to invading viruses or bacteria, his white blood cells lacked sufficient power and thus failed. Smoldering infections thrived inside his body as they gobbled up his best nutrients for their survival.

This cascade of mistakes crippled David. His broken defense stopped attacking some invaders, altogether. If he continued on this path, his cells would soon start to accidentally target his healthy cells. Yes, his own immune system could turn on him. The root of autoimmune dysfunction occurs when spy-white blood cells arise amongst the army of normal ones. The spies will attack the host instead of invaders. Messages from white blood cells get corrupted and mistakenly target the "good-guys." This error places the mark to kill on David's perfectly good cells. They aberrantly are programmed to destroy skin, thyroid, bowel, cartilage, blood vessels, muscles, or heart cells. The list could stretch as long as the list of tissues within his body. If the rogue system pecked away at his skin, we called it psoriasis, thyroiditis for thyroid attacks, lupus for blood vessels under siege, rheumatoid arthritis for the destruction of joints, and Crohn's or Ulcerative Colitis for bowels.

When the human immune system began destroying the person, one cell at a time, modern medicine threw the kitchen sink at the problem. Medical teams used steroids, immune modulators, pain meds, invasive surgery, and heavy metals. Radiologists offered radiation and oncologist infused chemicals to paralyze some cells while stimulating others. Gastroenterologists harvested poop from the healthy and squirted it into the bowels of ill patients.

These approaches failed to eliminate or reverse the core issue; it only slowed the progression. Reversal of autoimmune disorders only arrived on the back of ketones. Keto-chemistry sparked autophagy in David's immune system. The cells programmed to destroy his body depended upon his inflammation. Autophagy and ketones opposed his chronic grime and self-destruction.

Keto-chemistry repaired cells. A strict, well-formulated ketogenic diet reversed malnourishment in the obese and the skinny. Autophagy spun generations of new cells to seal the outpouring and stop the destruction from their immune system. Their body weight migrated toward healthy once their cellular injuries reversed. Scrawny ones eventually gained weight; plump ones shed it. The first step to reverse malnourishment was to eat fat. The second step required autophagy.

Dr Boz Ratio Predicted Autophagy

DR. BOZ RATIO
Glucose ÷ Ketones

Under 80: Might Get Autophagy
- Weight Loss

Under 40: Solid Chance of Autophagy
- Repair of Immune System

Under 20: Best Chance of Autophagy
- Goal for Cancer Patients

No blood test or biopsy proved when autophagy took place inside David's cells. Autophagic recycling of damaged proteins happened when he achieved ideal chemistry. It turned on and off based on David's chemical messages pulsating throughout his body. That preferred chemistry ignited the harvest of David's amino acids. The stale proteins in his leftover fascia, sagging tendons, lax ligaments, and unneeded blood vessels supplied ample resources. Empty fat cells, loose skin, and amino acids reshuffled into new proteins to repair and replace his damaged tissue.

David didn't know the difference between an amino acid and a free radical, but he knew something had worked. He looked different. His wrinkles softened, and his newly defined muscles flexed with youthful, toned skin. David hadn't imagined his fewer grey hairs. Photographs from the past year proved his reversed age.

The lower his Dr. Boz Ratio, the higher his chances of autophagy. The lower his Dr. Boz Ratio, the faster he gobbled up junky proteins and spat out valuable amino acids. Unlike his low-calorie starvation chemistry, high blood ketones protected his muscles from breaking down. Measuring his Dr. Boz Ratio gave David the confidence his muscles were safe from sacrifice. Keto chemistry ensured that he sacrificed his misfit proteins. That's autophagy.

A Dr. Boz Ratio under 20 practically guaranteed autophagy. However, that goal was tough for David to achieve. If his life depended upon it, he could reach that extreme, but why would he push that hard. Driving for that number destroyed too many sections of the rest of his life. Instead, David set a goal to hit a Dr. Boz Ratio of 40. This was a more reasonable goal for his situation. The more times he hit it, the faster he reversed his saggy skin, peppered-brain, and creaking joints.

When he followed ketoCONTINUUM #6 [Advanced 16:8.], his Dr. Boz Ratio hung around 150. Snacking sabotaged his progress, especially after sunset. Measuring his Dr. Boz Ratio put an end to that

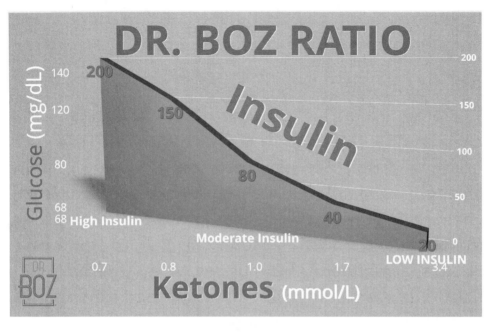

nibbling. Snitched food outside of his eating window jacked up his Dr. Boz Ratio. As his Dr. Boz Ratio decreased, his insulin regressed toward normal, and autophagy increased.

David's experiment at ketoCONTINUUM #8 pulled his ratios under 100. Limiting his calories to 60 minutes per day stressed his metabolism and exercised his mitochondria. Each day less glycogen nested in his liver, and more ketones swarmed his cells. His Dr. Boz Ratio ranged from 90-100 without exception. Every few days, the numbers notched down further. By the end of the second week, he satisfied his cellular hunger with stable, long-acting ketone-fuel and ratios in the 70s. Fasting for twenty-three hours daily flexed great numbers for David's metabolism. He also felt like he'd found a way to stretch time. Letting go of the number of times he ate opened up quite a bit of free time. He added two more hours to his day. He'd not realized how much time he spent thinking about food and planning his next meal.

ketoCONTINUUM #7 and #8 strained his mito-chondria as well as his marriage. It also meant he stepped away from social rituals rooted in eating. Even though, he had mastered how to eat keto while in the presence of others who weren't low-carb, fasting with them proved much harder. Sadly, too many social pressures pulled him back towards ketoCONTINUUM #6.

Even though he returned to the lesser metabolic stress of #6, his Dr. Boz Ratio stayed under 100. Some mornings it settled in the 80s despite expanding his eating window from 60 minutes to 4 to 5 hours. This ketoCONTINUUM fit his life.

Adding extended fasts to his baseline ketoCON-TINUUM further improved his metabolism. At the end of a 45-hour fast, his Dr. Boz Ratio decreased to his all-time-record of 29. The ratios trailing an extended fast rendered better numbers for days. Had he only mea-sured his morning fasting blood sugars, he'd have overlooked his improvements. His morning glucose readings hardly dropped. It was the rise in his ketones that made the most remarkable difference. Increasing them from 0.8 to 1.4 dropped his Dr. Boz Ratio by over a dozen points.

	ketoCONTINUUM	WHO DOES THE WORK?	TEST	GUIDELINES	NEXT STEP
STRESSING METABOLISM	#10. 36 Hour Fast without Celebration Meal	PSYCHOLOGY - USE TRIBE.	BLOOD STRIPS	After 36 hour fast, return to your normal pattern of eating without a splurge meal.	Offer a group fasting routine to others in your tribe. Fast together.
STRESSING METABOLISM	#11. 48 Hour Fast	PSYCHOLOGY - USE TRIBE.	BLOOD STRIPS	Fast for 48 hours. No calories. No sweeteners.	Safe to try twice a week. Unlike the 36-hour fast, this option keeps meals at the same time each day.

Brain Autophagy

On the day our story started, David's brain crept along like a slug on a dry sidewalk. Thirty years of bathing his mind in insulin clogged his circuits and slowed the signals. Chronic swelling and inflammation sent electrical sparks pinging around his grey matter. Free-radical electrons crashed into essential parts of his brain. The first few electrical farts bounced off of healthy cells causing minimal damage. David's youthful immune system squelched the rogue electrons into silence and rapidly mended any damage. Years of constant hare-brained electrons pestered his beautiful brain. Zaps of unexpected energy broke strands of DNA and aged his cells. Instead of healthy plump brain cells, some looked older than they should. Repeated blasts exposed more problems. These broken cells in David's brain eventually caused David's daily mental health struggles.

The curse of aging memory problems bombarded David's family history. His older sister lost her memory in her late 70s. His mother's memory faded her in her 80s. And several aunts and uncles had been robbed of retrievable thoughts in their last decade of life. Preventing this legacy depended upon David's ability to fix the cracks, wrinkles, and breaks inside his cells before they divided into a bigger problem. David was unaware that glucose-fed brain cells oozed an inflammatory byproduct that left clumps of plaque throughout his brain. Slimy proteins hovered around these brain-plaques and hardened each time his insulin surged. Through the years, these protein-plaques slowly added a layer on top of last season's grime. The trouble that brewed deep within the plaques of his neurons first started with inflammation. David's high insulin guaranteed the progression of his family's curse. Rubble cluttered within cells and neural spaces, further damaging his brain. Depending on the position of his piles of junk-proteins, David's future held the diagnosis of Parkinson's, Alzheimer's disease, dementia, or another age-related problem.

Becoming a real-life zombie worried David. Once his mind improved, he recognized that he'd had a problem. Before keto, he thought his brain worked fine, although his family would have argued otherwise. Ketone-chemistry siphoned the swelling out of his cerebrum and neutralized those wild electrons. He enjoyed improved energy, quicker memory, and a stable mood. Autophagy swept away the litter that accumulated within his brain. David's motivation came from the best brain performance of his life ... plus his fear of zombies.

Fast to Autophagy - Not to the Clock

David excelled using baseline metabolism keto-CONTINUUM #6 while fasting when his schedule allowed. Instead of measuring his length of fasting by the clock, David measured his success by how low his Dr. Boz Ratio sank during the fasts. Each fast emptied another layer of stored glucose, while ketoCONTINU-UM #6 prevented the return of excess glycogen. Each fast lowered his ratio quicker than the time before. The constant throttle using his baseline metabolism coupled with extended fasts, delivered visible improvements. Each fasting cycle reversed his age and strengthened his health. David won.

Chapter 30

ADVANCED METABOLIC BURSTS

F asting for 36 hours successfully sank David's Dr. Boz Ratios under 55. A block of time without food, combined with his baseline metabolism produced consistent numbers of autophagy. David's fasting skills matured; he stopped using time to measure the quality of his fast. Instead, he fasted until his metabolic goal was attained. The more fasting cycles he underwent the quicker he reached his goal. His spreadsheet containing a precise record of his Dr. Boz Ratios was private but *powerful*.

In a sense, his data offered a peek inside his mitochondria. He calculated his improvement. He progressed slowly, but the act of tracking his numbers delivered steady, confident improvement.

Each week at the keto support group, David watched participants ebb and flow along their keto-CONTINUUM. Some never participated long enough to "accidentally miss a meal." Others led the group with consistent number-driven progress as they healed from decades of chronic inflammation. ketoCONTINU-UM #12, the highest and ultimate level in the ketoCON-TINUUM program, beckoned David. He had his eye on the members who did that.

Gary, a 52-year-old man, had lost 100 pounds over the past year. Multiple Sclerosis was his dragon to slay. For years, he'd battled against it. Gary's brain had wandered into zombie-land before keto. At the start of keto-nutrition, he surrendered his job to a medical disability. He couldn't stay awake for more than a few hours before his brain simply shut down. It flickered on for a bit before dreamless slumber conquered him again. The entire room watched Gary's voyage as ketones, and weight loss restored his brain, and his hope.

Fasting for 72 hours each week, for eight consecutive weeks, was Gary's weapon to slay the MS beast. He had just reported to the room about his third week of ketoCONTINUUM #12 when David wondered aloud, "Should I fast for 72 hours?"

"Why?" I asked.

"To stress my metabolism."

"You already do that, David. Your autophagy numbers are solid. You've got a steady rhythm that fits into this season of your life. I wouldn't change a thing. Steady as it goes."

Months earlier, David's fat-built hormones had teetered on the edge of frustration. Since then, he had grown his whispering hormones to a victorious roar by eating fat and churning keto-nutrition through his body. The prerequisite for the 72-hour fast was a stream of ketones flowing from his liver. He had exercised his mitochondria into pretty good shape—his fat hormones circulated in healthy supply. Yet, David was shot down when he considered stepping up to the ultimate challenge of a 72-hour stress.

	ketoCONTINUUM	WHO DOES THE WORK?	TEST	GUIDELINES	NEXT STEP
STRESSING METABOLISM	#12. 72 Hour Fast	PSYCHOLOGY - USE TRIBE.	BLOOD STRIPS	Fast for 72 hours. No calories. No sweeteners.	When the timing is right, stress your metabolism with 8 weeks of a 72-hour fast. The rest of the week, return to your BASELINE METABOLISM. The best transitions happen through this challenge.

David had seen other keto-members fail when they jumped from ketoCONTINUUM #3 or #4 to the top bar of #12. That repeated mistake warned all those that watched them. But he wasn't at ketoCONTINUUM #4. He'd practiced his baseline metabolism for several weeks and was ready. The caution to stay away from the 72-hour fast bruised his pride. He was sure he could tackle the challenge. Why couldn't he join the elite fasters in the class?

ANSWER: He didn't need to. He needed to trust his Dr Boz Ratio—not the clock.

3 Advanced Stressors After Keto-Adaption

1:47 OMEOD: One Meal Every Other Day. This meant one satiating meal followed by 47 hours of fasting for two months.

Calorie-Restricted OMAD 23:1: Limit calories to under 900 in your solitary daily meal for two months.

ketoCONTINUUM #12: 72 hour fast: One 72-hour fast every week for eight consecutive weeks. For the remaining four days in the week, return to your preferred baseline metabolism.

These extreme stressors put forth robust improvements. But beware. These stressors don't fit into everyone's life.

1:47 OMEOD

OMEOD offered an eating pattern of **O**ne **M**eal **E**very **O**ther **D**ay. Like ketoCONTINUUM #8 [Advanced 23:1], the ideal time for that meal landed within 10 hours of sunrise. The closer the meal overlapped with the morning cortisol surge, the greater the benefit. Eating one meal every other day offers a very predictable schedule. This strict but stable rhythm tempted many to try it. Indeed, OMEOD rapidly evacuated fat, activated autophagy, and cranked up their metabolism. With 47 hours in between, they scheduled four satiating meals per week. For 60 minutes on Monday, Wednesday, Friday, and Saturday, they filled their bellies with ketogenic nourishment. Some people flourished with this plan. However, most fell victim to the inherent isolation as the schedule drew them away from their eating interactions. They hungered for relationships more than the food. By the end of week three, even introverts walked away from this plan. The metabolism created in the wake of OMEOD was incontestable, but rarely did they complete eight solid weeks of this schedule.

Calorie-Restricted 23:1

Another, advanced stressor limited calories and time. Using the schedule ketoCONTINUUM #8 [Advanced 23:1], they limited their keto-nutrition to less than 900 calories. Oncology teams used this protocol to maximize autophagy while pulverizing some of the most deadly cancers. Medical teams raced against the growth of cancers and applied the most powerful accelerator to the patients' metabolism. Success for these patients began with fat-based hormones in abundance. Keto-adaption was not a luxury all of these cancer patients had. However, it was required before the protocol could start. Once fat-adapted, patients were allotted 500 calories per day for the protocol's initial phase. Those first six weeks required careful supervision. Medical advisors stuffed vital nutrients into the limited calories eaten within that hour. Remarkable outcomes infused great hope into the cancer research field, but beware—don't do without medical supervision.

ketoCONTINUUM #12: 72 Hour Fast

The previous two options emerged in the scientific keto-literature and offered great promise. OMEAD and calorie-restricted 23:1 paled in comparison to the extensive literature surrounding the 72-hour fast. Although every step beyond ketoCONTINUUM #5 required fat-based hormones, none were as critical as ketoCONTINUUM #12. Without the support of the fatty endocrine system, the 72-hour fast did more damage than good. ketoCONTINUUM #12 marked the highest number on the continuum and the greatest level of metabolic stress. Like David, most never required this level of pressure. But when they did apply ketoCON-TINUUM #12, the reward was worth it.

Patients who reviewed and paid attention to their data unlocked the reason for their weight-reduction stall that occurred along the ketoCONTINUUM. A constant Dr. Boz Ratio over 100 guaranteed a plateau. Whether their goal was weight loss or autophagy, patients had to fire up their metabolism in order to push their Dr. Boz Ratio under 100. A quick study of David's chart revealed that most of his Dr. Boz Ratios were less than 100. His progress was slow but steady. And he was not experiencing a weight-loss stall.

If someone stalled at ketoCONTINUUM #4, it was a different puzzle to solve than a stall at ketoCONTIN-UUM #5. The apposed numbers, four and five, deceived people, "What is the difference, other than a single little step on the continuum?"

ANSWER: Fat-based hormones.

I cautiously and predictably watched patients stall if they rushed through the curriculum looking for the "magic elixir of ketones." Without the restoration of fat-based hormones, they would not be able to meet the longterm, chemical demands ahead. Ample fatty-hormones protected them from complications. Their presence almost guaranteed success.

Restored hormones carried David's metabolism forward. Once fat-based hormones flowed with abundance, he depended upon them. Even when bad habits snuck back into his evenings, these hormones carried David back to ketosis.

It had taken weeks of David's keto-chemistry to restore his dwindled endocrine system. But, once fat flowed along the endocrine vine, he relied on the presence of these hormones. Achieving the critical mass of these hormones protected David from missed steps. The gift of his ample, replenished supply meant it would take months of a bad habit to sink away. If David whimsically binged on carbs, his fat based hormones withstood the chemistry swing of that trip through the ditch. Practicing his baseline metabolism protected David. In his low-calorie, packaged-food diet, David never restored his fat-based hormones. One slip on that diet resulted in weeks of a setback. Not this time. His healthy supply of fat-based hormones protected against a bad day. Even during a weight loss stall, as long as he complied with one of the baseline metabolisms, he could readily accelerate his mitochondria and rely on his metabolism. keto-CONTINUUM #12 applied maximum metabolic stress.

David did not need any further metabolic stress yet. Others in the keto group did need that pressure applied to their metabolism. To rescue their metabolism, I instructed them to use eight weeks of 72-hour fasts to rev their mitochondria.

8 Weeks of ketoCONTINUUM #12

What will 8 weeks of ketoCONTINUUM #12 do?

-empty glycogen

-trigger autophagy

-ramp up norepinephrine

-spike growth hormone

-unlock the gift of fasting for a lifetime.

Empty Glycogen

Fasting for three days harbored a tipping point. Researchers tracked lean and obese patients who limited consumption to salt and water for 72-hours. Both sets of patients entered the fast from a standard diet, not in a state of ketosis. Like wringing a sheet of plastic bubble wrap, everyone popped glycogen bubbles in that block of time. Seventy-two hours with only salt and water, turned off their insulin and drained some sugar storage. Those patients without insulin resistance, most often found in the lean population, reached the bottom of their sugar-storage tank within the 72 hours. Obese patients with resistance to insulin did not.

"Doc, how long does it take to empty the glycogen bubbles from my liver?"

Answer: It depends upon the size of your liver and the state of your chemistry.

At the end of 72 hours, those with an empty liver were easy to spot. Test their blood glucose. The surest sign of an empty liver was a fasting blood sugar of 65mg/dl [3.6 mmol/L]. Livers with emptied glycogen-storage separated sharply from those with remaining glycogen. Without a stream of glucose unwinding from glycogen, their blood glucose hovered around 65.

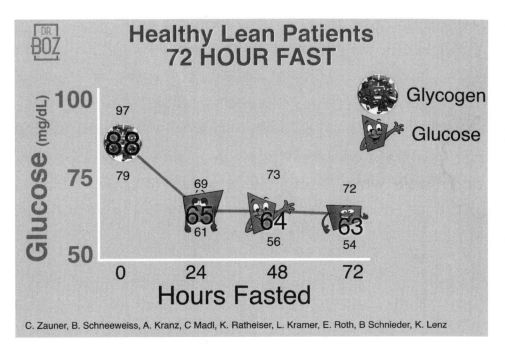

Healthy Lean Patients 72 HOUR FAST

C. Zauner, B. Schneeweiss, A. Kranz, C Madl, K. Ratheiser, L. Kramer, E. Roth, B Schnieder, K. Lenz

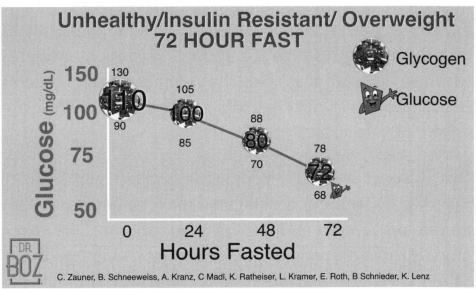

Unhealthy/Insulin Resistant/ Overweight 72 HOUR FAST

C. Zauner, B. Schneeweiss, A. Kranz, C Madl, K. Ratheiser, L. Kramer, E. Roth, B Schnieder, K. Lenz

Patients resistant to the clanging sound of insulin had blood sugars in the 70s-100s despite three days without calories. While their ketones surged on the second day of fasting, it took significantly longer to re-linquish the extra glucose. Severely insulin-resistant patients took over two weeks to hit the bottom of their storage. Their inflamed bodies held so much stored glycogen that their supply lasted up to ten times longer than lean patients. That's impossibly way too long to fast.

The time it took to hit glucose in the mid-60s varied from person to person. If patients started fasting with a liver overflowing with glycogen, their sugar supply took longer to empty. When lean athletes ate a plate of pasta the night before a competition, their glycogen offered hours of stored glucose. Their healthy systems released the stored energy about as quickly as they packaged it into glycogen. Athletes who ate high-fat, low-carb the night before they competed had fewer bubbles to pop. Their fasting glucose hit the 60s quicker.

If their liver spent months soaked with insulin, the king of endocrine delayed access again. Abundant insulin prevented millions of glycogen-bubbles from unlocking all at once. It took time to reveal the layers of old glycogen bubbles. Insulin had programmed the cells to lock the glycogen inside and stay there. Similarly, if their metabolism transmitted minimal energy for months, the gears to access more turned very slowly.

Deny food for 72 hours, and odd things happened inside the human body. Deny food for 72 hours when mitochondria have practiced keto-chemistry and have ample fat-based endocrine supply, and medical miracles occurred.

Stacking a 72-hour fast on top of a baseline ketoCONTINUUM turbocharged the greased wheels of metabolism. Insulin-resistant patients creaked their rusty parts into action during ketoCONTINUUM #2, #3, and #4. Their supporting cast of fat-based hormones trickled into place. Steady production of ketones corrected the dominant message of insulin while resurrecting fat-based hormones. Their mitochondria exercised during the baseline ketoCONTINUUMs, and they soon flaunted similar advantages as lean patients. Now, the slightest stress opened glycogen bubbles. Stretching their fast to 72 hours offered a rare opportunity for an insulin-resistant patient to reach the bottom of their storage bin.

Some with insulin resistance didn't sink into the 60s on their first 72-hour fast. It took three or four attempts to achieve that glucose reading. The oldest, most stubborn glycogen bubbles softened with every metabolic stress. The ancient, crusty bubbles popped during the final hours of the 72-hour fast. Upon eating, replacement glycogen formed. The newly formed ones were plump and flexible instead of hard and crystallized. Each fast strained their system. The phase following their fast recovered with healthier mitochon-

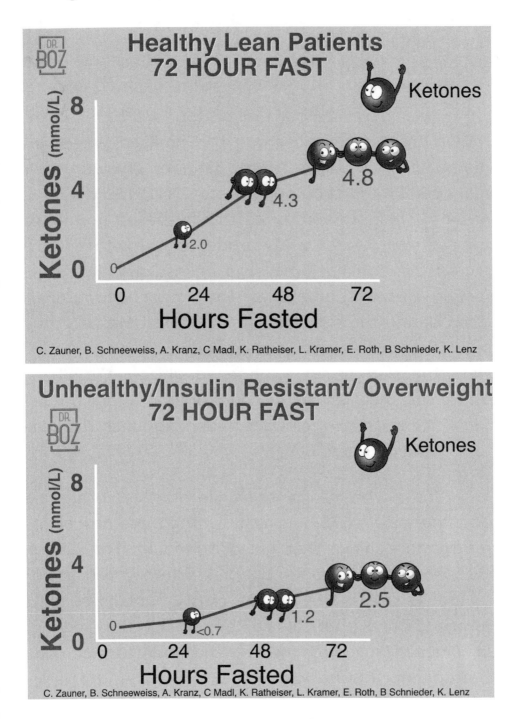

C. Zauner, B. Schneeweiss, A. Kranz, C Madl, K. Ratheiser, L. Kramer, E. Roth, B Schnieder, K. Lenz

C. Zauner, B. Schneeweiss, A. Kranz, C Madl, K. Ratheiser, L. Kramer, E. Roth, B Schnieder, K. Lenz

dria.

Repeating cycles for eight weeks chiseled closer to the bottom of the storage. The following week, freshly made glycogen bubbles emptied within hours of denying food. Hours later, fasting chipped away at more of their crusted layers. Fasting alternating with keto-chemistry reset their liver with young glycogen and robust ketogenic metabolism.

They didn't need to take my word on what was happening. Testing blood numbers along the way, empowered insulin-resistant patients. They saw it for themselves. They watched their fasting numbers draw closer to their goal of 65. Meanwhile, their ketone production spiked to a superior performance after each cycle.

Trigger Autophagy

The invisible, unmeasurable process of autophagy was predictable based on chemistry. The lower the Dr. Boz Ratio, the higher the confidence that autophagy had clipped defective proteins into amino acids at the sub-cellular level. Hitting a Dr. Boz Ratio of 80 triggered some autophagy, while a ratio of 40 sparked more recycling. The boosted chemistry found at ketoCONTINUUM #5- #8 spring-boarded them to confident autophagy numbers. Beginning each fast

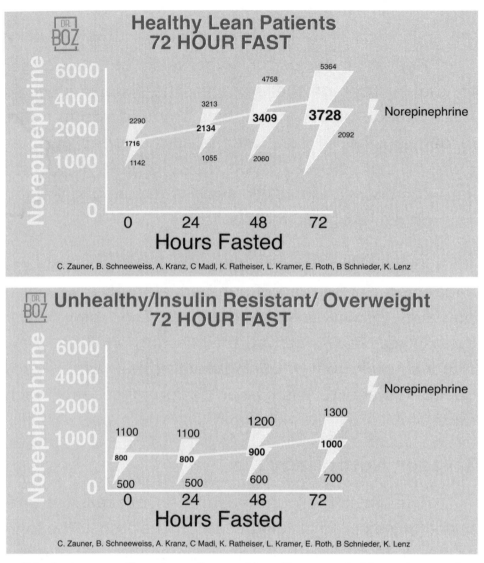

Healthy Lean Patients 72 HOUR FAST

Norepinephrine

2290	3213	4758	5364	
1716	2134	3409	3728	
1142	1055	2060	2092	

C. Zauner, B. Schneeweiss, A. Kranz, C Madl, K. Ratheiser, L. Kramer, E. Roth, B Schnieder, K. Lenz

Unhealthy/Insulin Resistant/ Overweight 72 HOUR FAST

Norepinephrine

1100	1100	1200	1300
800	800	900	1000
500	500	600	700

C. Zauner, B. Schneeweiss, A. Kranz, C Madl, K. Ratheiser, L. Kramer, E. Roth, B Schnieder, K. Lenz

with ketones flowing from the liver set the stage for faster repair.

Ramp Up Norepinephrine

Norepinephrine holds the bragging rights for boosting energy to the brain and body. This neuroendocrine hormone electrified messages when brains demanded it the most. During a fight or flight reaction, ancestors fled from predators, thanks to norepinephrine. They used this super-powered chemical to outsmart opponents and evade moments of danger. This unique molecule also got credit for feelings of enlightenment during prayer and fasting, and for sparking the flow of energy while connecting neurons for meditation-based euphoria. The claims of feeling smarter and wittier during extended fasts used norepinephrine as their supporting evidence.

Bursts of norepinephrine washed over healthy patients during the initial 72 hours of a fast. When fasts extended beyond three days, little benefit from norepinephrine occurred. Their norepinephrine production leveled off and declined, capturing ninety percent of the benefit in the first 72 hours.

Insulin-resistant patients with inflamed brains showed low levels of norepinephrine at the onset of their fast. By the end of 72 hours, their euphoric hormone had barely changed. Without hardy norepinephrine levels, they did not experience the exhilarated parallel universe described by the other fasters.

Spike Growth Hormone

As fasting-students practiced ketoCONTINUUM #12, their blood glucose reached 65 before the 72nd hour. Their liver emptied quicker on repeated fasts. Why not just quit fasting when the glucose hits 65?

ANSWER: Hormones! Specifically, growth hormone.

Human Growth Hormone, HGH, is a fat-based hormone released from your brain. HGH is like sprinkling pixie dust onto broken human bodies. It magically reverses chronic illness. HGH triggers fat cells to open up and release fat into your bloodstream. HGH improves energy, revs up metabolisms, brightens moods, and suppresses appetites. Growth hormone melts off pounds of fat, strengthens the density of bones, and reverses withered wrinkles. HGH heightens concentration, improves memory, and sparks your libido. Growth hormone gives you the power of an alchemist conjuring the fountain of youth.

Low HGH causes fatigue, decreasing stamina, depressed mood, dwindling muscle mass, weakening strength, thinning skin, increasing fat cells, slower thinking, and thinning bones. Higher insulin levels lock away the supply of fat as growth hormone crawls to a halt. Growth hormone lowers as insulin rises.

It's easy to see why syringes of HGH sell for big money. Dancers, actresses, and body-builders use this hack to grow muscles, look younger, and leaner. Please

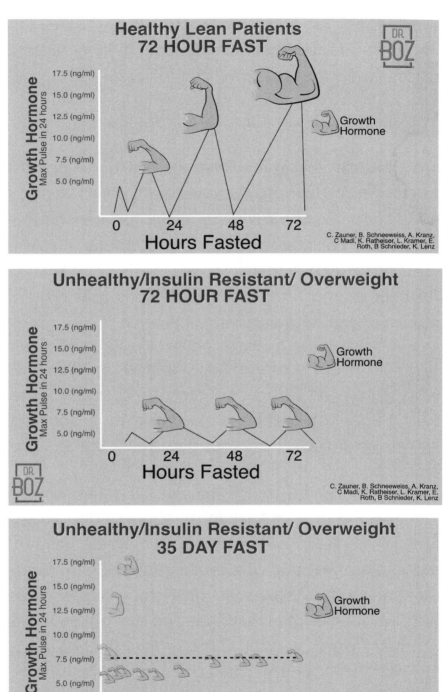

Healthy Lean Patients
72 HOUR FAST

Growth Hormone
Max Pulse in 24 hours

17.5 (ng/ml)
15.0 (ng/ml)
12.5 (ng/ml)
10.0 (ng/ml)
7.5 (ng/ml)
5.0 (ng/ml)

Growth Hormone

0   24   48   72

Hours Fasted

C. Zauner, B. Schneeweiss, A. Kranz, C Madl, K. Ratheiser, L. Kramer, E. Roth, B Schnieder, K. Lenz

Unhealthy/Insulin Resistant/ Overweight
72 HOUR FAST

Growth Hormone
Max Pulse in 24 hours

17.5 (ng/ml)
15.0 (ng/ml)
12.5 (ng/ml)
10.0 (ng/ml)
7.5 (ng/ml)
5.0 (ng/ml)

Growth Hormone

0   24   48   72

Hours Fasted

C. Zauner, B. Schneeweiss, A. Kranz, C Madl, K. Ratheiser, L. Kramer, E. Roth, B Schnieder, K. Lenz

Unhealthy/Insulin Resistant/ Overweight
35 DAY FAST

Growth Hormone
Max Pulse in 24 hours

17.5 (ng/ml)
15.0 (ng/ml)
12.5 (ng/ml)
10.0 (ng/ml)
7.5 (ng/ml)
5.0 (ng/ml)

Growth Hormone

0 1 3 5 7   14   21   28   **35**
                                 5 weeks

Days Fasted

C. Zauner, B. Schneeweiss, A. Kranz, C Madl, K. Ratheiser, L. Kramer, E. Roth, B Schnieder, K. Lenz don't shoot up with synthetic, costly HGH. Instead, once fat-adapted use the 72-hour fast as a safe and natural way to boost growth hormone.

STEP ONE: Ensure fat-adaption.

Notice the three images charting growth hormone during fasting. Researchers looked at the highest daily peak of growth hormone for lean, healthy patients and compared the levels to obese, insulin-resistant ones. Additionally, obese patients were studied for over a month of fasting. You read that correctly: A month of salt and water.

Growth hormone skyrocketed in lean patients who fasted for 72 hours. From the first day of fasting to the final hours, their growth hormone doubled. Not surprisingly, their lean young systems made a healthy amount of growth hormone at the start.

Insulin-resistant patients showed double trouble. Thanks to years of excess insulin, their growth hormone slumped out of normal range. Even when correcting for their age, their growth hormone measured well below the minimum needed for optimum health. As they fasted, very little happened to their hormone. The initial 72 hours caused no statistical change in their growth hormone production. As days of fasting stretched into weeks, their growth hormone nudged up slightly in the third week. By the final check on the 35th day of fasting, their growth hormone finally rose into the normal range. In comparison, the 35th day of growth hormone from insulin-resistant patients measured the same as the healthy group's 24-hour fasted level.

Why such a striking difference between the lean versus the obese?

ANSWER: Fat-based hormones versus insulin.

As long as insulin blocked the flow of fat, patients struggled. The fulcrum of rising insulin teetered between the presence of fatty-endocrine levels or not. Once that balance tipped in the wrong direction, they failed to produce growth hormone until their insulin regressed. As insulin drew closer to normal, fatty endocrine hormones like HGH began to flow. The reversal couldn't be forced as long as insulin remained high. The lack of food for 30 days did not strong-arm the production of hormones from lifeless endocrine cells. Time spent bathed in keto-chemistry could.

Unlock the Gift of Fasting for a Lifetime

David launched his fasts from his preferred baseline metabolism. He used ketoCONTINUUM #5 as his daily pattern to keep ketones in steady supply. David started each fast with adequate circulating ketones.

Keto-chemistry placed him at a chemical advantage over the healthy lean subjects mentioned in the previous studies. They didn't have ketones in supply for almost a day of fasting. In comparison, David's body seamlessly used glucose and ketones to power his body while fasting. His keto-chemistry mimicked a fasted state *before* he ever started his fast. David could reach the same Dr. Boz Ratio in the 40 hours of fasting as the healthy lean subjects achieved in 72 hours.

Each fast not only pumped hormones and chipped away at piles of junk proteins littering his brain and body; each fast squeezed the grime out of his system thoroughly and quicker than his healthy counterparts. The rewards of fasting multiplied even after David broke his fast. Cells that had triggered autophagy finished recycling the proteins that were breaking down. Autophagy swept up the crumbs as David relished the surging hormones of HGH, norepinephrine, and sex hormones that followed and flowed. His body reaped the benefits of the best hormone levels he had since his youth. And his metabolic stress also pulsed in slightly greater increments.

A successful fast wasn't measured by time but by the lack of complications. David gracefully fasted for about two days without medical hiccups or a rift in his social structure. He salted his way through his abstinence of food with pink crystals. The weekly keto support group kept him accountable, and he mentored others through their first fasts. David checked his Dr. Boz Ratio a couple of times per day when fasting. But when not fasting, he measured his numbers only a few mornings a week.

David's fasting success began with his support system. His greatest enemy was not his metabolism. It was the social consequences that fasting had. The first extended fast proved to David that he could do it—without dying. It also demonstrated to his family how fasting could fit into his life without severely impacting theirs. He used positive peer pressure from his family and the support group to succeed at his plan to fast for eight weeks. Instead of the rigid and strict rule of fasting for 72 hours, he used his blood sugars as his goal. When his blood sugar hit in the sixties before the 72 hours lapsed, he permitted himself to break the fast. Blood glucose in the sixties would have been an impossible goal for David six months prior. This number reflected that his liver worked to empty its storage in order to improve his health. David's organ no longer swelled with inflammation; nor was it crippled with maximum storage.

Every fast fortified David's confidence too. His success inspired all who watched him. Budding mirror neurons from the support group chirped, "If he can do it, I can too."

Eight weeks of spinning that whirlwind of chemistry reversed health problems. It was the gift David found at the end of those eight weeks that he treasured the most. This gift opened a new chapter of his life. For the first time in his life, he felt free, liberated from the shackles food had held over him. Freedom from carbs.

Eight weeks of fasting gifted freedom.

"The mind, once stretched by a new idea, never returns to its original dimensions."

— Ralph Waldo Emerson

TIPS FOR A 72 HOUR FAST

Don't attempt a 72 hour fast until you successfully fast for 48 hours with only water, black coffee (or tea), and salt.

If you attempt a 48 hour fast and needed bone broth or BHB supplements, do not advance to the 72 hour fast yet. Succeed at 48 hours before advancing. Once your metabolism is strong enough to fast for 48 hours without those crutches, then move to a 72 hour fast.

SUCCESS = strong metabolism + mature psychological state.

Sometimes these 2 characteristics don't overlap during a fast.

Solé Water: is water saturated with pink or red salt crystals. Solé water offers easy access to absorbable minerals. Consider adding a tablespoon to all your drinks even when you are not fasting. This tip has proven crucial for many of my students. Waves of hunger should pass with the help of salt and water. Sucking on salt crystals or drinking sole water buffers the changes of electrolytes. A special endorsement of Redmond's Salt. Their profile of micronutrients in their salt wins the gold medal.

Bone Broth is more than just salted, brown water. It's the second antidote I suggest when complications rattle your fast. Quality broth offers another layer of nutrients and takes fasting to an extended level. The more gelatinous the broth at room temperature, the greater the nutrients. I give many students my blessing to drink as much broth as they want for their first fast. Autophagy is rarely achieved when they overuse this, but a successful block of time without chewing is a win. As they mature in their fasting skills, the broth is thinned with sole water. Eventually, the broth is eliminated altogether. This gradual improvement also allows time for other healing.

All of my students on Calorie-Restricted OMEAD (One Meal Every Other Day —see Chapter 30) have daily high-quality bone broth with solé water.

Sip **BHB** is the third and final anecdote for new fasting students. If sole water did not help, and the bone broth didn't reverse symptoms of nausea or lightheadedness, I offer BHB as their final option before giving in. Start with a small dose of BHB. Within 15 minutes excess ketones circulate. The boost of ketone energy along with the solé water help the best.

Selecting days filled with busyness. The first two days are particularly keen for extra distraction.

Warning: There is predictable sleeplessness between the second and third nights. This correlates to robust production of ketones. The ketones flood the body as norepinephrine and growth hormone surge. Every hour of fasting after that surge is a bonus. Stay the course.

Break your fast gently. Start with bone broth, fermented foods, or nuts. Add food slowly. A huge celebration meal causes loose stools. Eating restarts your bowels. Food triggers your cells to produce the necessary digestive enzymes. Food and the secretions resume the squeezing of your colon. Even bone broth may result in loose stools upon breaking your fast. This is normal. Work toward eating a normal sized meal compliant with your chosen baseline metabolism.

Sometimes these 2 characteristics don't overlap during a fast.

Chapter 31

ROOM 2-125

On Sunday, October 25th, 2020 David received a text message, "Hi David, It's Dr. Boz, I need your help. Remember that picture you took of my mom in January 2018. I need a copy of it as soon as possible."

David's heart sank as he read the text message. For the past two weeks, he carefully watched for the messages on Facebook sharing updates from the ICU of room 2-125 —where Grandma Rose was fighting for her life. COVID-19 had swept across the country and his community.

David reflected upon the day he took Grandma Rose's picture in January of 2018. At 73 years old, she walked into his studio and he mistook her for Dr. Boz's sister. He expected a withered, chubby, fragile woman who'd been fighting cancer for a decade. Instead, he met the living version of Mary Poppins. Her light steps and vibrant energy captured his envy. He wanted what she had.

Grandma Rose served as an exemplar for David. He saw what was possible. Her example rescued him from the clouded life he was mired in. The moment she glided into his studio his brain was short-circuiting. Two and a half years later he had become as healthy as she was.

David had his fair share of struggles with the process. Improvement did not happen overnight. He tumbled into ketosis without caution; he failed to use enough salt, his body lacked magnesium, and he had fickle support. His urine contained ketones within 24 hours. This made David think he was "home free." But within days constipation caused his bowels to cease functioning. The "keto-flu" attacked and took him out of commission for several days while his cells scrambled to figure out how to use a ketone again.

By the grace of God and a bit of education, David made it to his first Keto support group three weeks into the transition. Since then he attended almost every weekly support group. His mirror neurons filled in the gaps as he watched others improve ... and watched them struggle. David came to terms with pricking his finger. He did not like the identity of being a diabetic, so he perished that self-image as he shed the pounds and cleaned up his metabolism. It took nearly 18 months to shave forty of the fifty pounds he had to lose to drop his obese BMI of 30 to an ideal number of 22. He slowly lost the final ten pounds over the next year, staying under 130 pounds.

When COVID swept the globe, the weekly support meetings moved to virtual attendance. David clicked into the meetings each week, but the remote participation cracked open opportunities for old, unhealthy habits to resurrect into his life. Instead of, "over-easy eggs, hold the toast," the toast "appeared" onto his plate. It was an oversight by the cook the first time. But a single bite became a half slice, and then an English muffin. The carbs tasted good, and the pandemic stress seemed easier to handle with carbs. He told himself it was, "Safe to eat that." By the end of the first wave of COVID David regained the 10 pounds he worked so hard to lose.

Despite increasing his carbs to over 50 grams per day, the promises about keto-chemistry reigned true. Even with the return of 10 pounds, his mitochondria performed well. His metabolism had strengthened over the past two years and even with some extra carbs, he peed ketones every time he checked. David continued to eat two meals or less per day without many cravings. He'd fallen victim to eating foods with the word keto on their marketing label— yet the fine print showed more carbs in one bar than he used to eat in one day. At first, when he lost the weight, every-one—and I mean every single person—remarked about his missing paunch. But then the real compliments began to trickle in.

How do you have so much energy?

What do you mean you never get sick anymore?

How do you look so much younger?

The same questions David had tossed at Grandma Rose the day of her photoshoot were now landing on his eardrums. In thirty-five months, he gifted over a hundred copies of ANYWAY YOU CAN. Initially, when people asked, he spewed out all the information he had learned about metabolism, energy, and campfires made from glucose versus ketones. However, that grew exhausting and most people had no idea what he was talking about. Eventually, he learned to keep copies of the book at the office. Whenever someone complimented him, he gifted them the book, "Just read it. You will see." David saved dozens of people's lives through his example.

John and Darlene rode the keto-wave of change for a while. Their waistlines shrunk and their scales read a lighter body weight. But without a strong WHY they did not have keto-chemistry pumping through their veins after a year and stalled out in their change. Each month at the mass-cards-and-friends event, they drew inspiration from David—yet not enough to change their PeeTone strip to pink. They claimed to be "dirty-keto" which turned out to mean they didn't count carbs, and they didn't measure ketones. In other words, they were not using keto-chemistry.

During the pandemic, David grew a better understanding of the connection between improved immune systems and ketosis. His friends and family who fueled their campfires with glucose and the lighter-fluid of chronically elevated insulin suffered the most. His eldest sister with memory problems and cancer passed away, another sister was diagnosed with pancreatic cancer, and several overweight friends suffered deadly consequences from the infection of COVID-19.

The pandemic crushed several businesses in the area, but David found opportunities where his skills proved valuable. With his creative brain fueling with logs, his mind stayed engaged and energized, instead of his gloomy astrocytes sinking into hibernation with all the stress. Long gone were the afternoons where he stared at the clock wondering ways to escape from himself. Ketone-fuel kept the sun shining and his glass half-full.

After four months of remote meetings, the keto support group provided the option to attend in-person. David's mirror neurons quickly activated again. Within a handful of meetings, he recognized the way he had inched backward in his choices. True to himself, he pledged to the group, "I need to get back on track. I am not in the ditch— but I have allowed little things slide back. And it's not okay." The group was entranced by his message. David saw he'd become a leader within the group and continued, "A cabinet gets full with one item at a time. I haven't fasted for nearly three months. Being here today and listening to all of you pushed me to step it up."

The live meetings reactivated David's Mirror Neurons and restored his accountability to the group. He fasted 36-hours twice the following week.

David lived most of his days at baseline keto-CONTINUUM #5 or 6. He often started his day with a cup of cream-filled coffee and had one or two high-fat meals each day. He stressed his metabolism with keto-CONTINUUM #9 using 36 hours with only black coffee, water, and pink salt crystals. It wasn't unusual for his 36-hour fast to stretch to ketoCONTINUUM #11 with 48 hours between meals. Several other members had shared setbacks due to COVID infections and other health problems. When they pledged to fast for an extended time, David joined them as his way to show his support. By the end of the month, he even completed a fast that lasted 62 hours—his longest one ever. At his check-in a month later he reported, "I am back to my baseline. The ten pounds are gone and I feel strong again -- both emotionally and physically."

Grandma Rose was one of those members of David's support group who was doing extended fasts for several weeks in a row. After 55 years of marriage, her husband, Richard, passed away from complications with kidney disease. A year of home dialysis strained Grandma Rose's and Richard's health. The added isolation due to COVID-19 marked a steep decline in Richard's health and on June 7th, 2020, he died.

Her doctor's appointment with the oncologist weeks following his funeral showed signs of fatigue. Although she had kept her weight down and was constantly in ketosis, Grandma Rose's body was tired, and her laboratory data also confirmed that. But she fought back with her pledge fast for 72-hour each week for, "As many weeks as I can." She used the group as accountability and documented ten consecutive weeks of fasting. On her non-fasting days, she lived at ketoCONTINUUM #8.

As the reality of being a widow settled into her soul, her health and her spirit healed measurably each week. During her hours of fasting, she prayed for God's favor and grace as she grieved the death of her husband. On the day Grandma Rose walked into the hospital with a positive diagnosis of COVID-19, she shooed her kids and grandkids away. "Go on, now. Don't come in here. I am healthy! I will be fine. I have over-come greater things than a virus." And she was healthy. Her mitochondria were in the best shape of her life. The ten weeks of stressing her metabolism with 72-hour-fasts built upon the five previous years of ketosis. She was strong.

But COVID won. On the Sunday afternoon of October 25th, Grandma Rose died.

As David sat at his computer remembering the day he took those photos, he recalled his wife saying, "She isn't headed for a coffin anytime soon!" The vibrant picture of Grandma Rose spoke that truth. Her eyes sparkled with life; her smile made him smile; her joy spread into his life. Grandma Rose lived and valiantly fought against the assumed death of her cancer. Grandma Rose used the power of ketones to restore her zombie-like body back to the magic of Mary Poppins. Grandma Rose made ketones for life and then shared that - her story, her journey - with thousands. She shared her improved health with David. His path - as well as the path of countless others - was better because of Grandma Rose.

David prayed a prayer of gratitude, "Lord, thank you for Grandma Rose."

Grandma Rose's health lives on in everyone who grew healthier because of her story. Including David.

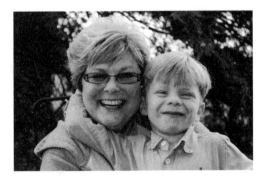
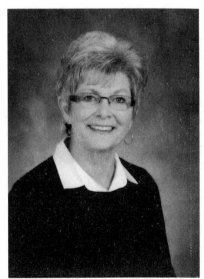

Author's Note:

Thank you, "David." David's name was changed for the book, but his story is real. Although not all of the teachable moments came from David's journey, most of them were his stumbles, restarts, and retries. He encouraged me to write this book sharing his private struggles with hope that it would help others. I pray it helped you.

This book teaches the art and science of staying consistently keto. Use the other tools to learn including the audiobook —where I read this book to you — the workbook, and the online course that contains mini-tutorial videos, all designed to support you. Use the book and workbook to help your physician track your progress. Follow my lead, by starting a keto-support group using this book and workbook. It's the entire curriculum you will need. That choice will improve your health - one ketone at a time.

"David" and I thank you for reading our book. The most powerful *thank you* happens when you leave an Amazon book review. The more FIVE STAR reviews, the more others see our story. Please take the time to write a review. Mark it with 5 stars if you think the book deserves it.

Finally, if you want to learn more about the keto diet from me connect with me at my website: www .BozMD .com

Annette Bosworth, MD

APPENDIX I

KETOSIS HEALS THE GUT

David did not suffer with symptoms of diarrhea, fat-malabsorption, or a leaky gut. But many people do. Adding a keto menu to an inflamed gut can scare the folks that need keto-chemistry the most. This appendix shares the progression of pathology that's taking place inside the lining of a gut that "leaks."

Leaky Gut Phase 1

Patients with a leaky gut secretly lose micronutrients like sodium, potassium, and magnesium. Unaware, they feel no symptoms. Initially, their body tries to replace the vital salts. Gradually, the lost volume becomes too much. Signs of fatigue and decreased concentration might prompt a doctor's visit. A routine physical exam and standard blood tests rarely reveal the problem. With colitis, low voltage warnings circulate from millions of cells lining their gut. These warnings are easily overlooked. The most astute professionals won't even notice the slight rise in inflammatory markers. A bug bite, bruise, or viral infection all cause similar signs that gradually reverse in several days.

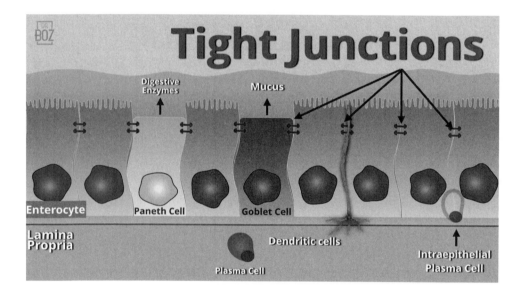

Tiny doorways between cells play an essential part in this intestinal drama. Much like staples, tight junctions seal adjacent cells to one another in a healthy patient. Inflammation loosens the staples and breaks the seal that keeps the useful particles in and the bad ones out. Swollen cells leak through these openings, and the patient's health declines. Long before they complained of gurgling, rumbling, or gas, colitis was already draining their energy, weakening their immune system and slowing down their brain's response time.

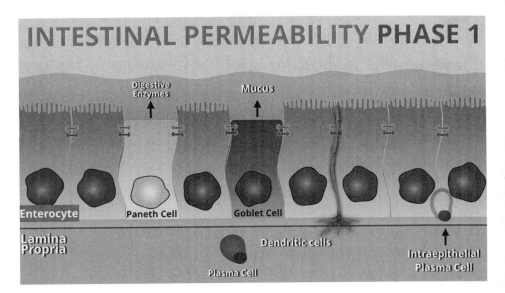

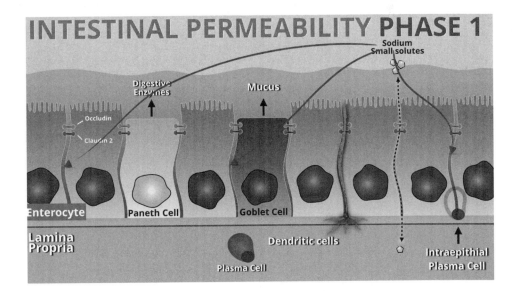

Leaky Gut Phase 2:

As the spaces widened, medical problems grew. Swollen, engorged cells failed to absorb essential nutrients while leaking out gobs of nutrients. Foreign food particles slip inside as they sneak past security. The immune cells policing the gut should have caught them. At first, those security cells defended against the invasion, and the immune system won. But excessive attacks from too many invaders wore down the gut's defenses, making the invaders victors.

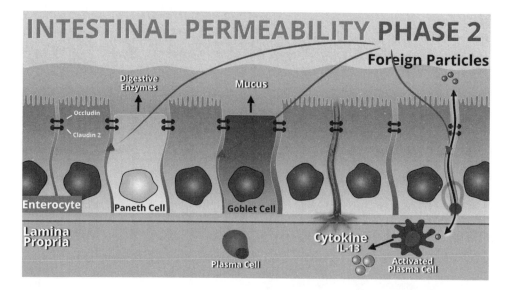

Leaky Gut Phase 3:

Again, their immune system further weakened, and the gaps widened. Larger-sized vitamins now slipped out while bacteria sneaked in. No antidote could make up for all the vanishing nutrients and invasion of unwanted particles. The system suffocated and stopped doing its job. Week after week, the patient's health flushed into the sewer.

"Doc, I feel tired."

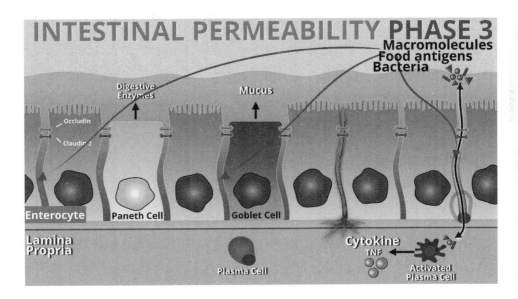

Leaky Gut Phase 4:

Finally, the distance between cells widened so much, it acted like a faucet draining the body. In desperation, the immune system flipped an emergency switch. Chemicals, called cytokines, defended the gut from foreign invasion. Cytokines worked like quarterbacks watching for problems and directing the attack towards the problem. However, when the alarm rang for too long, collateral damage occurred. The flood of cytokines signaled the death of healthy cells lining the intestine. As they perished, tiny openings gave way to larger holes called ulcers. These large gaping wounds, visible without magnification, tormented the patient. Severe malnourishment, via the leaking of nutrients through these bleeding holes, robbed them of life and vitality. The quality of life they had once had was now in decline.

"The only answer I've ever found to feel better was to stop eating." A Crohn's patient of mine said, "I stopped for a month. The first week sucked. But then, it felt like I didn't have Crohn's anymore. I wasn't sick. I had energy. I didn't hurt. It's the best I've felt in a decade."

At the time, this seemed ludicrous. I had no explanation for why he felt so energized and magically erased his chronic illness for those weeks of fasting.

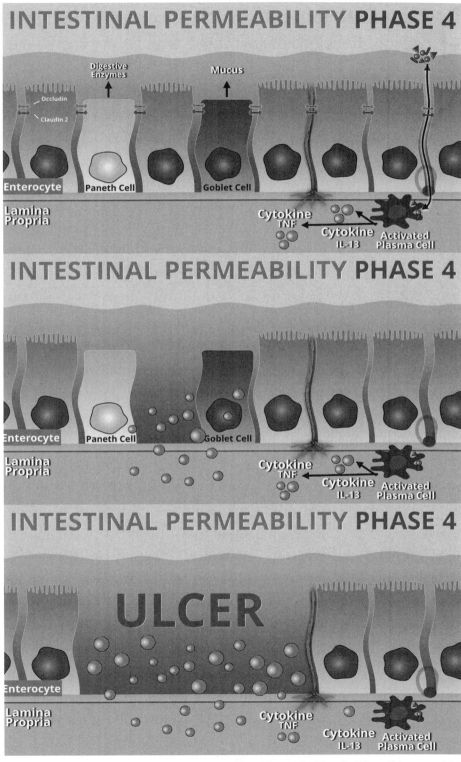

Why did that work? Only after studying the effects of ketosis did I appreciate what he was trying to tell me.

The early phases outlined above are called celiac, gluten intolerance, irritable bowel, depressed bowel, low-grade colitis, or leaky gut. Years of a faulty intestinal system lead to Alzheimer's disease, cancer, autoimmune problems, depression, psoriasis, and thyroid troubles.

Healing starts when they seal their gut with keto-chemistry.

LIMITED BIBLIOGRAPHY

1. Achanta, Lavanya B., and Caroline D. Rae. 'β-Hydroxybutyrate in the Brain: One Molecule, Multiple Mechanisms'. Neurochemical Research 42, no. 1 (January 2017): 35–49. https://doi.org/10.1007/s11064-016-2099-2.

2. Augustin, Katrin, Aziza Khabbush, Sophie Williams, Simon Eaton, Michael Orford, J. Helen Cross, Simon J. R. Heales, Matthew C. Walker, and Robin S. B. Williams. 'Mechanisms of Action for the Medium-Chain Triglyceride Ketogenic Diet in Neurological and Metabolic Disorders'. The Lancet. Neurology 17, no. 1 (2018): 84–93. https://doi.org/10.1016/S1474-4422(17)30408-8.

3. Azad, Meghan B., Ahmed M. Abou-Setta, Bhupendrasinh F. Chauhan, Rasheda Rabbani, Justin Lys, Leslie Copstein, Amrinder Mann, et al. 'Nonnutritive Sweeteners and Cardiometabolic Health: A Systematic Review and Meta-Analysis of Randomized Controlled Trials and Prospective Cohort Studies'. CMAJ: Canadian Medical Association Journal 189, no. 28 (17 July 2017): E929–39. https://doi.org/10.1503/cmaj.161390.

4. Barbanti, Piero, Luisa Fofi, Cinzia Aurilia, Gabriella Egeo, and Massimiliano Caprio. 'Ketogenic Diet in Migraine: Rationale, Findings and Perspectives'. Neurological Sciences: Official Journal of the Italian Neurological Society and of the Italian Society of Clinical Neurophysiology 38, no. Suppl 1 (May 2017): 111–15. https://doi.org/10.1007/s10072-017-2889-6.

5. Blackburn, Henry. 'The Seven Countries Study: A Historic Adventure in Science'. In Lessons for Science from the Seven Countries Study, edited by Ancel Keys, Hironori Toshima, Yoshinori Koga, and Henry Blackburn, 9–13. Tokyo: Springer Japan, 1994. https://doi.org/10.1007/978-4-431-68269-1_2.

6. Cahill, George F. 'Starvation in Man'. New England Journal of Medicine 282, no. 12 (19 March 1970): 668–75. https://doi.org/10.1056/NEJM197003192821209.

7. Cameron, Jameason D., Marie-Josée Cyr, and Eric Doucet. 'Increased Meal Frequency Does Not Promote Greater Weight Loss in Subjects Who Were Prescribed an 8-Week Equi-Ener-

getic Energy-Restricted Diet'. The British Journal of Nutrition 103, no. 8 (April 2010): 1098–1101. https://doi.org/10.1017/S0007114509992984.

8.Caraballo, Roberto Horacio, Santiago Flesler, Marisa Armeno, Sebastian Fortini, Ariela Agustinho, Graciela Mestre, Araceli Cresta, María Celeste Buompadre, and Nidia Escobal. 'Ketogenic Diet in Pediatric Patients with Refractory Focal Status Epilepticus'. Epilepsy Research 108, no. 10 (1 December 2014): 1912–16. https://doi.org/10.1016/j.eplepsyres.2014.09.033.

9.Cassiday, Laura. 'Big Fat Controversy: Changing Opinions about Saturated Fats'. INFORM: International News on Fats, Oils, and Related Materials 26 (1 June 2015): 342–77. https://doi.org/10.21748/inform.06.2015.342.

10.Castaldo, Giuseppe, Giovanna Galdo, Felice Rotondi Aufiero, and Emanuele Cereda. 'Very Low-Calorie Ketogenic Diet May Allow Restoring Response to Systemic Therapy in Relapsing Plaque Psoriasis'. Obesity Research & Clinical Practice 10, no. 3 (June 2016): 348–52. https://doi.org/10.1016/j.orcp.2015.10.008.

11.Castaldo, Giuseppe, Luigi Monaco, Laura Castaldo, Giovanna Galdo, and Emanuele Cereda. 'An Observational Study of Sequential Protein-Sparing, Very Low-Calorie Ketogenic Diet (Oloproteic Diet) and Hypocaloric Mediterranean-like Diet for the Treatment of Obesity'. International Journal of Food Sciences and Nutrition 67, no. 6 (September 2016): 696–706. https://doi.org/10.1080/09637486.2016.1186157.

12.Cervenka, Mackenzie C., Katlyn Patton, Ani Eloyan, Bobbie Henry, and Eric H. Kossoff. 'The Impact of the Modified Atkins Diet on Lipid Profiles in Adults with Epilepsy'. Nutritional Neuroscience 19, no. 3 (2016): 131–37. https://doi.org/10.1179/1476830514Y.0000000162.

13.Chen, I.-Ju, Chia-Yu Liu, Jung-Peng Chiu, and Chung-Hua Hsu. 'Therapeutic Effect of High-Dose Green Tea Extract on Weight Reduction: A Randomized, Double-Blind, Placebo-Controlled Clinical Trial'. Clinical Nutrition (Edinburgh, Scotland) 35, no. 3 (2016): 592–99. https://doi.org/10.1016/j.clnu.2015.05.003.

14.Cicero, Arrigo F. G., Maddalena Benelli, Marco Brancaleoni, Giuseppe Dainelli, Desiré Merlini, and Raffaele Negri. 'Middle and Long-Term Impact of a Very Low-Carbohydrate Ketogenic

Diet on Cardiometabolic Factors: A Multi-Center, Cross-Sectional, Clinical Study'. High Blood Pressure & Cardiovascular Prevention: The Official Journal of the Italian Society of Hypertension 22, no. 4 (December 2015): 389–94. https://doi.org/10.1007/s40292-015-0096-1.

15.Collins, J., C. Robinson, H. Danhof, C. W. Knetsch, H. C. van Leeuwen, T. D. Lawley, J. M. Auchtung, and R. A. Britton. 'Dietary Trehalose Enhances Virulence of Epidemic Clostridium Difficile'. Nature 553, no. 7688 (January 2018): 291–94. https://doi.org/10.1038/nature25178.

16.Craig, Courtney. 'Mitoprotective Dietary Approaches for Myalgic Encephalomyelitis/Chronic Fatigue Syndrome: Caloric Restriction, Fasting, and Ketogenic Diets'. Medical Hypotheses 85, no. 5 (November 2015): 690–93. https://doi.org/10.1016/j.mehy.2015.08.013.

17.Cussó, Lorena, Juan José Vaquero, Stephen Bacharach, and Manuel Desco. 'Comparison of Methods to Reduce Myocardial 18F-FDG Uptake in Mice: Calcium Channel Blockers versus High-Fat Diets'. PloS One 9, no. 9 (2014): e107999. https://doi.org/10.1371/journal.pone.0107999.

18.D'Agostino, Dominic P., Raffaele Pilla, Heather E. Held, Carol S. Landon, Michelle Puchowicz, Henri Brunengraber, Csilla Ari, Patrick Arnold, and Jay B. Dean. 'Therapeutic Ketosis with Ketone Ester Delays Central Nervous System Oxygen Toxicity Seizures in Rats'. American Journal of Physiology-Regulatory, Integrative and Comparative Physiology 304, no. 10 (15 May 2013): R829–36. https://doi.org/10.1152/ajpregu.00506.2012.

19.David, Lawrence A., Corinne F. Maurice, Rachel N. Carmody, David B. Gootenberg, Julie E. Button, Benjamin E. Wolfe, Alisha V. Ling, et al. 'Diet Rapidly and Reproducibly Alters the Human Gut Microbiome'. Nature 505, no. 7484 (23 January 2014): 559–63. https://doi.org/10.1038/nature12820.

20.De Feyter, Henk M., Kevin L. Behar, Jyotsna U. Rao, Kirby Madden-Hennessey, Kevan L. Ip, Fahmeed Hyder, Lester R. Drewes, Jean-François Geschwind, Robin A. de Graaf, and Douglas L. Rothman. 'A Ketogenic Diet Increases Transport and Oxidation of Ketone Bodies in RG2 and 9L Gliomas without Affecting Tumor Growth'. Neuro-Oncology 18, no. 8 (1 August 2016): 1079–87. https://doi.org/10.1093/neuonc/now088.

21. Derks, Terry G. J., and Margreet van Rijn. 'Lipids in Hepatic Glycogen Storage Diseases: Pathophysiology, Monitoring of Dietary Management and Future Directions'. Journal of Inherited Metabolic Disease 38, no. 3 (May 2015): 537–43. https://doi.org/10.1007/s10545-015-9811-2.

22. 'Diet Drink Consumption and the Risk of Cardiovascular Events: A Report from the Women's Health Initiative. - PubMed - NCBI', 31 January 2020. https://www.ncbi.nlm.nih.gov/pubmed/25515135.

23. Doksöz, Önder, Orkide Güzel, Ünsal Yılmaz, Rana İşgüder, Kübra Çeleğen, Timur Meşe, and Utku Uysal. 'The Short-Term Effect of Ketogenic Diet on Carotid Intima-Media Thickness and Elastic Properties of the Carotid Artery and the Aorta in Epileptic Children'. Journal of Child Neurology 30, no. 12 (October 2015): 1646–50. https://doi.org/10.1177/0883073815576793.

24. Erickson, N., A. Boscheri, B. Linke, and J. Huebner. 'Systematic Review: Isocaloric Ketogenic Dietary Regimes for Cancer Patients'. Medical Oncology 34, no. 5 (28 March 2017): 72. https://doi.org/10.1007/s12032-017-0930-5.

25. 'Fasting: The History, Pathophysiology and Complications. - PubMed - NCBI', 30 January 2020. https://www.ncbi.nlm.nih.gov/pubmed/6758355.

26. Feinman, Richard. The World Turned Upside Down: The Second Low-Carbohydrate Revolution by Richard Feinman. Nms Press - Duck in a Boat LLC, 1776.

27. Feinman, Richard D., Wendy K. Pogozelski, Arne Astrup, Richard K. Bernstein, Eugene J. Fine, Eric C. Westman, Anthony Accurso, et al. 'Dietary Carbohydrate Restriction as the First Approach in Diabetes Management: Critical Review and Evidence Base'. Nutrition (Burbank, Los Angeles County, Calif.) 31, no. 1 (January 2015): 1–13. https://doi.org/10.1016/j.nut.2014.06.011.

28. Felig, Philip, Errol B. Marliss, and George F. Cahill Jr. 'Metabolic Response to Human Growth Hormone during Prolonged Starvation', 1 February 1971. https://doi.org/10.1172/JCI106508.

29. Felton, Elizabeth A., and Mackenzie C. Cervenka. 'Dietary Therapy Is the Best Option for Refractory Nonsurgical

Epilepsy'. Epilepsia 56, no. 9 (2015): 1325–29. https://doi.org/10.1111/epi.13075.

30. Ferriss, Tim. 'Dom D'Agostino on Fasting, Ketosis, and the End of Cancer (#117)'. The Blog of Author Tim Ferriss, 3 November 2015. https://tim.blog/2015/11/03/dominic-dagostino/.

31. Fine, Eugene J., Anna Miller, Edward V. Quadros, Jeffrey M. Sequeira, and Richard D. Feinman. 'Acetoacetate Reduces Growth and ATP Concentration in Cancer Cell Lines Which Over-Express Uncoupling Protein 2'. Cancer Cell International 9, no. 1 (29 May 2009): 14. https://doi.org/10.1186/1475-2867-9-14.

32. Fine, Eugene J., C. J. Segal-Isaacson, Richard D. Feinman, Silvia Herszkopf, Maria C. Romano, Norica Tomuta, Amanda F. Bontempo, Abdissa Negassa, and Joseph A. Sparano. 'Targeting Insulin Inhibition as a Metabolic Therapy in Advanced Cancer: A Pilot Safety and Feasibility Dietary Trial in 10 Patients'. Nutrition (Burbank, Los Angeles County, Calif.) 28, no. 10 (October 2012): 1028–35. https://doi.org/10.1016/j.nut.2012.05.001.

33. Fine, Eugene, Cj Segal-Isaacson, Richard Feinman, and Joseph Sparano. 'Carbohydrate Restriction in Patients with Advanced Cancer: A Protocol to Assess Safety and Feasibility with an Accompanying Hypothesis'. Community Oncology 5 (1 January 2008). https://doi.org/10.1016/S1548-5315(11)70179-6.

34. Forsythe, Cassandra E., Stephen D. Phinney, Richard D. Feinman, Brittanie M. Volk, Daniel Freidenreich, Erin Quann, Kevin Ballard, et al. 'Limited Effect of Dietary Saturated Fat on Plasma Saturated Fat in the Context of a Low Carbohydrate Diet'. Lipids 45, no. 10 (October 2010): 947–62. https://doi.org/10.1007/s11745-010-3467-3.

35. Forsythe, Cassandra E., Stephen D. Phinney, Maria Luz Fernandez, Erin E. Quann, Richard J. Wood, Doug M. Bibus, William J. Kraemer, Richard D. Feinman, and Jeff S. Volek. 'Comparison of Low Fat and Low Carbohydrate Diets on Circulating Fatty Acid Composition and Markers of Inflammation'. Lipids 43, no. 1 (1 January 2008): 65–77. https://doi.org/10.1007/s11745-007-3132-7.

36. Gannon, Mary C., and Frank Q. Nuttall. 'Effect of a High-Protein, Low-Carbohydrate Diet on Blood Glucose Control in People with Type 2 Diabetes'. Diabetes 53, no. 9 (September 2004): 2375–82. https://doi.org/10.2337/diabetes.53.9.2375.

37.Gardner, Christopher, Judith Wylie-Rosett, Samuel S. Gid-
ding, Lyn M. Steffen, Rachel K. Johnson, Diane Reader, Alice H.
Lichtenstein, American Heart Association Nutrition Committee
of the Council on Nutrition, Physical Activity and Metabolism,
Council on Arteriosclerosis, Thrombosis and Vascular Biology,
Council on Cardiovascular Disease in the Young, and American
Diabetes Association. 'Nonnutritive Sweeteners: Current Use
and Health Perspectives: A Scientific Statement from the
American Heart Association and the American Diabetes Association'. Diabetes Care 35, no. 8 (August 2012): 1798–1808.
https://doi.org/10.2337/dc12-9002.

38.Ho, Kok-Sun, Charmaine You Mei Tan, Muhd Ashik Mohd
Daud, and Francis Seow-Choen. 'Stopping or Reducing Dietary
Fiber Intake Reduces Constipation and Its Associated Symp-
toms'. World Journal of Gastroenterology: WJG 18, no. 33 (7
September 2012): 4593–96. https://doi.org/10.3748/
wjg.v18.i33.4593.

39.Howard, Barbara, Linda Horn, Judith Hsia, JoAnn Manson,
Marcia Stefanick, Sylvia Wassertheil-Smoller, Lewis Kuller, et al.
'Low-Fat Dietary Pattern and Risk of Cardiovascular Disease:
The Women???S Health Initiative Randomized Controlled Di-
etary Modification Trial'. JAMA: The Journal of the American
Medical Association 295 (1 March 2006): 655–66. https://
doi.org/10.1001/jama.295.6.655.

40.Hursel, R., W. Viechtbauer, and M. S. Westerterp-Planten-
ga. 'The Effects of Green Tea on Weight Loss and Weight Maintenance: A Meta-Analysis'. International Journal of Obesity
(2005) 33, no. 9 (September 2009): 956–61. https://doi.org/
10.1038/ijo.2009.135.

41.Huynh, Karina. 'Heart Failure: Ketone Bodies as Fuel in
Heart Failure'. Nature Reviews. Cardiology 13, no. 3 (March
2016): 122–23. https://doi.org/10.1038/nrcardio.2016.22.

42.'Impact of a Ketogenic Diet Intervention during Radio-
therapy on Body Composition: I. Initial Clinical Experience with
Six Prospectively Studied Patients | BMC Research Notes | Full
Text', 31 January 2020. https://bmcresnotes.biomedcentral.-
com/articles/10.1186/s13104-016-1959-9.

43. 'JCI - A Ketogenic Diet Suppresses Seizures in Mice through Adenosine A1 Receptors', 31 January 2020. https://www.jci.org/articles/view/57813.

44. Jin, Zhicheng, Jessica M. Berthiaume, Qingling Li, Fabrice Henry, Zhong Huang, Sushabhan Sadhukhan, Peng Gao, Gregory P. Tochtrop, Michelle A. Puchowicz, and Guo-Fang Zhang. 'Catabolism of (2E)-4-Hydroxy-2-Nonenal via ω- and ω-1-Oxidation Stimulated by Ketogenic Diet'. The Journal of Biological Chemistry 289, no. 46 (14 November 2014): 32327–38. https://doi.org/10.1074/jbc.M114.602458.

45. Just, Tino, Hans Wilhelm Pau, Ulrike Engel, and Thomas Hummel. 'Cephalic Phase Insulin Release in Healthy Humans after Taste Stimulation?' Appetite 51, no. 3 (November 2008): 622–27. https://doi.org/10.1016/j.appet.2008.04.271.

46. Kelley, Sarah Aminoff, and Eric H. Kossoff. 'How Effective Is the Ketogenic Diet for Electrical Status Epilepticus of Sleep?' Epilepsy Research 127 (1 November 2016): 339–43. https://doi.org/10.1016/j.eplepsyres.2016.09.018.

47. Keys, Ancel & Margaret. Eat Well and Stay Well. Book Club Edition edition. Doubleday, 1959.

48. Kim, Do Young, Mohammed G. Abdelwahab, Soo Han Lee, Derek O'Neill, Roger J. Thompson, Henry J. Duff, Patrick G. Sullivan, and Jong M. Rho. 'Ketones Prevent Oxidative Impairment of Hippocampal Synaptic Integrity through KATP Channels'. PloS One 10, no. 4 (2015): e0119316. https://doi.org/10.1371/journal.pone.0119316.

49. Kindwall, Eric. Hyperbaric Medicine Practice, 3rd Edition by Eric P. Kindwall and Harry T. Whelan. Best Publishing Company, 1777.

50. Klement, Rainer J., Colin E. Champ, Christoph Otto, and Ulrike Kämmerer. 'Anti-Tumor Effects of Ketogenic Diets in Mice: A Meta-Analysis'. PLOS ONE 11, no. 5 (9 May 2016): e0155050. https://doi.org/10.1371/journal.pone.0155050.

51. Kolwicz, Stephen C., Sophia Airhart, and Rong Tian. 'Ketones Step to the Plate: A Game Changer for Metabolic Remodeling in Heart Failure?' Circulation 133, no. 8 (23 February 2016): 689–91. https://doi.org/10.1161/CIRCULATIONAHA.116.021230.

52.Kosinski, Christophe, and François R. Jornayvaz. 'Effects of Ketogenic Diets on Cardiovascular Risk Factors: Evidence from Animal and Human Studies'. Nutrients 9, no. 5 (19 May 2017). https://doi.org/10.3390/nu9050517.

53.Kratz, Mario, Ton Baars, and Stephan Guyenet. 'The Relationship between High-Fat Dairy Consumption and Obesity, Cardiovascular, and Metabolic Disease'. European Journal of Nutrition 52, no. 1 (February 2013): 1–24. https://doi.org/10.1007/s00394-012-0418-1.

54.Longo, Valter. 'The Longevity Diet', 31 January 2020. https://www.penguinrandomhouse.com/books/564866/the-longevity-diet-by-valter-longo-phd/.

55.Luis, Daniel de, Joan Carles Domingo, Olatz Izaola, Felipe F. Casanueva, Diego Bellido, and Ignacio Sajoux. 'Effect of DHA Supplementation in a Very Low-Calorie Ketogenic Diet in the Treatment of Obesity: A Randomized Clinical Trial'. Endocrine 54, no. 1 (October 2016): 111–22. https://doi.org/10.1007/s12020-016-0964-z.

56.Maalouf, Marwan, Jong M. Rho, and Mark P. Mattson. 'The Neuroprotective Properties of Calorie Restriction, the Ketogenic Diet, and Ketone Bodies'. Brain Research Reviews 59, no. 2 (1 March 2009): 293–315. https://doi.org/10.1016/j.brainresrev.2008.09.002.

57.Martin, Kirsty, Cerian F. Jackson, Robert G. Levy, and Paul N. Cooper. 'Ketogenic Diet and Other Dietary Treatments for Epilepsy'. The Cochrane Database of Systematic Reviews 2 (9 February 2016): CD001903. https://doi.org/10.1002/14651858.CD001903.pub3.

58.Masino, Susan, ed. Ketogenic Diet and Metabolic Therapies: Expanded Roles in Health and Disease. New York, NY, United States of America: Oxford University Press, 2017.

59.Masino, Susan A., and David N. Ruskin. 'Ketogenic Diets and Pain': Journal of Child Neurology, 16 May 2013. https://doi.org/10.1177/0883073813487595.

60.Mente, Andrew, Lawrence de Koning, Harry S. Shannon, and Sonia S. Anand. 'A Systematic Review of the Evidence Supporting a Causal Link between Dietary Factors and Coronary Heart Disease'. Archives of Internal Medicine 169, no. 7 (13

April 2009): 659–69. https://doi.org/10.1001/archinternmed.2009.38.

61.MHS, Dr Eric C. Westman MD. Adapt Program: A Low Carbohydrate, Ketogenic Diet Manual. 1 edition. CreateSpace Independent Publishing Platform, 2015.

62.'Migraine Improvement during Short Lasting Ketogenesis: A Proof-of-concept Study - Di Lorenzo - 2015 - European Journal of Neurology - Wiley Online Library', 30 January 2020. https://onlinelibrary.wiley.com/doi/abs/10.1111/ene.12550.

63.Moreno, Cesar L., and Charles V. Mobbs. 'Epigenetic Mechanisms Underlying Lifespan and Age-Related Effects of Dietary Restriction and the Ketogenic Diet'. Molecular and Cellular Endocrinology 455 (5 November 2017): 33–40. https://doi.org/10.1016/j.mce.2016.11.013.

64.Mullin, Gerard E., Sue J. Shepherd, Bani Chander Roland, Carol Ireton-Jones, and Laura E. Matarese. 'Irritable Bowel Syndrome: Contemporary Nutrition Management Strategies'. JPEN. Journal of Parenteral and Enteral Nutrition 38, no. 7 (September 2014): 781–99. https://doi.org/10.1177/0148607114545329.

65.Myette-Côté, Étienne, Helena Neudorf, Hossein Rafiei, Kieran Clarke, and Jonathan Peter Little. 'Prior Ingestion of Exogenous Ketone Monoester Attenuates the Glycaemic Response to an Oral Glucose Tolerance Test in Healthy Young Individuals'. The Journal of Physiology 596, no. 8 (2018): 1385–95. https://doi.org/10.1113/JP275709.

66.Nabbout, Rima. 'FIRES and IHHE: Delineation of the Syndromes'. Epilepsia 54 Suppl 6 (September 2013): 54–56. https://doi.org/10.1111/epi.12278.

67.Ness, Andy R. 'Diet, Nutrition and the Prevention of Chronic Diseases. WHO Technical Report Series 916. Report of a Joint WHO/FSA Expert Consultation.', 2004. https://doi.org/10.1093/ije/dyh209.

68.Nestle, M. 'Mediterranean Diets: Historical and Research Overview'. The American Journal of Clinical Nutrition 61, no. 6 Suppl (1995): 1313S-1320S. https://doi.org/10.1093/ajcn/61.6.1313S.

69.'Neurogenesis and Precursor Cell Differences in the Dorsal and Ventral Adult Canine Hippocampus. - Abstract - Europe PMC', 31 January 2020. https://europepmc.org/article/med/25778416.

70.Newport, Mary T. Alzheimer's Disease: What If There Was a Cure?: The Story of Ketones. 2 edition. Basic Health Publications, Inc., 2013.

71.'Nobel Prize in Medicine Honors Autophagy Discovery | Cancer Discovery', 30 January 2020. https://cancerdiscovery.aacrjournals.org/content/early/2016/10/16/2159-8290.CD-NB2016-127.article-info.

72.Özdemir, Rahmi, Orkide Güzel, Mehmet Küçük, Cem Karadeniz, Nagehan Katipoglu, Ünsal Yılmaz, Murat Muhtar Yılmazer, and Timur Meşe. 'The Effect of the Ketogenic Diet on the Vascular Structure and Functions in Children With Intractable Epilepsy'. Pediatric Neurology 56 (March 2016): 30–34. https://doi.org/10.1016/j.pediatrneurol.2015.10.017.

73.Ozdemir, Rahmi, Mehmet Kucuk, Orkide Guzel, Cem Karadeniz, Unsal Yilmaz, and Timur Mese. 'Does Ketogenic Diet Have Any Negative Effect on Cardiac Systolic and Diastolic Functions in Children with Intractable Epilepsy?: One-Year Follow-up Results'. Brain & Development 38, no. 9 (October 2016): 842–47. https://doi.org/10.1016/j.braindev.2016.03.009.

74.Phinney, Stephen D., and Jeff S. Volek. The Art and Science of Low Carbohydrate Living: An Expert Guide to Making the Life-Saving Benefits of Carbohydrate Restriction Sustainable and Enjoyable. 1st edition. Beyond Obesity LLC, 2011.

75.'Plasma Glucose and Insulin Response to Macronutrients in Nondiabetic and NIDDM Subjects | Diabetes Care', 30 January 2020. https://care.diabetesjournals.org/content/14/9/824.

76.Puchalska, Patrycja, and Peter A. Crawford. 'Multi-Dimensional Roles of Ketone Bodies in Fuel Metabolism, Signaling, and Therapeutics'. Cell Metabolism 25, no. 2 (07 2017): 262–84. https://doi.org/10.1016/j.cmet.2016.12.022.

77.Pw, Siri-Tarino, Sun Q, Hu Fb, and Krauss Rm. 'Meta-Analysis of Prospective Cohort Studies Evaluating the Association of Saturated Fat with Cardiovascular Disease.' The American

Journal of Clinical Nutrition 91, no. 3 (00:00 1AD). https://doi.org/10.3945/ajcn.2009.27725.

78.Rahman, Mahbubur, Sajjad Muhammad, Mahtab A. Khan, Hui Chen, Dirk A. Ridder, Helge Müller-Fielitz, Barbora Pokorná, et al. 'The β-Hydroxybutyrate Receptor HCA2 Activates a Neuroprotective Subset of Macrophages'. Nature Communications 5 (21 May 2014): 3944. https://doi.org/10.1038/ncomms4944.

79.Reeves, Sue, Jörg W. Huber, Lewis G. Halsey, Yasmin Horabady-Farahani, Mehrnaz Ijadi, and Tina Smith. 'Experimental Manipulation of Breakfast in Normal and Overweight/Obese Participants Is Associated with Changes to Nutrient and Energy Intake Consumption Patterns'. Physiology & Behavior 133 (22 June 2014): 130–35. https://doi.org/10.1016/j.physbeh.2014.05.015.

80.Ketogenic Forums. 'Richard Morris & Carl Franklin (Aka the 2 Keto Dudes)', 23 March 2018. https://www.ketogenicforums.com/t/richard-morris-amp-carl-franklin-aka-the-2-keto-dudes/35578.

81.Silva-Nichols, Helena B., Eric C. Woolf, Loic P. Deleyrolle, Brent A. Reynolds, and Adrienne C. Scheck. 'ATPS-77THE KETONE BODY ß-HYDROXYBUTYRATE RADIOSENSITIZES GLIOBLASTOMA MULTIFORME STEM CELLS'. Neuro-Oncology 17, no. suppl_5 (1 November 2015): v35–v35. https://doi.org/10.1093/neuonc/nov204.77.

82.Skodje, Gry I., Vikas K. Sarna, Ingunn H. Minelle, Kjersti L. Rolfsen, Jane G. Muir, Peter R. Gibson, Marit B. Veierød, Christine Henriksen, and Knut E. A. Lundin. 'Fructan, Rather Than Gluten, Induces Symptoms in Patients With Self-Reported Non-Celiac Gluten Sensitivity'. Gastroenterology 154, no. 3 (2018): 529-539.e2. https://doi.org/10.1053/j.gastro.2017.10.040.

83.Staverosky, Tom. 'Ketogenic Weight Loss: The Lowering of Insulin Levels Is the Sleeping Giant in Patient Care'. The Journal of Medical Practice Management: MPM 32, no. 1 (September 2016): 63–66.

84.Stephen, Alison M., and J. H. Cummings. 'Water-Holding by Dietary Fibre in Vitro and Its Relationship to Faecal Output in Man'. Gut 20, no. 8 (August 1979): 722–29.

85.Stubbs, James, Stephen Whybrow, and Nik Mamat. 'Macronutrients, Feeding Behavior, and Weight Control in Humans', 295–322, 2008. https://doi.org/10.1201/9781420047844.

86.Swithers, Susan E. 'Artificial Sweeteners Produce the Counterintuitive Effect of Inducing Metabolic Derangements'. Trends in Endocrinology and Metabolism: TEM 24, no. 9 (September 2013): 431–41. https://doi.org/10.1016/j.tem.2013.05.005.

87.The Fasting Method Team. 'Blog - The Fasting Method'. The Fasting Method (blog), 30 January 2020. https://thefastingmethod.com/blog/.

88.Tóth, Csaba, and Zsófia Clemens. 'Halted Progression of Soft Palate Cancer in a Patient Treated with the Paleolithic Ketogenic Diet Alone: A 20-Months Follow-Up'. American Journal of Medical Case Reports 4, no. 8 (14 September 2016): 288–92. http://pubs.sciepub.com/ajmcr/4/8/8/.

89.Tóth, Csaba, Andrea Dabóczi, Madhvi Chanrai, and Zsófia Clemens. 'Comment on "Systematic Review: Isocaloric Ketogenic Dietary Regimes for Cancer Patients" by Erickson et Al'. Journal of Cancer Research and Treatment 5, no. 3 (29 July 2017): 86–88. https://doi.org/10.12691/jcrt-5-3-2.

90.Tóth, Csaba, Mária Schimmer, and Zsófia Clemens. 'Complete Cessation of Recurrent Cervical Intraepithelial Neoplasia (CIN) by the Paleolithic Ketogenic Diet: A Case Report'. Journal of Cancer Research and Treatment 6, no. 1 (5 January 2018): 1–5. https://doi.org/10.12691/jcrt-6-1-1.

91.Triantafyllou, Konstantinos, Christopher Chang, and Mark Pimentel. 'Methanogens, Methane and Gastrointestinal Motility'. Journal of Neurogastroenterology and Motility 20, no. 1 (January 2014): 31–40. https://doi.org/10.5056/jnm.2014.20.1.31.

92.Turnbaugh, Peter J., Ruth E. Ley, Michael A. Mahowald, Vincent Magrini, Elaine R. Mardis, and Jeffrey I. Gordon. 'An Obesity-Associated Gut Microbiome with Increased Capacity for Energy Harvest'. Nature 444, no. 7122 (December 2006): 1027–31. https://doi.org/10.1038/nature05414.

93.Vergati, Matteo, Eriseld Krasniqi, Girolamo D. Monte, Silvia Riondino, Doriana Vallone, Fiorella Guadagni, Patrizia Ferroni, and Mario Roselli. 'Ketogenic Diet and Other Dietary Intervention Strategies in the Treatment of Cancer'. Current Medicinal

Chemistry 24, no. 12 (2017): 1170–85. https://doi.org/10.2174/0929867324666170116122915.

94.Villamizar-Schiller, Ives T., Laudy A. Pabón, Sophia B. Hufnagel, Norma C. Serrano, Gabriela Karl, John L. Jefferies, Robert J. Hopkin, and Carlos E. Prada. 'Neurological and Cardiac Responses after Treatment with Miglustat and a Ketogenic Diet in a Patient with Sandhoff Disease'. European Journal of Medical Genetics 58, no. 3 (March 2015): 180–83. https://doi.org/10.1016/j.ejmg.2014.12.009.

95.Volek, Jeff, Erin Quann, and Cassandra Forsythe. 'Low-Carbohydrate Diets Promote a More Favorable Body Composition Than Low-Fat Diets'. Strength and Conditioning Journal 32, no. 1 (February 2010): 42–47. https://doi.org/10.1519/SSC.0b013e3181c16c41.

96.Volek, Jeff S., Kevin D. Ballard, Ricardo Silvestre, Daniel A. Judelson, Erin E. Quann, Cassandra E. Forsythe, Maria Luz Fernandez, and William J. Kraemer. 'Effects of Dietary Carbohydrate Restriction versus Low-Fat Diet on Flow-Mediated Dilation'. Metabolism 58, no. 12 (1 December 2009): 1769–77. https://doi.org/10.1016/j.metabol.2009.06.005.

97.Wheless, James W. 'History and Origin of the Ketogenic Diet', 2004. https://doi.org/10.1007/978-1-59259-808-3_2.

98.Wyatt, Holly R., Gary K. Grunwald, Cecilia L. Mosca, Mary L. Klem, Rena R. Wing, and James O. Hill. 'Long-Term Weight Loss and Breakfast in Subjects in the National Weight Control Registry'. Obesity Research 10, no. 2 (2002): 78–82. https://doi.org/10.1038/oby.2002.13.

99.Yki-Järvinen, Hannele. 'Nutritional Modulation of Non-Alcoholic Fatty Liver Disease and Insulin Resistance'. Nutrients 7, no. 11 (5 November 2015): 9127–38. https://doi.org/10.3390/nu7115454.

100.Zinn, Caryn, Matthew Wood, Mikki Williden, Simon Chatterton, and Ed Maunder. 'Ketogenic Diet Benefits Body Composition and Well-Being but Not Performance in a Pilot Case Study of New Zealand Endurance Athletes'. Journal of the International Society of Sports Nutrition 14 (12 July 2017). https://doi.org/10.1186/s12970-017-0180-0.

www.BozMD.com

Make smart choices, Not sacrifices.

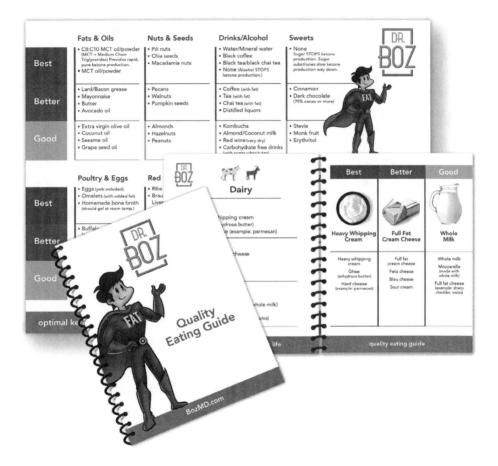

To enter ketosis, you need to know which foods and beverages will spark your body's natural energy production. This Pocket Guide & Fridge Chart will step you through foods that are good Better and BEST for your keto journey. At the grocery story or dining out, this reference will help you make better choices one decision at a time.

Quality Eating Pocket Guide & Fridge Chart

<u>Quality Eating Guide</u>: [Size:4 x 5.5 inch] Take this handy pocket guide with you on every trip to the market or restaurant. There are 30 pages of Good, Better, and Best food options. Let me walk you through the gradual improvement of your food choices. This guide is printed on water resistant, non-tearable, synthetic paper for maximum dura-bility. Change happens one decision at a time. Use this guide to move to the next best decision.

<u>Fridge Magnet</u>: [Size:11 x 8.5 inch] Feature this lami-nated eating guide on your refrigerator – or any magnetic service – as an easy-to-use reminder of your successful keto-journey. My favorite reviews of this tool have come from those who hung this in the kitchen area at work. Watch the discussions begin!

A special thanks to the thousands of patients that have blessed my life by inviting me into theirs.